A HISTORICAL DICTIONARY OF
Psychiatry

A HISTORICAL DICTIONARY OF Psychiatry

EDWARD SHORTER

OXFORD
UNIVERSITY PRESS
2005

OXFORD
UNIVERSITY PRESS

Oxford University Press, Inc., publishes works that further
Oxford University's objective of excellence
in research, scholarship, and education.

Oxford New York
Auckland Cape Town Dar es Salaam Hong Kong Karachi
Kuala Lumpur Madrid Melbourne Mexico City Nairobi
New Delhi Shanghai Taipei Toronto

With offices in
Argentina Austria Brazil Chile Czech Republic France Greece
Guatemala Hungary Italy Japan Poland Portugal Singapore
South Korea Switzerland Thailand Turkey Ukraine Vietnam

Published by Oxford University Press, Inc.
198 Madison Avenue, New York, New York 10016

www.oup.com

Library of Congress Cataloging-in-Publication Data
Shorter, Edward
A historical dictionary of psychiatry / Edward Shorter.
p. cm.
Includes bibliographical references and index.
ISBN-13 978-0-19-517668-1
ISBN 0-19-517668-5
1. Psychiatry—History—Dictionaries. I. Shorter, Edward.
[DNLM: 1. Psychiatry—history—Dictionary—English. WM 13 H673 2005]
RC438.H524 2005
616.89'003—dc22 2004049507

For Tom Ban

from one of his students

Preface

This is the first-ever historical dictionary of psychiatry. It is needed because clinical psychiatry today, as well as all the mental health-care specialties, is emerging from a period of turmoil. The past 40 years have seen the virtual death of one of the great intellectual paradigms that guided psychiatry—psychoanalysis—and its replacement by a starkly different kind of paradigm, one emphasizing brain biology in the understanding of illness and psychopharmacology as the leading edge of treatment. Inevitably, amidst this vast change of paradigms, a number of psychiatry's key concepts and diagnostic traditions have undergone a kind of unhitching from the continuity of history and float in conceptual confusion: What does psychiatry still owe to Freud? Where does all this emphasis on pharmaceuticals come from? Who was Kraepelin (and how does one pronounce the name)?

This dictionary will enable quick reference to these questions and many others, arranged as it is alphabetically, with a comprehensive index to give information about historical figures and concepts not included in the main alphabetical listing. The book also takes many key concepts, such as "depression" and "psychotherapy," and traces their evolution in chronological order (the concepts themselves appear alphabetically). The *Dictionary* is designed for the edification of clinicians and scientists today as well as for general readers who wish to know the origins of currently familiar concepts; it is not conceived as an encyclopedia of important events in the history of psychiatry, and much of history that has somehow not left its mark on the present is left out.

The entries in a dictionary of this nature will lend flesh to the skeleton of change adumbrated in the following Introduction. However, the reader is advised that several areas are covered rather poorly if at all. My intent has been to make this dictionary useful to today's mental health professionals, and so much of the history of psychiatry that is important to historians—and celebrated in their academic annals—does not really appear here. I have included almost nothing on psychiatry before the mid-eighteenth century, a shame given that medical writing on mental illness stretches back to the Ancients. The asylums of the nineteenth century, which bequeathed relatively little to today's psychiatry, also receive short shrift in these pages. On the other hand, such issues as the development of diagnosis, a matter of really intense interest in today's medicine, receive extensive coverage, likewise the origins of psychopharmacology, again for reasons that are evident. In terms of personalities, the most important psychiatric thinkers have been given independent entries; many other leading psychiatrists of the past are mentioned in the diagnosis narratives, and readers may find them through the index.

Readers will soon discover my preference for the biological approach to psychiatry in contrast to the doctrines that previously prevailed. Yet, I bear in mind that biologism too represents a kind of fad, and the reductionism of the biological model—meaning the assumption that clinical illness is reducible to malfunctioning molecules—will almost certainly yield pride of place to other approaches that lie yet undiscovered before us. It is thus important to approach today's biological psychiatry tentatively, with the mere suspension of disbelief, rather than trumpeting neurotransmitter hypotheses as though they represented the Rosetta Stone of human misbehavior.

The selections in this dictionary inevitably reflect the subjective tastes of the author, for there is no preordained measure of what was important in the past. It is mainly casting back from what one finds important today, and on that, opinions will vary widely. So the choices made are one man's view, the choices of an author who has spent years of research in the history of psychiatry, to be sure, but nonetheless they are inevitably somewhat arbitrary. In any event, given limited space, much that is significant has been left out, and readers who make a good case for the inclusion of a beloved figure or concept may have their wishes granted in future editions.

Despite the most meticulous editorial attention, it is inevitable in a work of this nature that errors will creep in. That they may be expunged from successive printings, sharp-eyed readers are invited to contact me at the History of Medicine Program, University of Toronto, 88 College Street, Toronto, Canada, or to send an e-mail to history.medicine@utoronto.ca.

Susan Bélanger, the world's best research assistant, was terribly helpful in bringing together material for this dictionary. Andrea Clark, the administrative assistant in the History of Medicine Program of the University of Toronto, deserves special mention for her efficiency and patience. Heather Dichter and Ellen Tulchinsky dug ably in the University of Toronto's tremendous libraries. For comments on earlier drafts, Susan Abbey, Gemma Blok, Gabrielle A. Carlson, Max Fink, Colin Gale, Cyril Greenland, Jeremia Heinik, Donald Klein, Walter Kucharczyk, Isaac Marks, Harry Oosterhuis, and Robert Spitzer must be thanked. Oxford University Press could not have made a better choice for outside readers than Joel Braslow, Mark Micale, and Simon Wessely, and the work is much richer for their thoughtful and painstaking comments. I would like to acknowledge the help of Jeffrey House and Fiona Stevens at Oxford University Press who are, how can one put this, simply wonderful to work with. Literary agent Beverly Slopen eased the hull into the water. This book was forged in many long conversations with Tom Ban about individual entries. Tom shared with me his enormous knowledge of the history of psychiatry. Some of his suggestions for change were accepted, others were not. For my recalcitrance, I have only myself to blame.

Contents

A HISTORICAL DICTIONARY OF

Psychiatry

Introduction

Psychiatry is the medical specialty concerned with mental symptoms caused by disorders of the brain and mind. Because medical attention to such symptoms stretches back to the Ancients, psychiatry has a long history indeed, moreover a history thoroughly interleaved with the culture and society of the day. This kind of connectiveness to culture makes psychiatry particularly vulnerable to social changes, and the history of psychiatry is associated with discontinuities that do not necessarily occur in the history of other medical specialties. Yet, this highly eventful nature also gives the history of psychiatry its charm. What are the major moments in the evolution of the discipline?

THE HISTORY OF PSYCHIATRY

The history of psychiatry may be divided into roughly three periods: the asylum period of the years 1770–1870, in which biological concepts held sway; the psychotherapy period of the years 1870 to around 1970, in which Freud's doctrine of psychoanalysis came increasingly to the fore; and the second biological psychiatry, from the 1970s to the present, in which biology has come rushing back with a vengeance and psychodynamic explanations have largely been unhorsed, psychotherapy sliding from the psychiatrists to the psychologists.[1]

Inevitably, cutting history at the joints in this manner vastly oversimplifies, for even as psychoanalysis became all the rage in community psychiatry, the number of patients in mental hospitals continued to rise. And even in the heyday of American psychoanalysis, the 1950s and 1960s when every department chair lay in the hands of an analyst, centers of excellence in psychopharmacology and neuroscience were establishing themselves. Yet, *grosso modo* the image of the pendulum swinging from biology to psychogenesis and then back to biology does capture the main trend.

Psychiatry as a discipline began in the last quarter of the eighteenth century with the founding of a new kind of asylum—the therapeutic rather than the custodial asylum. The world had known asylums since the Middle Ages, hospices in which the insane were thrown together willy nilly with the halt, the diseased, the senile, and the impoverished. Such hospices made no pretense of therapeutics and existed merely for the convenience of removing psychotic and demented individuals, those whose families were unable to care for them, from the streets of the big cities.

It goes without saying that since the days of Hippocrates, medicine has always been interested in psychiatric illness, recognizing its forms and prescribing remedies against it. As one of the Hippocratic writers in the fifth or fourth century B.C. suggested, "Most melancholics usually also become epileptics, and epileptics melancholics. One or the other prevails according to where the disease leans: if towards the body, they become epileptics, if towards reason, melancholics."[2] (This quote gives a good opportunity to warn the reader that in the past, terms such as "melancholia" and "epilepsy" did not mean exactly what we understand by them today. I, however, attempt to signpost these pitfalls throughout the text.)

As for therapeutics, since the Greeks, physicians had administered white hellebore, or veratrum viride, to open the bowels and slow the pulse. As Oxford's Robert Burton tells us in *The Anatomy of Melancholy*, published in 1621, "[White hellebore] helps melancholy, the falling-sickness [epilepsy], madness, gout, et cetera, but not to be taken of old men, youths, such as are weaklings, nice or effeminate."[3] So psychiatric illnesses have always existed, and individual doctors have always struggled to confront them.

Yet, psychiatry as a medical speciality arises only with the birth of the therapeutic asylum late in the eighteenth century because only then was a corps of trained physicians established to run these new institutions, persons knowledgeable about administering a mental hospital in a way that would prove beneficial to the patients, as opposed merely to safeguarding society from them. That implied some knowledge of psychiatric illness, an understanding of mental therapeutics, and some sense of the beneficent use of the environment. This is first adumbrated by William Battie in London in the 1760s, then Vincenzo Chiarugi in Florence in the 1780s, and finally Philippe Pinel in Paris on the cusp of the new century.

In the early nineteenth century, asylums rapidly increased in number, as an urbanizing society became more sensitive to the presence of psychotic individuals in the public thoroughfares; as civic values became more humane toward the suffering of people who previously had been quite outcast; and finally as the number of mentally ill themselves increased. An actual increase in the incidence of insanity seems to have occurred as a result of rising alcoholism (the nineteenth century saw drastic declines in the price of liquor), as a result of rising rates of neurosyphilis, and possibly as a result of a rise in schizophrenia, though this latter point is somewhat controversial.[4] In any event, the asylum population soared; ever more of these vast bins of brick and mortar went up; and the public accounts wheezed under the expenditure of institutionalizing large numbers of individuals.

Simultaneously, for the sake of well-to-do and aristocratic patients, private nervous clinics, sanatoriums, and residential treatment centers in spas pullulated.

Many private psychiatric clinics sailed under the banner of "hydrotherapy," others under "physical and dietetic therapy," still others under such euphemisms as "institutes for nervous disease," whereby everybody understood that nerves meant psychiatry. So the explosion in institutionalization was by no means confined to the poor and the less favored.

In the years before 1870, the discipline of psychiatry was thus confined largely to institutions: asylums for the poor, private clinics for the wealthy. Private practice psychiatry, to be sure, went on, but under the aegis of "hydrotherapy specialist," "electrotherapist," or "specialist in physical therapies." That these specialties for the most part no longer exist (except in places such as Austria) is evidence of the triumph of private-practice psychiatry.

In the last quarter of the nineteenth century, private practice took off as psychiatry acquired increasing psychological understanding. The first systems of medical psychotherapy were brought in by such figures as the Philadelphia neurologist S. Weir Mitchell, who described the "rest cure," or the Swiss psychiatrist Paul Dubois, who anticipated with his "rational psychotherapy" what is today called cognitive-behavioral therapy.

Yet, the key to opening a Main Street private practice and escaping from the asylum was offered by Sigmund Freud. Freud's psychoanalysis made little sense in an asylum. It was a one-on-one talking therapy that demanded a psychiatrist interested enough in what his patients were saying to spend hours on end listening to them talk—and patients who were wealthy enough to afford the fees. By the late 1920s, medical psychology was almost entirely dominated by psychoanalysis. It would lose its grip on the urban middle-classes and their private-practice psychiatrists only in the 1970s.

So even though the numbers of asylum patients continued to rise until well after the Second World War, the center of gravity of psychiatry as a discipline was slowly shifting from the asylum to Main Street. And the discipline's therapeutics were gradually wheeling from the array of sedatives proposed by the chemical industry to psychotherapy.

The rise of the pharmaceutical industry represents a major chapter in the history of psychiatry. Hellebore was left at the roadside after the 1870s with the advent of synthetic chemicals from coal tar. The new industry was centered primarily in German-speaking Central Europe, specifically in the industrial centers of the Rhine Valley stretching north from Basel (Roche, Geigy, Ciba, and Sandoz), along the course of the great Rhine river past Ludwigshafen (BASF) and Leverkusen (Bayer), to the wharves of Rotterdam, where ships would carry Bayer's barbiturates and Roche's bromide-based Sedobrol to the homes of middle-class America. Chloral hydrate was the first product of the organic-chemical industry to find application in psychiatry (in 1869), but by the First World War, a whole world of hypnotics and sedatives lined the shelves of the apothecaries. Thus, it is a mistake to think of pharmaceuticals arriving in psychiatry only in the 1950s.

Yet after the 1920s, the self-concept of the discipline became increasingly psychotherapy rather than psychopharmacology, and the theories of causation ever more stressed Freud's model of psychogenesis rather than the brain-biological theories of the nineteenth century with their emphasis upon degeneration and genetics.

Psychoanalysis, of course, arose in Freud's Vienna around 1900. It quickly turned into a kind of movement, in which junior practitioners would learn the ropes in the course of training analyses from seniors, rather than from textbooks or public lectures. One can grasp the fervor with which psychoanalysis was preached—particularly in American psychiatry—only in understanding it as a kind of secular religion; it was a religion in which articles of faith in such concepts as "the Oedipus complex" were laid down despite the inability of their adepts to demonstrate them empirically in any fashion save anecdotally.

The success of psychoanalysis in the New World was greatly accelerated by the tragedy of the Hitler regime and the Holocaust, in which the leaders of German psychoanalysis found refuge in New York, Washington, D.C., and Los Angeles. Such was the prestige of these internationally known figures that they virtually captured control of American psychiatry. Sándor Radó, Franz Alexander, and Hilde Bruch acquired immense authority within the discipline in the United States, and by the 1950s—even though the number of actual psychoanalysts was rather small—psychoanalytic ideas informed virtually every training program in the country except that of Washington University in St. Louis and one or two others.

Meanwhile, a counter-assault was brewing, fueled by advances in psychopharmacology and the neurosciences. One of the signal events in the history of psychiatry was the discovery in 1952 of the antipsychotic effects of the drug chlorpromazine. Launched as Largactil in much of the world and as Thorazine in the United States, chlorpromazine initiated a virtual revolution as it showed that the florid symptoms of psychosis and schizophrenia—the delusions, hallucinations, and agitation—could be brought under control chemically without unduly sedating the patients yet making them more or less functional again, or making them accessible to psychotherapy as the doctrine of the day had it. (Even the drug companies said in their ads, laughing up their sleeves of course, that the phenothiazine antipsychotics—of which chlorpromazine was one—did not in themselves cure but made patients accessible to psychotherapy, the only "true cure" in psychiatry.) Chlorpromazine was the beginning of a great wave of phenothiazine antipsychotics, a wave further powered by the advent in the 1960s of other chemical classes of antipsychotic medication, such as haloperidol (marketed as Haldol, of the butyrophenone class).

The 1950s had seen the launch of a number of successful "antineurotic" drugs, such as meprobamate (Miltown) and methylphenidate (Ritalin). Yet in 1960, one of the most successful drug groups in history made its debut: the benzodiazepine class of antianxiety drugs, of which Librium (chlordiazepoxide) was the first. Valium (diazepam), arguably next to Prozac the single most successful drug in the history of psychopharmaceuticals, was launched in 1963. Many other "benzos" followed, edging the barbiturates from the scene.

As a third important development in psychopharmacology, following chlorpromazine and the antineurotics, from 1957 on, drugs effective in hospital depression began to appear. Though community anxiety-depression had been treatable since the 1940s with the amphetamines, and the amphetamine–barbiturate combinations,[5] melancholic hospital depression remained a condition for which there was no remedy except electroconvulsive therapy (ECT)—and that only available after 1938. Swiss psychiatrist Roland Kuhn's discovery in 1957 of the efficacy of the "tricyclic" antidepressant imipramine (Tofranil) in "vital" depression opened up the whole area of mood disorders to pharmacotherapy. The tricyclics gave way in time to other classes of antidepressants, such as the selective serotonin reuptake inhibitors (SSRIs) of the 1980s and 1990s.

Yet, the success of these chemical strategies against such conditions as depression and psychosis—believed by the psychoanalysts to be "psychogenic"—caused a massive rethinking about what actually caused psychiatric illness: Was it a psychogenic disorder of mind, arising from unconscious conflicts of a sexual nature? Or was it a neurogenic disorder of brain, arising from "chemical imbalances"? The great wheel of fashion in psychiatry, arrested for years at psychoanalysis and depth psychiatry, began to turn slowly on, toward brain biological theories for which pharmaceutical strategies were indicated.

Spurred by these pharmaceutical successes, interest in the neurosciences began to revive, having been in the deep freeze since the discrediting of the "brain mythology" of the nineteenth century. Here, for the first time, American scientific figures started to take the baton from the Europeans. From 1955 on, at the National Institute of Mental Health (NIMH) and the National Heart Institute—both part of the federal National Institutes of Health (NIH) centered in Bethesda, Maryland—fundamental advances started to be made in cerebral chemistry: understanding the metabolism of adrenalin, or the nature of the neurotransmitters and how the brain used them. In the mid-1950s, NIMH scientists developed a spectrophotofluorimeter for detecting the presence of neurotransmitters in brain tissue. All these developments in basic science were essential to pushing drug development forward on the basis of a firm platform of rational discovery.

Finally, the scientific revolution in psychiatry rolled forward in the area of clinical diagnostics and of nosology (the theory behind the grouping of diagnoses). To backtrack for a second: in the nineteenth century, during the period of the first biological psychiatry, there were a multitude of diagnostic systems: each psychiatry textbook proposed a different one. Then, beginning in 1893, the Heidelberg psychiatry professor Emil Kraepelin suggested a system of his own, and such was his authority—or such was the inherent logic of his system—that it swept most of the others from the board and became for decades the dominant international system. Kraepelin grouped the many different psychosis diagnoses into one category, which he called "Dementia praecox" (in 1908, Zurich psychiatry professor Eugen Bleuler renamed it schizophrenia). As well, Kraepelin took the many different diagnoses for mood disorders and lumped them into a single category, which he called "manic-depressive illness." All the while, he insisted that these were totally separate diseases. The French were reluctant to embrace Kraepelin's system in its entirety, but elsewhere the adjective "Kraepelinian" acquired great staying power.

Now we race forward in time. Psychoanalysis triumphs, and the psychoanalysts had little interest in the refinement of diagnosis. They considered that most people had a psychic state located at some point on a continuum from well to ill, and that it made little sense to categorize patients' symptoms into boxes because the underlying psychic conflicts that caused the symptoms were of greatest interest. In the middle third of the twentieth century, psychopathology, meaning symptoms that communicate the manifestations of illness, languished. It was once said that the study of symptoms represented the least interesting aspect of American psychiatry.

In the early 1970s, the American Psychiatric Association decided that it was time for a revision of its diagnostic handbook, the *Diagnostic and Statistical Manual* (*DSM*), of which the second edition had appeared in 1968. Robert Spitzer, a Columbia University psychiatrist whose main interest was the measurement and classification of illness, was asked to head the task force in charge of the revision. Spitzer and his collaborators produced in *DSM-III*, published in 1980, a handbook dramatically different from previous editions. *DSM-III* attempted to put diagnosis on a scientific footing by specifying operational criteria that a patient would have to meet to qualify for a given diagnosis. Also, *DSM-III* brought back the firewall that Kraepelin had erected between mood disorders and schizophrenia and set up vast basket-diagnoses similar to Kraepelin's: in this case, "major depression" and schizophrenia. With *DSM-III* and its successors, the hope of achieving scientific diagnoses once again loomed in the forefront of the discipline's attention.

If nosology was one factor in distancing post-1970s psychiatry from its psychoanalytic past, the other was psychopharmacology. Psychopharmacology in a strict sense means the study of the differential response to drugs, using medications as a pharmacological torch to delineate new disease entities. In a wider sense, it means simply studying the clinical response to medication. In any event, medication became the new accent in psychiatry after the success of chlorpromazine, imipramine, the benzodiazepines, and numerous other drug classes.

With the arrival of effective medications, the discipline became increasingly oriented toward the prescribing of pharmaceuticals rather than the provision of psychotherapy. The "couch," for example, began disappearing from psychiatrists' offices, and the "*PDR*," the *Physician's Desk Reference* for the use of American doctors in prescribing, became instead a steady companion. By the 1990s, the vast majority of consultations in psychiatry would end with a prescription, a practice unusual before the 1970s. The manufacture and promotion of psychoactive medication became a big business, with annual sales of popular drugs such as fluoxetine (Prozac) and paroxetine (Paxil) running into billions of dollars. Accordingly, psychiatrists increasingly became the objects of attention of the drug companies, and industry funds became essential to the financing of large psychiatry meetings. This great involvement with industry has a positive side—the swifter development of new drugs—as well as a negative side (efforts of industry to steer psychiatric diagnosis in the direction of the drugs a company has on offer). Yet, by the beginning of the new millennium, psychiatry as a discipline would extensively be intertwined with the corporate sector.

These massive changes in the nature of psychiatry proved disorienting for many practitioners. As early as 1924, Heidelberg psychiatrist Willi Mayer-Gross deplored the tendency of the discipline to throw out past discoveries completely with the advent of each new orientation: "It has unfortunately almost become a rule in psychiatry that we begin everything again from zero after a new viewpoint appears [he was almost certainly referring to psychoanalysis], and we simply throw the past overboard."[6] The biological psychiatrists of the nineteenth century, who prided themselves on their careful descriptions of patients' symptoms, felt bewildered as the psychoanalysts rushed past them without so much as a glance at the profession's accumulated knowledge of 100 years. The psychoanalysts themselves felt suddenly adrift in the 1980s as *DSM-III* trashed such valued concepts as "neurosis," bringing an end to "neurotic depression," which had been the profession's single most valued diagnosis. The advocates of social and community psychiatry, whose voices in the 1950s and 1960s had sounded so strongly on behalf of progressive social policies, felt wounded as the discipline's energies flowed into pharmacology rather than cleaning up the slums. And even the psychopharmacologists today, who otherwise sit so firmly in the saddle, become uneasy as the psychologists point out that in the treatment of nonhospital depression, psychotherapy seems every bit as effective as antidepressant drugs.[7]

Thus, the story ends provisionally with the triumph of biology. Yet even a biologized psychiatry pulled back from seeing itself merely as an extension of neurology—for which latter discipline the mind really does not intervene between brain and behavior. What remained distinctive about psychiatry was its interest in the mind rather than in synapses and neurotransmitters. As Paul McHugh and Philip Slavney of Johns Hopkins University point out, "Psychiatrists cannot go directly from knowing the elements of brain (neurons and synapses) to explaining the conscious experiences that are the essence of mental life." "In other words, psychiatry cannot be replaced by neurology because brain facts cannot be substituted for mind facts."[8]

The essential message of this review of the discipline during the past 200 years is that historically, psychiatry has been subject to jolting changes and discontinuities that are less common in other medical specialties such as cardiology or nephrology. This is because so little is understood about the underlying causes of psychiatric illness. Not having a solid "pathophysiology," or understanding of the mechanisms of disease, psychiatry cannot rigorously delineate disease entities on the basis of anatomical pathology, as other medical fields do. Thus, the discipline is subject to faddism—anything could be true, nothing can be disproven. During the years, time and again psychiatry has been held hostage by trendy new ideas that cannot be invalidated on the basis of scientific evidence but that must either be the objects of disbelief or of sectarian enthusiasm. Readers of the *Dictionary* will immediately be struck, in the diagnosis narratives of "depression" and "schizophrenia," or "psychotherapy" and "personality disorders," at how little building on the past seems to take place, how little accumulation of wisdom and experience there has been during the years. Instead, bold new ideas rush onto center stage, strut and fret for their half-hour in the limelight, and then disappear. A dictionary of this nature can at least point out what now forgotten ideas lie in the rubble of the past that might merit reexamination.

NATIONAL TRADITIONS

"If French is the language of diplomacy, German may be said to be the language of psychiatry," wrote one senior British psychiatrist in 1962.[9] In truth, the history of psychiatry until the Hitler regime is dominated by German-speaking authors from the various small states that came together in 1871 to form the German Empire, additionally by psychiatrists in the Austro-Hungarian Empire, and in German-speaking Switzerland. Even leading authorities in Hungary (such as Ladislaus von Meduna who described metrazol convulsion therapy) and from Scandinavia (such as geneticist Erich Strömgren) wrote in German. Today, in a world of scientific communication dominated by English, the primacy of the German language seems inconceivable, but that simply shows how the world has changed.

Even though the French pride themselves as the founders of psychiatry, a primacy they share partly with the Italians, France ceased relatively soon to be a psychiatric Great Power, while it was to Vienna and Berlin that eager young American and English clinicians would flock in the years around 1900 to learn the secrets of microscopy and the flair of differentiating schizophrenia from psychotic depression. Indeed, as early as 1854, after returning from a tour of German asylums, French psychiatrist Jacques-Joseph Moreau ("Moreau de Tours") conceded the German advance, talking of "the great scientific movement in German psychiatry."[10] What accounts for the German lead, the French and English lag?

For one thing, there was the sheer bulk of German academic psychiatry, 34 medical schools teaching psychiatry in the German language, from Prague in the Austro-Hungarian Empire to Strasbourg (which after 1871 had become German again), from Graz in Austria to Greifswald in the north of Germany.[11] Psychiatry in Basel, Switzerland, was marked by close ties to the pharmaceutical industry; Heidelberg was characterized by the phenomenological movement; Munich by its history of research in brain anatomy and the German Psychiatric Research Institute in addition to the university department of psychiatry (such departments are usually centered in psychiatric hospitals, or "clinics"); Vienna supplied the world with distinguished psychiatrists and psychoanalysts far out of proportion to its population;[12] and from Zurich's Burghölzli, the cantonal mental hospital and university psychiatric clinic, comes the term "schizophrenia."

In France, by contrast, there was really just one big center of excellence: the Paris University; the few provincial universities that acquired departments of psychiatry late in the nineteenth century were not really on anybody's radar. Of course, a world of distinguished contributions comes to us from Paris: from Pinel in 1800 to Jean Delay and his gifted co-workers after the Second World War. Yet, in quantitative terms, the French are overwhelmed; to see this within medicine in general, one can take a medical dictionary such as *Dorland's*, open it to entries under "signs," and encounter page after page of German and German-Jewish surnames but relatively few French.

But it was not just the brute size of the German academic establishment. There were in Germany incentives to do research that were muted elsewhere. To qualify for university teaching, for example, German M.D.s and Ph.D.s had to prepare a Habilitation, a very substantial postdoctoral thesis (in addition to the doctoral dissertation, which they would have done earlier), whereas the French had merely to pass an exacting exam, the Agrégation. There is a world of difference between cramming the knowledge of others for an exam and producing new knowledge of one's own. Then, once on the ladder of promotion, German academic psychiatrists tended to be advanced on the basis of publication rather than through the old-boys' network—although there was also a good deal of the latter, as everywhere. Yet it was simply infeasible—it could not be justified to the Ministry of Education—to promote complete dullards to professorships. Because there were so many professorships, many of the brightest in the German-speaking universities were selected for academic leadership. The French Agrégation, and the many other competitive exams in the French system, tend to select bright people too, of course, but they may lack that deep scientific curiosity that research requires.

In the hydra-headed German system, therefore, the many centers of excellence meant that it was impossible for a single academic to dominate an entire discipline at the national level. In the highly centralized French system, this did happen, and if that individual happened to be eccentric, or a mediocrity, there would be a national scholarly disaster. This occurred late in the nineteenth century in France in psychiatry and neurology, in the form of Jean-Martin Charcot, the master of the Salpêtrière; although Charcot was certainly not a dullard, his doctrine of "hysteria," which crumbled with his death in 1893, probably set French psychiatry and neurology back by about 30 years.

Britain until the 1930s lagged far behind the Continent. As an official of the Rockefeller Foundation noted in 1933, apropos a request from Edward Mapother, superintendent of the Maudsley Hospital in London, for a small grant, "There are not enough scientific papers being turned out in England to fill one small journal whereas lesser countries like Belgium and Italy support several journals of comparable quality. . . . Outside London there is hardly a place where any research in psychiatry is being done. . . . I feel a litle disappointed myself at the Maudsley show. The laboratory facilities are limited, and there is hardly any provision for animal experimentation."[13]

What accounted for the British delay? Although medical education was decentralized, as in Germany, psychiatry played little role in the British academic curriculum, and the psychiatric hospitals received almost nothing in the way of government money, as opposed to Germany, where the university hospitals were largely state-funded. The differences in 1908 between undergraduate education in psychiatry in Germany and Great Britain are instructive: of the 16 British universities offering medicine, a goodly number including Oxford, Cambridge, and London set no questions in psychiatry in the final exams of the medical students; only 3 had a separate oral and clinical exam in psychiatry. Of the 19 medical faculties in the German Empire, all required a 6-month rotation in a psychiatric clinic and required questions on psychiatry in the examinations. In addition, many students would garner 3 months or more experience in a mental hospital after qualifying, and any physician wanting to work as coroner or district medical officer had to pass a special exam in psychiatry.[14] Clearly, English physicians were little exposed to psychiatry and so had little opportunity to make research contributions to it.

Finally, the Germans cultivated the art of close clinical observation in the interest of defining new diseases. In the 1990s, English psychopharmacologist Malcolm Lader recalled, "We always used to say if you go back far enough and look at German literature at the turn of the century, you're sure to find that someone described panic disorder and everything else."[15] The Germans prided themselves on extensive case histories in their publications and on teasing out fine psychopathological differences between one syndrome and another, in the hopes that these differences might lead at the end of the day to different disease entities. It is not that the English were not careful clinical observers; internationally, they were known for their shrewdness at the bedside, but in the spirit of English empiricism they pulled back from constructing daring disease entities (the disproval of which is the motor of scientific progress), and in the disease narratives of this dictionary there are somewhat fewer English contributions, whereas there is German all over the page.

Before the Second World War, the United States was scarcely on the map of contributions to world psychiatry. "In the four quarters of the globe, who reads an American book?" sneered English critic Sydney Smith in the nineteenth century, and the answer was as valid for American psychiatry as for literature. Before Adolf Meyer became head of psychiatry at Johns Hopkins University in 1910, it was unusual for an American psychiatrist to be quoted abroad, and Meyer's influence was mainly among his former students in Britain. (George Miller Beard, who in 1869 proposed the diagnosis "neurasthenia," was an electrotherapist; S. Weir Mitchell, who launched the famous "rest cure," was a neurologist.) Set against the German heavyweights and the French systematizers, the clinicians of the young Republic were like the proverbial country mice.

All this changed after the Second World War. First of all, Germany vanished as a psychiatric Great Power. Having murdered or driven out their Jewish clinicians and scientists, the Germans had doused some of the brightest lights in the academy. The migration to the United States of their world-famous psychoanalysts has already been noted. But the Germans lost many important Jewish clinicians and basic scientists, who reappeared at places like the Rockefeller Institute and

Columbia University, ready to train coming generations of young Americans. Yet, there were many non-Jews who went into "internal exile" during the Nazi years and ceased to be productive. The Heidelberg school of "phenomenology," for example, simply disintegrated after 1933. Then, the chaos of war and reconstruction further hobbled German science, so that German ceased to be a language of international scientific discourse. Indeed today, almost all German psychiatrists and neuroscientists publish in English, not German, and the lead Central European journals appear in English.

In France and Germany alike after the war, such basic components of psychiatry as psychopathology and psychopharmacology received considerable setbacks with the vogue for psychoanalysis that set in during the 1960s, at a time when psychoanalysis had started to ebb in the United States. Now in the new millennium, when psychoanalysis has virtually vanished from United States psychiatry, it remains strong in Europe, a telling component of the European lag.

A better way to pose the question is not to ask why Europe remained "behind," but why the United States bounded so suddenly to world leadership in psychiatry. The answer has two components, aside from the above-noted migration of European leaders to escape the Holocaust. The first concerns the enormous sums of money that the American government began shoveling into psychiatry research after the National Institute of Mental Health opened its doors in 1949. Government funding was less generous elsewhere, and science thrives as the dew of mammon is sprinkled upon it.

Second, the pharmaceutical industry began to pay for significant amounts of academic research. Even though industry money often goes to fund drug trials that are scientifically uninteresting—although required for regulatory purposes—lots of basic psychopharmacology and neuroscience was sustained with industry money. Many of the drugs—as well as the scientific publications—that resulted from this enterprise have unquestionably benefited the public health. (Industry money has flowed much more to America than to Europe because the American market is the largest in the world, and companies can charge what they wish for new products, unlike elsewhere.)

Finally, it is interesting to speculate that the Americans and British were able to hack so much hard, useful science from the coalface because they have traditionally been tone-deaf to the kind of philosophical speculation that has infused European psychiatry since Immanuel Kant and Georg W. F. Hegel started writing late in the eighteenth century. "Even the word psychopathology is not well understood in the United States," lamented Spanish psychiatrist Juan J. Lopez Ibor.[16] Heinz Lehmann, a pioneer psychopharmacologist trained in Germany who had something of a philosophical bent, recalled a plane trip back from Zurich to North America in 1957 in which he sat beside his English colleague, Aldwyn Stokes: Everybody was making so much of a fuss about existentialism, said Stokes, who then asked Lehmann, "What is this whole thing?"

Lehmann thought, "Well, here is a captive audience; he wants to hear about it, he is a professor, he is obviously quite bright so I'll start. Then for about two hours I talked about it—Husserl and Heidegger and so on. He listened carefully and very attentively and at the end he said, 'well the whole thing is really just a symphony of words, isn't it?' So ever since I have given up trying to explain existentialism to anyone outside Europe. . . . "[17]

This Anglo-Saxon empiricism that resisted ratiocination about the real meaning of the patients' symptoms produced a harvest of useful drugs, a more promising psychiatric nosology—the *DSM-III* now widely adopted in Europe—and some innovative new psychotherapies that broke with psychoanalysis.

It is perhaps the new, humanistic psychotherapies that arose in the years after the Second World War from such popular bases as the "mind-cure" movement of the nineteenth century that have been the greatest contribution of the United States to mental health. They came more from psychologists, not psychiatrists. From 1946, psychologist Carl Rogers developed his "client-centered therapy" that would have an enormous impact on the psychotherapy scene. Gregory Bateson was, to be sure, an anthropologist—and Donald Jackson a psychiatrist—yet the "family therapy" they began to elaborate in the mid-1950s had a substantial impact on the management of schizophrenia. And Aaron Beck's "cognitive therapy," in the public forum from 1963 on, became widely adopted by psychologists and psychiatric social workers. All were distinctively American products that owed nothing to psychoanalysis and that, in their turn, would go on to colonize much of the global psychotherapy scene.

The grand history of psychiatry, then, provides some striking changes in international dominance. The nosological fervor of the years 1860–1920, in which almost all current diagnostic concepts were laid down, was largely a German–French phenomenon. In terms of psychotherapy, psychoanalysis came to us from Vienna and Berlin, but the humanistic psychotherapies of the mid-twentieth century emphasizing personal growth were homegrown in America. The French have been in the forefront of diagnostic systems that seek to separate delusions and hallucinations from personality deterioration—and thus to dismantle schizophrenia into what might possibly be treatment-responsive subgroups. (A German current of research, termed here "the Wernicke–Kleist–Leonhard pathway," has also sought to do this, yet its members have achieved much less familiarity.) In keeping with the pragmatism of the British, their contributions to the story have been of a more practical nature, featuring epidemiology and child psychiatry. The British led the world during the whole era of asylum building, which reached its apogee in the nineteenth century. But because the asylums left almost no footprint on today's psychiatry (save for the German passion for microscopy, which originated in the asylum rather than the university clinic), many British contributions have unjustly been forgotten.

In sum, the history of psychiatry is hallmarked by continual shifts in national dominance, as well as by profound changes in the discipline's diagnostic schema and its therapeutics. It is certain that much more of both lies ahead.

ARRANGEMENT

The *Dictionary* has been arranged into main entries that are alphabetical, and subentries that are chronological. Readers will find the main historic figures in psychiatry at their alphabetical location, but will be able to follow chronologically the development of diagnostic concepts and procedures, such as neuroimaging or psychotherapy. Thus depression as a master concept unfolds over the years in terms of neurotic depression, major depression, psychotic depression, and so forth—and the Depression entry offers a handy overview of these changes. All concepts, institutions, individuals, and diagnoses are included in the index, and extensive use is made of cross-referencing to permit readers to hop back and forth between "depression" and "melancholia," for example, or between "Vienna" and the scads of individual psychiatrists who made that city an epicenter. Unusual for a dictionary, this one mentions the journals in which important contributions appeared, and gives the page numbers of quotations taken from them, without deploying the whole scholarly apparatus of citation. Finally, extensive use is made of boldface to direct readers to main entries. Please note that in the United Kingdom the degree "M.B.," for "Bachelor of Medicine," is equivalent to the "M.D." of the United States. The degree "M.D." in the United Kingdom is the same as a Ph.D. but is only open to physicians.

NOTES

1. Readers will find this brief account fleshed out in Shorter, Edward. (1997). *A History of Psychiatry from the Era of the Asylum to the Age of Prozac*. New York: John Wiley & Sons.

2. Quoted in Jackson, Stanley. (1986). *Melancholia and Depression From Hippocratic Times to Modern Times* (p. 31). New Haven: Yale University Press.

3. Burton, Robert. (1621). *The Anatomy of Melancholy*. (Reprint edition based on text of 1651, New York: Tudor, 1948, p. 575).

4. See Hare, Edward. (1988). Schizophrenia as a Recent Disease. *British Journal of Psychiatry, 153*, 521–531.

5. See Legge, D., & Steinberg, H. (1962). Actions of a Mixture of Amphetamine and a Barbiturate in Man. *British Journal of Pharmacology, 18*, 490–500.

6. Mayer-Gross, W. (1924). *Selbstschilderungen der Verwirrtheit: die oneiroide Erlebnisform* (p. 111). Berlin: Springer.

7. See, for example, Greenberg, Roger P., & Fisher, Seymour. (1997). Mood-mending medicines: probing drug, psychotherapy, and placebo solutions. In S. Fisher & R. P. Greenberg (Eds.), *From Placebo to Panacea: Putting Psychiatric Drugs to the Test* (pp. 115–172). New York: Wiley; see also Kirsch, Irving, & Sapirstein, Guy. (1998). Listening to Prozac but hearing placebo: a meta-analysis of antidepressant medication. *Prevention and Treatment*, article 0002a. From http://journals.apa.org/prevention/volume1/pre0010002a.html

8. McHugh, Paul R., & Slavney, Phillip R. (1998). *The Perspectives of Psychiatry*, 2nd ed. (p. 12). Baltimore: Johns Hopkins University Press.

9. Anderson, E. W. Foreword to Fish, Frank J. (1962). *Schizophrenia* (p. ix). Bristol: Wright.

10. Moreau, Jacques-Joseph P. (1854). Notes sur les établissements d'aliénés de Siegburg. *Annales médico-psychologiques*, 2nd ser., *6*, 428–439 (quote p. 430).

11. See Eulner, Hans-Heinz. (1970). *Die Entwicklung der medizinischen Spezialfächer an den Universitäten des deutschen Sprachgebietes* (pp. 670–680). Stuttgart: Enke.

12. For a listing of distinguished psychoanalysts, see Mühlleitner, Elke. (1992). *Biographisches Lexikon der Psychoanalyse: die Mitglieder der Psychologischen Mittwoch-Gesellschaft und der Wiener Psychoanalytischen Vereinigung, 1902–1938*. Tübingen: Diskord.

13. Quoted in Angel, Katherine. (2003). Defining psychiatry: Aubrey Lewis's 1938 Report and the Rockefeller Foundation. In Katherine Angel et al. (Eds.), *European Psychiatry on the Eve of War: Aubrey Lewis, the Maudsley Hospital, and the Rockefeller Foundation in the 1930s* (pp. 39–56). London: Wellcome Trust Centre for the History of Medicine at UCL.

14. Crammer, John L. (1996). Training and education in British psychiatry, 1770-1970. In Hugh Freeman & German E. Berrios (Eds.), *150 Years of British Psychiatry, vol. II: the Aftermath* (pp. 209–242). London: Athlone.

15. Interview with Malcolm Lader. (1996). In David Healy (Ed.), *The Psychopharmacologists: Interviews* (vol. I, pp. 463–481). London: Chapman and Hall.

16. Interview with Juan Lopez-Ibor. (1998). In David Healy (Ed.), *The Psychopharmacologists: Interviews* (vol. II, pp. 431). London: Chapman and Hall.

17. Interview with Heinz Lehmann. (1996). In David Healy (Ed.), *The Psychopharmacologists: Interviews* (vol. I, p. 169). London: Chapman and Hall.

A

AFFECTIVE DISORDERS. *See* DEPRESSION: EMERGENCE; DEPRESSION: RECENT CONCEPTS; HYPOMANIA; MANIC-DEPRESSIVE ILLNESS.

AGORAPHOBIA. *See* ANXIETY AND PHOBIAS (1870 and after).

AKATHISIA, OR INABILITY TO REMAIN IN A SITTING POSTURE.

First description of akathisia (1880). In his *Practical Treatise on Nervous Exhaustion (Neurasthenia)*, New York neurologist and electrotherapist George Beard (1839–1883) described as a characteristic of neurasthenia, "Fidgetiness and inability to keep still—a sensation that amounts to pain—is sometimes unspeakably distressing. . . . When the legs feel this way, the sufferer must get up and walk or run. . . . A gentleman once under my care could not sit still in the chair long enough to take an application of electricity" (pp. 41–42).

Naming the syndrome akathisia (1901). From Greek "a" (neg.) + "kathisis" (sitting down). In November 1901, Ladislav Haskovec (1866–1944), a neurologist from Prague who had previously studied with **Jean-Martin Charcot**, demonstrated to the Paris Neurological Society two patients who were unable to remain seated. At the time he did not know what to make of it and suggested it was close to "astasia-abasia [hysterical ataxia] of the French school." Yet, as he continued in his paper, published in 1901 in the *Neurological Review* (*Revue neurologique*), "If this phenomenon is encountered more commonly . . . one might give it the name 'akathisia.'" The following July, **Pierre Janet** highlighted yet a further patient with this "bizarre nervous disease" and published the case in a psychiatric journal (*La Nouvelle Iconographie de la Salpêtrière*), thus lending his own authority to the neologism. Haskovec, said Janet, had deemed the disorder the exact opposite of hysterical astasia-abasia. But Janet was dubious: These patients are dysphoric while standing as well. "What the patient wants to do, in sum, is unlimited walking, drifting here and there with no particular destination" (Janet, *Les Obsessions*, II, 80). In other words, akathisia was a symptom that could not be controlled by will.

A result of psychoactive medication (from 1947). Although Parkinson's disease had always been associated with akathisia, in 1947 in the *Revue neurologique* Jean Sigwald (1903–) and co-workers at the Brousse Psychiatric Hospital in Paris reported that one of the early phenothiazine-type (*see* **CHLORPROMAZINE**) drugs, diethazine hydrochloride (Rhône-Poulenc 2987), caused akathisia in patients with Parkinsonism. The advent of more powerful antipsychotic medications in the early 1950s created interest in the subjective feelings of restlessness in akathisia, as well as in the motor component. "Neuroleptic-induced acute akathisia" entered the *Diagnostic and Statistical Manual* (***DSM***) series in ***DSM-IV*** (1994), in the category of diagnoses provided "for further study." According to the *Manual*, "The subjective complaints include a sense of inner restlessness, most often in the legs; a compulsion to move one's legs . . . dysphoria and anxiety." It also noted that, "Akathisia may be associated with dysphoria, irritability, aggression, or suicide attempts" (pp. 744–745). According to the *Manual*, antidepressants as well as antipsychotics could induce the syndrome. For neurologists, akathisia is often seen as a first sign of Parkinsonism.

In the 1990s and after, concern arose that the **selective serotonin-reuptake inhibitor** (SSRI)-style drugs could induce in a select subgroup of patients the kind of akathisia that might lead to violent acts including suicide. For details, the reader may consult David Healy, *Let Them Eat Prozac* (2003).

ALCOHOLISM. (*See also* **SUBSTANCE ABUSE.**) Since the beginning of modern times, medicine has considered alcoholism a disease rather than a moral failing. In the nineteenth century, with the advent of inexpensive, industrially distilled alcohol, alcoholism became a colossal social problem, filling the asylums with victims of alcoholic dementia and delirium. **Emil Kraepelin**, himself teetotal, in the fourth edition of his textbook (1893) rather puritanically classed alcoholism among the "poisonings," next to ergotism, and spoke of "misuse" rather than addiction. In his *Outline of Psychiatry* (*Grundriss der Psychiatrie*, 1900), Carl Wernicke (1848–1905), professor of psychiatry in Breslau, devoted an entire lecture to "alcoholic delirium," especially delirium tremens. (*See* **WERNICKE–KLEIST–LEONHARD PATHWAY**.) For the pioneers of psychiatry, alcoholism was thus very much on the radar.

In the late twentieth century, however, the medical emphasis in alcohol came to fall on its addictive rather than toxic qualities. In ***DSM-I*** (1952), the accent was mainly on poisoning: delirium, hallucinosis, and alcoholic dementia. Yet, a section on "alcoholism" was added to the *Manual*: "cases in which there is well established addiction to alcohol without recognizable underlying disorder" (p. 39). ***DSM-II*** (1968) enlarged the classification of "alcoholism" considerably, admitting not only "addiction," as before, but "episodic excessive drinking" and "habitual excessive drinking." The pathology thus lay in the pattern of consumption rather than in the brain consequences.

Then, a sea change: ***DSM-III*** (1980) included the usual brain consequences of ethanolic intoxication yet added a concept going beyond "addiction" that permitted classifying alcoholism among all the other "substance use disorders." That word was "dependence." What the substance-use disorders had in common was the induction of dependence: "The essential features of Alcohol Dependence are either a pattern of pathological alcohol use or impairment in social or occupational functioning due to alcohol, and either tolerance or withdrawal" (p. 169). (One knew that one was dependent—as opposed to having brain toxicity—if one kept upping the dose to get the same effect [tolerance] or if one suffered "withdrawal" symptoms.) By ***DSM-III-R*** in 1987, "alcohol dependence" had become a "psychoactive" substance use disorder.

DSM-IV (1994) further augmented the range of alcohol pathology, differentiating between the disorders that alcohol touched-off (ranging from brain toxicity to depression) and those inherent in its use: abuse and dependence. This massed array of pathology was in a sense neo-Kraepelinian, returning to the teetotal spirit of the founder of modern psychiatry.

ALZHEIMER, ALOIS (1864–1915). Known for describing the type of presenile **dementia** named after him, Alzheimer was born in a small town in Lower Franconia, Germany, the son of a local bureaucrat. After completing his medical studies in 1888 at the University of Würzburg—and after orienting himself toward neurohistology in a short spell of research in the lab of Rudolf Albert Kölliker (1817–1905) in Würzburg—Alzheimer took a post later in 1888 as assistant physician at the Frankfurt City Asylum, where the director Emil Franz Sioli (1852–1922) at least tolerated scientific work with a microscope. Shortly thereafter **Franz Nissl**, another young psychiatrist with an interest in central-nervous tissue, joined Alzheimer at the Frankfurt asylum. (Nissl had studied with Bernhard von Gudden [1824–1886] in Munich and was terribly keen on pressing forward with studies of the microanatomy of the brain.) For the next 7 years, Nissl and Alzheimer worked in close cooperation, Nissl doing research on stains for CNS tissues (one of which is named after him) and Alzheimer doing the postmortems on patients who had suffered from psychiatric and neurological disorders. In 1894, Alzheimer began to report his work on the histology of neurosyphilis, an early step in the differentiation of the organic **dementias**. He collaborated on much of this histological work with Nissl, and in 1898, Alzheimer discovered some unusual changes in the brain tissue of a patient with senile dementia.

In 1895, **Emil Kraepelin** had invited Nissl to come and work at the university psychiatry clinic in **Heidelberg**, where Kraepelin was chief; in March 1903, Alzheimer followed Nissl to Heidelberg. Kraepelin was now following attentively the research of both men.

In October 1903, Alzheimer went with Kraepelin to Munich, where Kraepelin had just become professor of psychiatry. (Nissl had initially joined them but returned to Heidelberg to become professor of psychiatry there.) Three years later, in 1906, Alzheimer gave a paper on a patient with presenile dementia in which he described what would later be called "tangles and plaques." In 1907, Alzheimer's much-cited paper "On a Distinctive Disease of the Cerebral Cortex" ("Über eine eigenartige Erkrankung der Hirnrinde") appeared in the *General Journal of Psychiatry* (*Allgemeine Zeitschrift für Psychiatrie*). Kraepelin found these findings so interesting that in the next edition of his psychiatry textbook, the eighth edition (the volume published in 1910), he created the disease category "presenile insanity" that later became known as "Alzheimer's disease": severe dementias with characteristic histological changes but no cerebral arteriosclerosis. For all of these researchers, identifying dementias was marginal to their true interests: finding anatomical differences between dementia praecox and manic-depressive illness, which they never discovered.

ALZHEIMER'S DISEASE. *See* DEMENTIA: **Alzheimer's presenile dementia** (1906, 1910).

AMPHETAMINES. *See* NARCOLEPSY; ANTIDEPRESSANT: **First-generation antidepressants: the amphetamines.**

ANDREASEN, NANCY COOVER (1938–). Known for introducing new imaging techniques in the study of schizophrenia, Andreasen was born in Lincoln, Nebraska, and earned a Ph.D. in English literature at the University of Nebraska in 1963. She taught English at several institutions in Nebraska and then, after a harrowing encounter with a postpartum infection (and after being inspired by the life-saving powers of antibiotics), decided to study medicine. She received her M.D. from the University of Iowa in 1970, trained as a psychiatrist, and remained at Iowa—a university that already was a powerhouse in biological psychiatry—for the rest of her career. In 1981, she was appointed professor of psychiatry and later became chair of the department. In 1992, she became the eleventh editor of the *American Journal of Psychiatry*—a publication founded in 1844—and the first woman to fill that office. In 1986, she led the first quantitative magnetic-resonance study of schizophrenia (*see* **NEUROIMAGING**), reinforcing the hypothesis that schizophrenia was a neurodevelopmental disease associated with "hypofrontality" rather than being psychogenic or a result of toxic exposure in adult life. (*See* **SCHIZOPHRENIA: RECENT CONCEPTS.**) She is also known for developing a scale for the measurement of negative symptoms in schizophrenia, work published in the *Archives of General Psychiatry* in 1982 that became a "citation classic." (*See* **POSITIVE VS. NEGATIVE SYMPTOMS.**)

ANHEDONIA (1896 and later). Although loss of interest in pleasure had always been seen as one of the symptoms of depression, it was only in 1896 that Théodule-Armand Ribot (1839–1916), professor of experimental psychology at the University of Paris, coined in *The Psychology of Sentiments* (*La Psychologie des Sentiments*) the term "anhédonie," meaning "insensibility relating to pleasure alone" (p. 53). Yet Ribot's coinage had little immediate impact.

Anhedonia became launched into the German world of psychopathological thinking as **Karl Jaspers** in 1913 used the expression "the feeling of loss of feelings" ("das Gefühl, man habe keine Gefühle mehr"). "The patients complain that they are unable to experience pleasure or pain" (*General Psychopathology* [*Allgemeine Psychopathologie*], p. 67). In 1922, Boston psychiatrist Abraham Myerson (1881–1948) defined anhedonia in the *American Journal of Psychiatry* to mean the loss of interest in everything pleasurable plus "the disappearance of the energy feeling": "life itself lacks desire and satisfaction" (p. 91). Myerson's broader definition became the standard in American psychiatric writing. (During the years, the belief established itself that in schizophrenia there is no feeling; this is sometimes called "anhedonia" as well.)

"ANNA O." Pseudonym for Josef Breuer's patient Bertha Pappenheim (1859–1936), and described in **Freud** and Breuer's *Studies in Hysteria* (1895). (*See* **FREUDIAN PSYCHOTHERAPY: TECHNIQUE: cathartic method** [1893, 1895].)

ANOREXIA NERVOSA. *See* **BODY IMAGE, DISTURBANCES OF.**

ANTIDEPRESSANT. The concept of drugs thought to work specifically against a disease called depression is probably a misnomer because depression often includes anxiety and other symptoms as well. Yet, "antidepressant" has claimed a firm place in the nomenclature of psychopharmacology, and drugs called antidepressants have evolved over the arc of several generations.

First-generation antidepressants: the amphetamines and mixed amphetamine–barbiturates. There is a good deal of evidence that the amphetamines, launched in 1936 with Smith Kline & French's Benzedrine (racemic amphetamine sulfate), have efficacy in community (nonhospital) depression. The firm began advertising Benzedrine for "mild depression" in 1942. In 1946, Smith Kline brought out dextro-amphetamine sulfate (Dexedrine) for mild depression, among other indications, and 2 years later they were billing the compound—used widely as well in weight reduction—as "the antidepressant of choice." In 1950, Smith Kline launched a combination product, Dexamyl—a mixture of dextro-amphetamine and Lilly's amobarbital (Amytal) (*see* **BARBITURATES**), informing medical readers of its "smooth and profound antidepressant action": the "smooth" was emphasized because many patients found unpleasant the revved-up feeling they got from amphetamines alone. (This was not mere marketing hype. In 1963, Ruth Rushton and Hannah Steinberg, members of the Department of Pharmacology, University College London, found that, "The combined effect of the two drugs can be regarded as true potentiation, since the maximal effects produced by the mixtures are considerably greater than the maximal effects produced by . . . either constituent alone and are greater than would be expected from simple addition" [*British Journal of Pharmacology*, p. 304].) (*See* **WOMEN IN PSYCHIATRY: Steinberg.**)

Finally, the member of this first generation of antidepressants later to be the most deeply stigmatized was methamphetamine, launched by several firms in 1950 (Burroughs Wellcome's "Methedrine"; Endo Products' "Norodin": "psychomotor stimulant and antidepressant").

Subsequently, indications for all of the amphetamines became tightly circumscribed, and methamphetamine vanished entirely from the pharmacopoeia. Yet, for more than a decade they represented the beginning of "antidepressant" therapy. The amphetamines started to become drugs of abuse when they were widely prescribed for obesity; an article in 1938 by Mark Falcon Lesses (1903–), a research associate at Boston State Hospital, and Abraham Myerson (1881–1948), director of research at the hospital, on "Benzedrine Sulfate as an Aid in the Treatment of Obesity" in the *New England Journal of Medicine* launched this rather fateful evolution.

Second-generation antidepressants: the monoamine oxidase inhibitors (MAOIs) and tricyclic antidepressants (TCAs). The MAOIs, the first of which was **iproniazid,** were introduced for tuberculosis in 1952 (Roche's Marsilid) and used in psychiatry after 1957. **Imipramine,** the first of the tricyclic antidepressants (Geigy's Tofranil), was first marketed in Switzerland in 1957; in the United States in 1959. (For details, *see* the main entries for these two drugs.) Here it is reminded that iproniazid was initially billed as a "psychic energizer," only later as an antidepressant; Geigy brought out imipramine (Tofranil) as a "thymoleptic, specific in depression."

Third-generation antidepressants: the first compounds developed on the basis of neurotransmitter theories about "reuptake inhibition." The Organon company developed (but did not design) the antidepressant drug mianserin with a view to inhibiting the reuptake of the monoamine **neurotransmitters** serotonin and norepinephrine. It was patented in The Netherlands in 1967 and by 1979, when the company launched it in France as Athymil (Norval in the United Kingdom), Organon realized that it inhibited the reuptake of monoamines. Because of confusion surrounding several American trialists who submitted fraudulent data, it was never registered in the United States.

The Italian pharmacologist Bruno Silvestrini in Rome synthesized the antidepressant drug trazodone; he speculated that it might affect serotonin but did no biochemical or pharmacological testing. It was patented in the United States in 1968 by the Italian firm Angelini Francesco, who developed it as an anxiolytic. The license for the United States was sold to the Mead Johnson company, and by the time the company marketed it as Desyrel in 1982, the penny had dropped about reuptake inhibition, and the company claimed that it "selectively inhibits serotonin uptake in the brain." (In fact, its effect on serotonin is weak.)

Also in 1968, Ciba patented their antidepressant drug maprotiline. It was launched in France in 1975 as Ludiomil and in the United States in 1981 under the same name: "Acts primarily by blocking re-uptake of norephinephrine [*sic*] at nerve endings to produce a significant therapeutic response on depressed mood," the company said. (The misspelling in the ad copy shows how new these concepts were.)

All three of these third-generation antidepressants, and other compounds as well, were developed as designer drugs, tested clinically with specific neurohumoral actions in mind; namely, inhibiting the reuptake of the monoamine neurotransmitters serotonin, norepinephrine, and dopamine.

Fourth-generation antidepressants. *See* **SELECTIVE SEROTONIN REUPTAKE INHIBITORS.**

ANTIPSYCHIATRY MOVEMENT. Early in the 1960s, as part of the general intellectual tumult of the time, a protest movement arose against psychiatry. Members of the movement were by no means all in agreement about doctrine; some argued that there was no such thing as psychiatric illness, others that adverse sociocultural conditions exposed members of marginalized groups to political repression conducted under the guise of medical diagnosis, still others that treating mental patients against their will was unethical, and that **electroconvulsive** therapy was brain-destroying rather than therapeutic. This grab bag of diverse claims and objectives came together under the banner "antipsychiatry." The movement crystallized around a number of prominent intellectual spokespersons.

Thomas Szasz (pronounced SASS) (1920–). The credit for launching antipsychiatry among a mass audience goes to Szasz. Born in Budapest, Hungary, the son of a businessman, he emigrated to the United States at 18 years of age and in 1944 graduated in medicine from the University of Cincinnati. He trained in psychiatry in that city, then a hotbed of psychoanalytic thinking, and at the University of Chicago where a similar clime prevailed. From 1947 to 1950, Szasz studied at the Chicago Institute for Psychoanalysis, then went on staff there until serving 2 years of active duty in the U.S. Navy. In 1956, Szasz moved to the Veterans Administration hospital in Syracuse, where he remained as professor of psychiatry at the State University of New York Upstate Medical Center. While in the Navy, Szasz said, he had reflected about "what had long been on my mind," which turned out not to be psychoanalysis (although he already had a long publication record in the area of psychosomatic illness), but a dramatically libertarian conception of patients' rights and a conviction of the uselessness of psychiatry as a discipline. For Szasz, there was really no such thing as psychiatric illness apart from organic brain disease; there were only "problems of living." This attack, first in a 1960 article on "The Myth of Mental Illness" published in the *American Psychologist*, then in a 1961 book of the same title, disputed the legitimacy of psychiatry's claim to be a discipline. "'Mental illness' is a metaphor," he said. "Strictly speaking, disease or illness can affect only the body; hence, there can be no mental illness." Moreover, "Psychiatric diagnoses are stigmatizing labels, phrased to resemble medical diagnoses and applied to persons whose behavior annoys or offends others" (p. 267 of revised ed.).

In 1969, Szasz became cofounder of the Citizens Commission on Human Rights of the Church of Scientology. As the steam started to go out of the antipsychiatry movement itself, a good deal of the popular agitation against psychiatry in the 1970s and after was funded by Scientology.

Erving M. Goffman (1922–1982). It is ironic that the antipsychiatry movement should have received its launching shove among intellectuals from Goffman, one of the most luminious sociologists of the twentieth century whose research specialty was everyday behavior, what Goffman called "micro-sociology." Goffman tossed off his classic book *Asylums* almost as a second thought; certainly the book had less impact on sociology and anthropology than his other writings on such subjects as "the presentation of self in everyday life" (1959)—meaning day-in and -out behavior almost as a performance, stigma (1963), and social interaction (a series of works from 1963). The story: Born of a shopkeeper's family in a small town in Alberta, Canada, Goffman received his Ph.D. from the University of Chicago in 1953, where he first heard the term "total institution" from sociologist Everett Hughes (1897–1983). Between 1954 and 1957, Goffman was the holder of a visiting scientist award at the **National Institute of Mental Health** in Bethesda, Maryland, and in 1955–1956 he did a year's field work, masquerading as an assistant to the athletics director, at St. Elizabeths Hospital, affiliated with the Public Health Service and having then more than 7000 beds. The book *Asylums: Essays on the Social Situation of Mental Patients and Other Inmates* (1961) emerged from that experience (as did a 1959 article on "The Moral Career of the Mental Patient" published in *Psychiatry*). Goffman's argument was that mental hospitals exercised an ominous kind of control over patients because they functioned as "total institutions." "Their encompassing or total character is symbolized by the barrier to social intercourse with the outside and to departure that is often built right into the physical plant, such as locked doors, high walls, barbed wire, cliffs, water, forests, or moors" (p. 4). The new recruit to such an establishment "begins a series of abasements, degradations, humiliations, and profanations of self" (p. 14).

That St. Elizabeths functioned as such an institution there could be no doubt in Goffman's mind: "Like the neophyte in many of these total institutions, the new inpatient finds himself cleanly stripped of many of his accustomed affirmations, satisfactions, and defenses, and is subject to a rather full set of mortifying experiences: restriction of free movement, communal living, diffuse authority of a whole echelon of people, and so on" (p. 148). The book was highly influential in the subsequent unfolding of the antipsychiatry movement, and Franco Basaglia and Ronald Laing (*see below for both*), for example, often referred to it. Goffman thus counts as the intellectual godfather of antipsychiatry. He went on to become professor of sociology at the University of California at Berkeley, and from 1968 until his death from cancer he was Benjamin Franklin Professor of Anthropology and Sociology at the University of Pennsylvania.

Michel Foucault (1926–1984). Born in Poitiers, France, into a surgeon's family, Foucault became an influential practitioner of theory-based history and an important philosopher. In 1946, he was admitted to the prestigious École Normale Supérieure in Paris, an elite training school outside the university system, and in 1952 he received a graduate degree in psychopathology. He taught abroad for the remainder of the 1950s, returning to France as the head of the philosophy department at Clermond-Ferrand university. Among his many interests was the history of psychiatry, and in 1961 he published *Folie et déraison* (*Madness and Unreason*), which in 1964 came out in an abridged paperback edition under the title *Histoire de la Folie à l'âge classique*. It was that abridged edition that was translated into English in 1965 as *Madness and Civilisation: A History of Insanity in the Age of Reason*. The book rocketed into prominence in 1967 with an enthusiastic review by Ronald Laing (*see below*) published in the *New Statesman*. Thereupon, Foucault became the name to conjure with in the antipsychiatry movement.

Foucault's idea was that the discipline of psychiatry served as an agency of social control, imposing order upon those who did not fall in line behind the capitalist factory system. The function of the hospices and workhouses during the "grand confinement" of the seventeenth century was clear: "It was no longer merely a question of confining those out of work, but of giving work [in the hospices] to those who had been confined and thus making them contribute to the prosperity of all. The alternation is clear: cheap manpower in the periods of full employment and high salaries; and in periods of unemployment, reabsorption of the idle and social protection against agitation and uprisings" (p. 51). There was also the role of the asylum in the imposition of industrial work discipline: "In the classical age [seventeenth century], for the first time, madness was perceived through a condemnation of idleness. . . . This [industrial] community acquired an ethical power of segregation, which permitted it to eject, as into another world, all forms of social uselessness. It was in this other world, boxed in by the sacred powers of labor, that madness would assume the status we now attribute to it" (p. 57). These ideas exercised great influence upon the intellectual class in the late 1960s and 1970s and became the bowsprit of the antipsychiatry movement.

In 1968, the year of revolution in Paris, Foucault returned from Tunisia, where he had been living with a lover, to Paris to become head of the philosophy department of the University of Paris at the Vincennes campus. In 1970, he was elected to the Collège de France, and in 1984 he died of AIDS, one of the first prominent intellectuals to be thus stricken.

Franco Basaglia (1924–1980). Born in Venice, Basaglia served for 12 years as an assistant at the university psychiatric clinic in Padua before becoming superintendent in 1961 of the asylum in Gorizia (Görlitz) at Italy's eastern border with Yugoslavia. He was already much inclined against institutional psychiatry from the work of Erving Goffman on "total institutions" (*see above*) and resolved to implement in Gorizia the kind of therapeutic community he had learned of in visiting Maxwell Jones in England. (*See* **PSYCHOTHERAPY: therapeutic community** [from 1939].)

Basaglia believed in the reality of psychiatric illness but thought it should be treated in the community rather than in isolated mental hospitals that functioned as prisons. In Gorizia, Basaglia implemented a system of humane care, an open-door policy, and implemented the discharge of many patients into the community. Yet, these measures seemed halfhearted to many of the radical young men and women who were streaming to Gorizia from all over Italy, some being admitted as patients.

Thus, Basaglia left Gorizia in 1968; from this period resulted his book *Refusing the Institution* (*L'istituzione negata*; 1968).

After a sojourn in Parma, in 1971 Basaglia became director of the psychiatric hospital in Trieste. Now he directed his efforts to the actual abolition of the institution, and by 1978 he was able to announce its closing, except for 300 "guests" still remaining on the premises for whom no community placement could be found. Thereupon, Basaglia left Trieste for Rome to implement in the capital region a national law abolishing psychiatric hospitals that was passed in 1978, the so-called law 180. (The law mandated community treatment and the end of compulsory admissions to any institution save a general hospital.) In the meantime, the Italian antipsychiatry movement hooked up with the political Left to form a large political party, "Democratic Psychiatry" (Psichiatria Democratica) that explained diagnosis and confinement of psychiatric patients in terms of the Marxist theory of class. For his efforts, Basaglia became a virtual idol of antipsychiatric forces across Europe. His writings were collected by his widow, Franca Ongaro Basaglia, and were made available in a two-volume *Scritti* (*Writings*); volume one treating the period 1953 to 1968 ("from phenomenological psychiatry to the time of Gorizia" ["Dalla psichiatria fenomenologica all'esperienza di Gorizia"]), and volume two treating the period 1968 to 1980 ("from the opening up of the asylum to the new law on psychiatric care" ["Dall'apertura del manicomio alla nuova legge sull'assistenza psichiatrica"]), with both volumes published in 1981. His biographer, Anzel Finzen, in a 1980 obituary published in *Psychiatrische Praxis*, believes that it is unfair to refer to Basaglia as "the father of antipsychiatry," because he was not really antipsychiatric; he merely sought to overthrow the imbalance of political power that left patients defenseless in the face of arbitrary and autocratic institutional force (Basaglia: "Science is always at the service of the ruling class").

Ronald D. Laing (1927–1989). Raised in Glasgow, Laing graduated with an M.D. from Glasgow University in 1951, training as a psychiatrist in the army and at Glasgow; from 1956 to 1960, he prepared as a psychoanalyst at the **Tavistock Clinic** in London, then came on staff at the Tavistock Institute of Human Relations. Between 1962 and 1967, he was director of the Langham Clinic. In 1964, he founded the Philadelphia Association, a network of group homes for schizophrenic patients in the community, its most celebrated being Kingsley Hall in the East End of London. Although he was the most prominent of English intellectuals in the antipsychiatry movement, he himself disclaimed the term. In a series of books that began with *The Divided Self* in 1960, Laing articulated the view that schizophrenia was not a disease in the classic sense, having no anatomical or biochemical lesion, but rather a reaction to a hopeless situation, such as in family life. The young man or woman chooses the symptoms as an exit from this intolerable pain. (One of the conflictual families described in the book was his own.)

Laing became an icon of the New Left with his Marxist-style theory that the ego of the schizophrenic patient disintegrates as a result of revolution against the exploitative forces of the superego. In *The Politics of Experience* (1967), Laing called schizophrenia "a label that some people pin on other people under certain social circumstances. The 'cause' of 'schizophrenia' is to be found by the examination . . . of the whole social context in which the psychiatric ceremonial is being conducted" (p. 103). As Alec Jenner, a biochemically oriented psychiatrist, said later, "I knew Ronnie Lang very well. . . . He wasn't totally antipsychiatry in what he said when he was talking to me. . . . The truth is that the medical world had almost no time for him. The arts faculty and the literary world were enamoured by him and the revolutionary attitude of students—the don't-change-your-mind-there's-a-fault-in-reality type of philosophy" (Healy, III, *Psychopharmacologists*, p. 154).

David G. Cooper (1931–1986). Psychiatrist David Cooper revived the term "antipsychiatry"—first used in Germany at the turn of the century—in his 1967 book *Psychiatry and Anti-psychiatry*. Born in Cape Town, South Africa, into a pharmacist's family, he graduated in medicine there in 1955, then gained a diploma in psychological medicine in England in 1960. After the end of his training, he served at a number of English mental hospitals, then, inspired by the experiences of **Tavistock** psychiatrists during the Second World War with therapeutic communities, from 1962 to 1966 at Shenley Hospital in Hertfordshire he administered "Villa 21," a therapeutic community housed in a converted insulin-coma unit mainly for schizophrenic young males, where power roles were inverted and the patients became the equals of the doctors and nurses in a complete leveling of hierarchical relationships. As this experiment was winding down—the result of the collective exhaustion of the medical staff—in 1965 Cooper joined Ronald Laing's Philadelphia Association at its hostel, Kingsley Hall. The experiment was short-lived. In general, Cooper believed that the symptoms of schizophrenia were metaphorical representations of social relationships rather than symptoms of illness. Psychiatrists themselves, he said in his 1976 book, *The Grammar of Living*, were merely "a small part in an extensive system of violence." He saw the family in particular as a seedbed of failed communication and wrote in his 1970 book, *The Death of the Family*, that "the family must be abolished to enable people to love each other."

In response to the antipsychiatry movement, at least in the United States, Canada, and the United Kingdom, the power of psychiatrists to commit people to hospital and to treat them under compulsion has been restricted by legislation. In many jurisdictions, independent boards or tribunals have been established to protect the civil rights of detained patients. Whether this restriction represents a plus or a minus for those with serious psychiatric illness remains a matter of debate.

ANTIPSYCHOTICS. Antipsychotics represent a class of drug for the treatment of psychotic illness, particularly in schizophrenia. They are also known as "neuroleptics" and were previously called "major tranquilizers" and "ataractics." (*See* **CHLORPROMAZINE AND THE PHENOTHIAZINE CLASS OF ANTIPSYCHOTICS.**) **Heinz Lehmann** coined the term "antipsychotic" in 1961 in the *Canadian Medical Association Journal*: "Antipsychotic drugs are defined as pharmacological agents which have a therapeutic effect on symptoms of a specifically psychotic nature, such symptoms as hallucinations, paranoid delusions or the autistic thought disorder which is present in many patients with schizophrenia" (p. 1145).

ANXIETY AND PHOBIAS. Anxiety and phobic thinking may be normal emotions, distinct clusters of symptoms ("syndromes"*), or diseases in the sense of distinct illness entities. In psychoanalysis, "anxiety" is used as a theoretical term, the presumed unconscious

---

* For example, heart failure or jaundice are syndromes caused by a variety of factors.

state that triggers such defense mechanisms as repression (banishing unacceptable ideas from consciousness), sublimation (substituting an unacceptable drive for something more socially acceptable), and displacement (transferring psychic energy from one set of ideas to another). Symptoms of anxiety are common in most psychiatric illnesses, and anxiety occurs together with depression so frequently as to represent a distinct illness entity of its own (which English psychiatrist Peter Tyrer [1940–] calls "cothymia"). Yet, there are some landmarks in the attempts of medical practitioners to come to grips with this protean concept. In the literature, phobias have been somewhat arbitrarily differentiated from anxiety, though clinically all these forms tend to flow together without sharp delineation.

Physicians during the centuries have recognized the subjective symptoms of anxiety (fearfulness), as well as the objective, or somatic, symptoms (racing heart, loose bowels), as medical syndromes attached to larger diseases but not as diseases in themselves. In his *Textbook of the Disturbances of Mental Life* (*Lehrbuch der Störungen des Seelenlebens*), Leipzig psychiatry professor Johann Christian August Heinroth (*see* **GERMAN "ROMANTIC" PSYCHIATRY: Heinroth**) described the disease "quiet fury" (mania melancholica) as having among its characteristics "anxious, oppressive, inconsolable despondency." "The anxiety and depression mount from hour to hour. . . . He seems to have lost the gift of speech, or else keeps saying, 'it is all up with me, nobody can help me any longer' " (p. 206).

The use of "phobia" to mean fear of something goes back to the classifiers (nosologists) of the eighteenth century. **William Cullen**, for example, had used "hydrophobia" for what was later called rabies (supposed fear of water amidst convulsions), and the Philadelphia psychiatrist **Benjamin Rush** later parodied this sense of phobia in a contribution to a newspaper in 1798: "The CAT PHOBIA. It will be unnecessary to mention instances of the prevalence of this distemper. . . . The SOLO PHOBIA; by which I mean the dread of solitude . . . the HOME PHOBIA. This disease belongs to all those men who prefer tavern, to domestic society" (quoted in Macalpine and Hunter, *300 Years*, pp. 669–670). Some landmarks in the evolution of anxiety diagnoses follow.

Morel's délire émotif (1866). **Bénédict-Augustin Morel** described in the *General Archives of Medicine* (*Archives générales de médecine*) in 1866 "emotional delusions" (délire émotif), by which he understood a mixture of what would later be considered anxiety, panic, and obsessive-compulsive behavior. (Individuals may be delusional not just in their thinking, in other words, but in their emotions.) He found a common denominator for these various symptom pictures in disturbances of the "visceral ganglionary nervous system," especially at its "epigastric center." In describing this "neurosis," Morel said, "One is struck at the rapidity with which maladaptive emotions arise, at the instantaneous nature with which certain fixed ideas are implanted in the mind, leading to unmotivated fears, to impulsions that are virtually irresistable, to ridiculous fears that sometimes take the proportion of a kind of generic fearfulness [une véritable panophobie]" (p. 704). This may be considered the beginning of a rather broadly constructed "anxiety neurosis."

Agoraphobia (Platzschwindel) as a concept (1870). Platzschwindel, explained Vienna neurologist Moritz Benedikt (1835–1920) in an article in the *General Viennese Medical Newspaper* (*Allgemeine Wiener Medizinische Zeitung*), meant fear of open spaces.

"This unusual condition concerns individuals who are well so long as they remain in doors or in narrow streets; yet as soon as they enter a boulevard, or especially a public square, they are seized by dizziness, so that either they fear falling down or are seized by such anxiety that they do not even dare to cross the space" (p. 488). Benedikt later said in his autobiography that he came up with the diagnosis one evening in 1867 at a scientific meeting in Frankfurt am Main as he, **Griesinger**, and **Ernest Lasègue** were sitting together discussing "the obscure disorders of the brain and the mind." The three of them agreed on Platzschwindel as a disorder, which Benedikt then wrote up 3 years later (p. 125). Benedikt believed that it was caused by masturbation. The term, although an early description of agoraphobia, did not catch on.

The first anxiety syndrome described: "irritable heart" (1871). During the U.S. Civil War, Jacob M. DaCosta (1833–1900), an army doctor, had seen a number of patients such as "Henry H.": "He did a great deal of hard duty with his regiment. Some time before the battle of Fredericksburg, he had an attack of diarrhoea; after the battle he was seized with lancinating pains in the cardiac region, so intense that he was obliged to throw himself down upon the ground, and with palpitation. These symptoms . . . were attended with dimness of vision and giddiness." The symptoms went away after the soldier was seconded to police duty (p. 21). DaCosta, misattributing the symptoms to cardiac disorder, called the syndrome "irritable heart," later also known as "soldiers' heart." But the dizziness, headache, sweaty hands, palpitations, "precordial" pain (epigastric region and lower thorax), insomnia, and "nervous" symptoms that the young troopers complained of ("one solider spoke often of dreaming that he was falling off high buildings") are generally considered the somatic symptoms of anxiety. DaCosta wrote up his findings in 1871 in the *American Journal of Medical Sciences*, by which time he had become a physician in the Pennsylvania Hospital in Philadelphia.

Westphal's agoraphobia-panic (1872). "For a number of years patients have been coming to me," wrote Carl Westphal (1833–1890), then head of the Division for Psychiatric and Nervous Illnesses of the Charité Hospital in Berlin, "with the singular complaint that it is not possible for them to walk across open places or to go down certain streets and that the fear of such places constrains their freedom of movement." Westphal suggested the coinage "agoraphobia," calling it additionally in German, Platzfurcht. He emphasized the "feelings of anxiety" that overcame his patients as they contemplated these various itineraries. In the same article, Westphal also described sudden feelings of panic that came unexpectedly over others of his patients, such as a salesman who "four years ago, when engaged in writing, suddenly suffered an attack of powerful anxiety and feelings of oppressiveness in the stomach area, so that he had to run out into the street. From this moment on, he dates his complaints about all kinds of abnormal and fluctuating sensations that he localizes here and there, and about a certain anxiety in various situations. Sometimes he develops anxiety if his wife leaves their home by even just a few steps." Recently, agoraphobia had begun complicating the panicky anxiety attacks of this patient. (Westphal penned this classical description of agoraphobia and panic in 1872 in the *Archive of Psychiatry and Nervous Diseases* [*Archiv für Psychiatrie und Nervenkrankheiten*].) There had been, of course, previous descriptions in medicine of agoraphobia and panic, yet Westphal elevated agoraphobia to paradigmatic status with his term.

Lasègue's "mental vertigo" (1877). The syndrome begins, **Ernest-Charles Lasègue** said in an article in the Paris *Hospital Gazette* (*Gazette des hôpitaux*), with a feeling of compressive precordial anguish, then a sensation of being about to faint; the visual field becomes cloudy. There are mental feelings of anxiety, blanching of the visage, anxious respiration, and cold sweats. In one form of the syndrome, dizziness is the overwhelming sensation; in another, fearfulness. The patient is aware that there is no reason for his anxiety yet is unable to help himself. These attacks of anxiety may coincide with a fear of open spaces. The term "mental vertigo" itself was not widely taken up, yet it is a clear precursor of **panic disorder.**

Beard's neurasthenia: 1880 version. When New York electrotherapist George Miller Beard (1839–1883) coined the term "**neurasthenia**" in 1869 in an article published in the *Boston Medical and Surgical Journal,* he had nothing to say about anxiety. Yet, in his influential 1880 book, *A Practical Treatise on Nervous Exhaustion* (*Neurasthenia*), Beard dilated at length about anxiety as a cardinal symptom of neurasthenia, or lacking nerve force. On "morbid fears," he wrote: "A healthy man fears; but when he is functionally diseased in his nervous system he is liable to fear all the more; to have the normal, necessary fear . . . descend into an abnormal pathological state, simply from a lack of force in the disordered nervous system" (p. 26). Among the fears Beard enumerated were "topophobia," a general fear of places (Beard spoke belittlingly of Westphal's agoraphobia), "anthropophobia" (a general fear of social encounters later labeled "social anxiety disorder"), and "pantaphobia," or "fear of everything" (pp. 29–36). Later interpretations of neurasthenia emphasized "irritable weakness," a fatigue state rather than anxiety. Yet at the beginning, anxiety was important to Beard.

Hecker's description of somatic anxiety as a separate syndrome (1893). Ewald Hecker (1843–1909), a previous collaborator of **Kahlbaum's** (*see* **SCHIZOPHRENIA: EMERGENCE: hebephrenia** [1871]), was by 1893 director of a private nervous clinic in Wiesbaden. In an article "On Masked and Partial Anxiety Conditions in Neurasthenia" ("Über larvirte und abortive Angstzustände bei Neurasthenie") published in the *Central Journal for Nervous Diseases* (*Zentralblatt für Nervenheilkunde*), he said: "For many [neurasthenia] patients there may be just a single anxiety attack [Angstanfall] in the course of the entire illness; others may have a considerable number of anxiety attacks. As with agoraphobia and similar phobias they occur either on quite specific occasions with always the same triggering circumstances, or they occur spontaneously without exterior causation." In still further cases, "mild and to some extent chronic anxiety becomes manifest not in the form of self-contained attacks, but dominates the patient's entire day" (p. 565). Hecker found it of interest that the patients did not always perceive these anxiety conditions as being consciously "anxious" in nature (i.e., they were somatic anxiety). He analogized to the syndrome of "dizziness in public spaces" (Platzschwindel), whereby the patients did not always feel "dizzy" but rather anxious. His conclusion: "Among neurasthenics, it happens with surprising frequency that instead of complete anxiety attacks a number of possible physical symptoms of anxiety may appear individually in pronounced attacks, without being accompanied by psychological feelings of anxiety" (p. 567).

Freud differentiates "actual" neuroses, including anxiety neurosis, from psychoneuroses (1895). The beginning of much psychoanalytic speculation about anxiety was **Sigmund Freud's** paper "On the Justification for Differentiating a Certain

Syndrome from Neurasthenia as 'Anxiety Neurosis,'" which appeared in the *Neurological Central Journal* (*Neurologisches Centralblatt*) in 1895. Freud said that he had believed his conception of an anxiety syndrome (Symptomenkomplex) was original until he came across Hecker's 1893 paper. Freud's paper did, however, differentiate anxiety neurosis from Beard's neurasthenia. Freud's analysis of the presumed cause was, for adult women, the failure to achieve orgasm in intercourse as a result of the husband's premature ejaculation or use of withdrawal as a means of birth control. For men, it was coitus interruptus that produced anxiety neurosis, mixed together with neurasthenia. (Freud conceded that overwork and exhaustion could also elicit anxiety neurosis.) The mechanism of the sexually produced variety: "The psychic diversion of somatic sexual arousal and a consequently abnormal application of this arousal" (*Gesammelte Werke*, I, p. 334). Both anxiety neurosis and neurasthenia had in common, however, that they arose from current problems (an Aktualneurose), meaning coitus interruptus (anxiety) and masturbation (neurasthenia), rather than being "psychoneuroses" such as hysteria with roots in intrapsychic conflict.

Wernicke's anxiety psychosis (Angstpsychose) (1895, 1900). First in a brief note published in 1895 in the *General Journal of Psychiatry* (*Allgemeine Zeitschrift für Psychiatrie*), then in his clinical lectures *Outline of Psychiatry* (*Grundriss der Psychiatrie*) in 1900, Carl Wernicke (1848–1905), professor of psychiatry in Breslau (*see* **WERNICKE–KLEIST–LEONHARD PATHWAY**), proposed psychotic anxiety as a separate illness entity, differentiated from affective melancholy and from "acute psychoses with perplexity." Acoustic hallucinations were frequently present in psychotic anxiety, he said, along with delusions. "The basic symptom is anxiety, frequently in the thorax and in particular the heart and the epigastrium. . . . This anxiety regularly eventuates in the emergence of certain conceptions [Vorstellungen] of an anxious nature" (*Outline*, p. 239). Prominent in the disorder was physical (motor) agitation; the patients were impossible to keep in bed. Wernicke said that so-called agitated melancholy represented a subform of psychotic anxiety and was not further related to melancholy. The prognosis of anxiety psychosis was favorable.

Hartenberg describes "timidity" (1901). Parisian psychiatrist Paul Hartenberg's (1871–1949) book *The Timid and Timidity* (*Les Timides et la timidité*; 1901) is sometimes seen as being the ancestor of the ***DSM-III*** diagnosis "social phobia," later also called "social anxiety disorder." He defined timidity as "a complex state of agitation [trouble], confusion, embarrassment, fear, scrupulousness, shame etc. . . . accompanied clearly by such symptoms as heart palpitations, anxiety, cold sweating, tremor, blushing etc." Hartenberg considered these symptoms the result of "two fundamental emotions": fear and shame. "For a young man," explained Hartenberg, "it is a big deal just to enter a salon. He imagines that everybody is looking at him and he dies of the fear that there might be something in his outfit that is not absolutely impeccable" (quote from fourth ed., pp. 3–4).

Stekel differentiates "hysterical anxiety" (Angsthysterie) from Freud's "anxiety neurosis" (Angstneurose) (1908). At Freud's suggestion, Vienna family doctor and psychoanalyst Wilhelm Stekel (pronounced SHTAY-kel) (1868–1940) separated hysterical anxiety, the core of which was various phobias, from the larger illness entity anxiety neurosis. Stekel's 1908 book, *Nervous Anxiety Conditions and Their Treatment* (*Nervöse Angstzustände und ihre Behandlung*), argued that unlike anxiety neurosis, hysterical anxiety had psychic causes. Stekel could never accept the idea that Freud's anxiety neurosis—if it was in fact an "actual neurosis"—was caused by current sexual problems. He deviated from the master's view and insisted that anxiety neurosis must be psychogenic. This disagreement caused Stekel to be thrown out of the psychoanalytic movement just before the First World War, and until his death by suicide in 1940, Stekel continued to insist on intrapsychic conflict as the genesis of all neuroses. In the third edition of the book (1921), he also abandoned the distinction between hysterical anxiety and anxiety neurosis and said that only hysterical anxiety existed, although he continued to use the term "anxiety neurosis." By this point, he was confining the clinical use of the term "hysterical anxiety" largely to phobias: "We always note in all parapathias [Parapathien = neuroses] a disorder of affective life, meaning a struggle between two affects. It is never a question of a struggle between two thoughts but rather between two feelings. (Religious feeling fights against the sex drive, which expresses itself as love, and the other way around)" (third ed., p. 276).

The category hysterical anxiety survived for many years in the psychoanalytic movement. New York psychoanalyst Otto Fenichel (pronounced PHEN-ih-kel) (1898–1946), a Freud pupil and Viennese emigré, had a large section on it in his textbook, *The Psychoanalytic Theory of Neurosis* (1945), though, of course, without any reference to Stekel, who by then had long been branded a heretic.

Freud's conception of anxiety collapses many previous subdivisions (1926). As the psychoanalytic movement gained in influence, Freud's concepts increasingly displaced previous distinctions in psychopathology. In Freud's 1926 book, best known in English as *The Problem of Anxiety* (*Hemmung, Symptom und Angst*), he argued that, "Anxiety is a reaction to the danger of object loss" (*Gesammelte Werke*, XIV, p. 202). Thus anxiety, next to mourning, became one of the great motors of the dynamics of the psyche, and in the psychoanalytic tradition anxiety is more a mechanism than a symptom. Thus, the psychopathologic study of anxiety initiated by Morel in 1866 came to a provisional end.

Leonhard describes "anxiety-ecstasy psychosis" (Angst-Eingebungspsychose) (1939). Working at Karl Kleist's clinic in Frankfurt (*see* **WERNICKE–KLEIST–LEONHARD PATHWAY**), Karl Leonhard differentiated from **Emil Kraepelin's** great bloc diagnosis dementia praecox (*see* **SCHIZOPHRENIA: EMERGENCE: Kraepelin** [from 1893]) a circular disorder in which patients alternated between anxiety psychosis and an unreal sense of ecstasy: "The anxiety phase (paranoid anxiety psychosis) deviates from anxiety psychosis through the presence of perplexity, ideas of reference [paranoid thinking], and sensory hallucinations; the ecstatic phase (Kleist's Eingebungspsychose) is accompanied by an ecstatic mood [and] boundless personal grandiosity." Leonhard said in his article in the *Journal of Combined Neurology and Psychiatry* (*Zeitschrift für die gesamte Neurologie und Psychiatrie*) that the circular disorder had heavy hereditary roots and a good prognosis, including full remission between episodes.

Anxiety and phobia disorders in *DSM* "One" (1952). The first edition of the ***DSM*** series gave "phobic reaction" a category of its own (following the World Health Organization's *International Classification of Diseases* in 1947); the guide also included "anxiety reaction," putting it and phobia under the category "psychoneurotic disorders." "The chief characteristic of these [psychoneurotic] disorders," the guide noted, "is 'anxiety' which may be directly felt and expressed or which may be unconsciously . . . controlled by . . . various psychological defense mechanisms" (p. 31).

Anxiety and phobic disorders in *DSM-III* (1980). There had been no change in the classification of anxiety and phobia from ***DSM-I*** (1952) to ***DSM-II*** (1968), except to rename the "reactions" of *DSM-I* as "neuroses." ***DSM-III***, however, recast the nosology substantially, calling all the entities "disorders" rather than "neuroses." As the "Research Diagnostic Criteria" of 1978 in the *Archives of General Psychiatry* by **Robert Spitzer**, Jean Endicott (a Columbia University psychologist, born in 1936), and **Eli Robins** had forecast (*see* **PANIC DISORDER**), anxiety neurosis was split into panic disorder and generalized anxiety disorder. Phobic neurosis was subdivided into five categories: agoraphobia with and without panic, "social phobia" (or fear of doing certain activities in public), "simple phobia" (a residual category), and "separation anxiety disorder (childhood)." ***DSM-III-R*** (1987) and ***DSM-IV*** (1994) made no major changes to this schema, aside from suggesting in the 1994 edition "social anxiety disorder" as a synonym for "social phobia," and "specific phobia" for the former "simple phobia." (These may sound like trivial changes, but they are important, for example, in the marketing of pharmaceuticals.)

The distinction between somatic and psychological anxiety is reactivated (2003). "The sympathetic nervous system has been forgotten by psychiatry," said Conrad M. Swartz (1946–), head of psychiatric research at Southern Illinois University in Springfield, in 2003. In *Psychiatric Times*, Swartz called attention to "jumpiness, startle, agitation, restlessness and muscle pain" as symptoms of somatic anxiety (once called anguish [angoisse] in the psychiatric literature). To decrease the effects of neurotransmitters epinephrine and norepinephrine, he recommended prescribing such "beta-blockers" as propranolol for the treatment of somatic anxiety, leaving the **selective serotonin reuptake inhibitors** for the psychological variety.

See **PANIC DISORDER: anxiety, panic, and phobic disorders in *ICD-10*** (1992).

ATTENTION DEFICIT HYPERACTIVITY DISORDER (ADHD). Historically, a small group of children has always been seen as pathologically restive and unable to pay attention. In 1845, Heinrich Hoffmann (1809–1894), then a family doctor in Frankfurt am Main (later a psychiatrist), wrote an amusing little collection of children's stories that featured, among other characters, "Struwwelpeter," a very bad boy who let his fingernails grow uncut for a whole year. Around 1900, Mark Twain translated the book (originally *Der Struwwelpeter: oder lustige Geschichten und drollige Bilder für Kinder von 3-6 Jahren*) as *Slovenly Peter or Cheerful Stories and Funny Pictures for Good Little Folks*. Struwwelpeter has always been considered a poster boy for hyperactivity, and here is Twain's rendering of Hoffmann's verse:

> See this frowsy 'cratur'
> Pah! It's Struwwelpeter
> On his fingers rusty,
> On his two-head musty,
> Scissors seldom come;
> Lets his talons grow a year
> Do any loathe him? Some!
> They hail him 'Modern satyr–
> Disgusting Struwwelpeter.'

ADHD: Diagnosis (from 1902). "Hyperactivity" in children was to become a familiar medical concept. In 1902, George F. Still (1868–1941), working at the Hospital for Sick Children in Great Ormond Street, London, and pioneer of the study of pediatrics as a discipline in England, described in the *Lancet* a group of children showing "a marked inability to concentrate and to sustain attention." One boy of 6 years was "unable to keep his attention even to a game for more than a very short time, and, as might be expected, the failure of attention was very noticeable at school. . . ." Still ascribed this syndrome, and numerous other "abnormal psychical conditions in children," to "defective moral control" (p. 1166).

But it was only in the epidemic of encephalitis in Europe after the First World War that hyperactivity as a syndrome in children truly got on the medical radar, one of the symptoms of encephalitis often being hyperkinesis.

There were subtler brain injuries than encephalitis also causing hyperactivity. The concept of children suffering behavioral consequences of real but scarcely detectable central nervous lesions was familiar even before Arnold Lucius Gesell (1880–1961), the Yale pediatrician, suggested in 1941 in his textbook, *Developmental Disease*, "minimal cerebral injury" as a cause of pathological behavior in children. Without making specific reference to hyperactivity, Gesell wrote: "It must be granted that a child may inherit motor weaknesses, motor eccentricities, even motor demeanors. But when these are highly atypical one is tempted to think of injury instead of inheritance" (p. 237).

In the 1950s, various permutations of the phrases "minimal cerebral injury" or "minimal brain dysfunction" became associated with hyperactivity. In 1962, an Oxford conference organized by Ronald MacKeith (1908–1977), a pediatrician who was medical-education director of the Spastic Society and had an appointment at Guy's Hospital in London, and Martin Bax (1933–), a psychiatrist also at Guy's, recommended that "minimal brain dysfunction" replace "minimal brain damage." As for hyperactivity, the participants recommended: "In a child who has no history of a devastating cerebral illness, it cannot be stated with confidence that 'brain damage' is a necessary and constant precursor of hyperkinetic behaviour disorder" (*Minimal Cerebral Dysfunction*, p. 88).

It was indeed the increasing implausibility—or social unacceptability—of the notion that the growing numbers of children with the diagnosis "MBD" had some kind of brain injury that led to the recasting of hyperactivity. In 1954, Maurice W. Laufer (1914–), Eric Denhoff (1913–), and Gerald Solomons at the Emma Pendleton Bradley Home in Riverside, Rhode Island, in a paper at a child psychiatry meeting in Toronto (and published in 1957 in *Psychosomatic Medicine*) proposed the "hyperkinetic impulse disorder" in children who were basically nonretarded but who could not sit still and manifested "short attention span and poor powers of concentration." The authors said, "It is necessary to emphasize that the hyperkinetic syndrome is a very specific entity. It does not account for the majority of children's behavior disturbances" (p. 48).

This language reappeared in ***DSM-II*** in 1968 as the "hyperkinetic reaction of childhood (or adolescence) . . . characterized by overactivity, restlessness, distractibility, and short attention span" (p. 50). In ***DSM-III*** (1980), the diagnosis became Attention Deficit Disorder (ADD), followed by the subcategory "with hyperactivity." And in

DSM-III-R (1987), "ADHD" was born: The diagnosis became "Attention Deficit Hyperactivity Disorder."

In 2003, Elizabeth R. Sowell (1965–), a member of the neurology department of the medical school of the University of California at Los Angeles (UCLA), and co-workers, using high-resolution magnetic resonance imaging (MRI), found in research published in the *Lancet*, that compared to controls, children with ADHD had smaller inferior dorsolateral aspects of the frontal cortices. There were other findings as well in regions that are "thought to form a broadly distributed action-attentional system that supports the maintenance of attentional focus and successful inhibitory control of unwanted impulses" (p. 1705). Although this study was not the first use of MRI in children with hyperactivity, it was the first worldwide, carried out at the UCLA Laboratory of Neuro Imaging, to computer-map the entire cortical surface.

ADHD: Treatment (from 1937). Disruptive children have long been medicated: in the nineteenth century with opium and in the early twentieth century with barbiturates. Specific medication for hyperactivity, however, surfaced only with the amphetamines in the 1930s (Smith Kline & French introduced Benzedrine [racemic amphetamine sulfate] in 1936. *See* **ANTIDEPRESSANTS.**) In 1937, Charles Bradley (1902–1979), a child psychiatrist who was medical director of the Emma Pendleton Bradley Home in Riverside (East Providence), Rhode Island, described the use of Benzedrine in nonretarded children who had "neurological and behavior disorders." "Fifteen of the 30 children responded to benzedrine by becoming distinctly subdued," he reported in the *American Journal of Psychiatry* (p. 579).

In the days of the first psychiatric drug set of the 1950s, numerous antipsychotics such as **chlorpromazine** were indicated for children who presented "behavioral problems," in the absence of a specific psychiatric diagnosis. Yet, the definitive moment in the treatment of ADHD occurred in 1970 when the Ciba company began advertising its drug methylphenidate (Ritalin), a compound introduced in Europe in 1954 (in the United States in 1956) for depression, as effective for the " 'hyperactive' problem child." Although not an amphetamine, methylphenidate was chemically close to that drug class and similarly counted as a "stimulant." Stimulant medication went on to become the treatment of choice in ADHD.

AUTISM. This term refers to either a symptom of schizophrenia or, more commonly, a developmental disorder in children beginning in the first 3 years of life. In children, the brain disability involves a qualitative impairment in social interaction, significant impairment in communication, and behavior that is often rigid, obsessional, and ritualistic.

The term "autism" (der Autismus) was coined by **Eugen Bleuler** in 1910 in an article on "Schizophrenic Negativism" in the *Psychiatrisch-Neurologische Wochenschrift* (p. 185f). In his 1911 book, *Schizophrenias*, Bleuler amplified that autism was a basic symptom of schizophrenia involving the inability to distinguish an internal phantasy world from reality. "We term autism the loss of contact with reality together with the relative and absolute predominance of an interior life" (*Schizophrenien*, p. 52). In his later *Textbook of Psychiatry* (*Lehrbuch der Psychiatrie*), published in 1916, Bleuler abandoned the term "autism" because it had created too much confusion about "egoism" and substituted the term "dereistic" thinking: whenever the patient's fantasy world conflicted with reality, it was the fantasies that received preference: "The laborer who's engaged to a princess is simply no longer a laborer but ruler of the world or some other grand figure" (quote from eighth ed., p. 24).

Yet, in his original *Schizophrenia* book in 1911, Bleuler allowed that autism could occur in non-schizophrenic individuals as well, especially children: "There is a normal style of autistic thinking, that takes no consideration of reality and is guided by emotions [Affekten]. The child plays with a piece of wood that one day is a baby for him, another day a house" (p. 305).

In 1943, Leo Kanner (1894–1981), a psychiatrist at Johns Hopkins University who is considered the father of child psychiatry in the United States (he wrote the first American textbook on the subject, *Child Psychiatry*, in 1935), described in the journal *Nervous Child* "autistic disturbances of affective contact." "The outstanding, 'pathognomonic,' fundamental disorder is the children's inability to relate themselves in the ordinary way to people and situations from the beginning of life. . . . There is from the start an extreme autistic aloneness that, whenever possible, disregards, ignores, shuts out anything that comes to the child from the outside" (p. 242). Kanner emphasized that they were not feebleminded but had "strikingly intelligent physiognomies. Their faces at the same time give the impression of serious-mindedness." He noted their "astounding vocabulary" and "good intelligence." The disorder further entailed elaborate repetitive routines. It was caused, said Kanner, by a chilly home environment: "In the whole group, there are very few really warmhearted fathers and mothers. . . . Even some of the happiest marriages are rather cold and formal affairs" (p. 250). Kanner dwelt upon how some of the children had been constrained to recite from the "Presbyterian Catechism." (In a personal communication, Gabrielle A. Carlson, director of child and adolescent psychiatry at Stony Brook University, suggests that Kanner may have been seeing genetic similarities and misattributing the resultant child to the coldness of the parents rather than to the genetic contribution.) Kanner later termed the condition "early infantile autism." Kanner's observation about cold parents got the field off onto the wrong foot for many years. Yet, many of his observations were accurate.

Meanwhile in Vienna, pediatrician Hans Asperger (1906–1980), who remained unaware of Kanner's work, was describing in 1944 in the *Archive for Psychiatry and Nervous Diseases* (*Archiv für Psychiatrie und Nervenkrankheiten*) virtually the same condition but calling it "autistic psychopathy." "While people normally live in a continuous reciprocal relationship with the surrounding world, constantly reacting to it, for these 'autistic' [children] these relationships are grossly disrupted, contracted. The autistic child is only 'he himself' . . . not a living part of a larger organism that continuously influences him and is influenced by him" (p. 84). Asperger described avoidance of eye contact, an unnatural almost caricatural mode of speaking directed not at the listener but off into the distance, and an intelligence marked often by startling originality yet substantially learning-disabled. The author was also struck by the artistic creativity of these children.

Asperger's contribution (it was his Habilitation), published in German in the final years of a long war, went virtually unnoticed abroad until 1981, when English child psychiatrist Lorna Gladys Wing (1928–)—then at the Social and Community Psychiatry Unit of the **Maudsley**—decided to baptize as "Asperger's Syndrome" a population of children with many of the characteristics that Asperger had described. She took issue with Asperger's description of the group as creatively gifted: "It would be more true to say that their thought processes are confined to a narrow, pedantic, literal, but logical, chain of reasoning." She also doubted his assessment that many patients were of high intelligence: "Those with the syndrome are conspicuously lacking in common sense." In her view, "Asperger's Syndrome" was a helpful term for "explaining the problems of children and adults who have autistic features but who talk grammatically and are not socially aloof" (p. 124). (This was not exactly the population that Asperger described.) Her paper, appearing in *Psychological Medicine*, suggested that Asperger's syndrome and "typical Kanner's autism" were situated somewhere within a "triad" of problems affecting early child development that involved (1) "absence or impairment of two-way social interaction," (2) impairment of linguistic comprehension and of language, and (3) impairment of imagination, substituting rituals instead.

Psychoanalyst Bruno Bettelheim (1903–1990), director of the Orthogenic School at the University of Chicago, created a boomlet for the concept of autistic children as badly damaged by concentration-camp–like trauma—above all in his 1967 book, *The Empty Fortress*. (*See* **PSYCHOTHERAPY: milieu therapy** [from 1925].)

In 1992, Christopher L. Gillberg (1950–), professor of child psychiatry at the University of Goteborg, Sweden, proposed in the *Journal of Child Psychology and Psychiatry* the term "disorders of empathy" for a spectrum of autistic-like conditions that included autism and Asperger's syndrome.

In ***DSM-I*** (1952) and ***DSM-II*** (1968), "autistic thinking" appeared as a symptom of **schizoid personality**. (*DSM-I*: "As children, they are usually quiet, shy, obedient, sensitive and retiring.") "Infantile autism" entered ***DSM-III*** in 1980 under the class of "pervasive developmental disorders." Among its essential features were disturbed ability to communicate and to respond to others, in addition to "bizarre responses to various aspects of the environment"—all occurring within the first 30 months of age. Many of the children had **mental retardation** as well. In the *Manual*, it was described as "very rare." Alongside infantile autism was a second diagnosis—"childhood onset pervasive developmental disorder"—that sounded a good deal like previous definitions of autism ("profound disturbance in social relations and multiple oddities of behavior") and was also "extremely rare."

DSM-III-R in 1987 considerably expanded the number of symptoms that would qualify someone for the diagnosis of autism, requiring 8 out of a possible 16. Autism, the guide said, was "merely the most severe and prototypical form of the general category Pervasive Developmental Disorders" (p. 34). In this edition, childhood onset pervasive developmental disorder became folded into autism, thus widening considerably the scope of autism.

DSM-IV (1994) arrayed a number of pervasive developmental disorders, including "Childhood Disintegrative Disorder," "Asperger's Disorder," and "Autistic Disorder." "In most cases, there is an associated diagnosis of mental retardation," as described in the *Manual* (p. 67). These additional diagnoses had the effect of again narrowing the scope of autism, yet raising awareness of the concept of an autism spectrum.

B

BARBITURATES (1903 and after). Although the organic-chemical industry had introduced numerous sedatives before the barbiturates (chloral hydrate, for example, was first used in psychiatry in 1869), the barbiturates enjoyed great popularity for half a century because they tasted better, had fewer side effects, and were less toxic than their predecessors.

In 1903, Emil Fischer (1852–1919), professor of chemistry in Berlin who had extensive contacts with industry, and Joseph von Mering (1849–1908), professor of internal medicine at Halle University, announced in *Today's Therapeutics* (*Therapie der Gegenwart*) their discovery of the therapeutic use of the barbiturates as sedatives and hypnotics. Fischer had suggested to the Bayer company of Leverkusen, Germany, the improved production of diethylbarbituric acid (the parent barbiturate)—a compound first synthesized in 1863—opening the door to the pharmaceutical use of the barbiturate class. Barbital sodium, a "substituted" form of diethylbarbituric acid that was synthesized in 1882, was the first of the barbiturates and was marketed in 1903 by the Bayer company as Veronal and by the Schering company as Medinal: both brand names soon became household words. In 1911, Bayer patented phenobarbital (Luminal), an even more powerful sedative and anticonvulsant, bringing it out the following year.

During the next 40 years, more than 2500 different barbiturate preparations followed, including pentobarbital sodium (patented by Bayer in 1916; Abbott introduced it in the United States in 1941 as Nembutal), amobarbital sodium (patented in 1924; Lilly introduced it as Sodium Amytal), butabarbital sodium (patented by Lilly in 1932; McNeil introduced it as Butisol Sodium), secobarbital sodium (patented in 1934; Lilly introduced it in 1945 as Seconal Sodium), and thiopental sodium (patented in 1939; Abbott introduced it as Pentothal Sodium).

See **DEEP-SLEEP THERAPY AND BARBITURATES.**

Narcotherapy and barbiturates (1930 and after). In 1930, William J. Bleckwenn (1895–1965), assistant director of the Wisconsin Psychiatric Institute, proposed in the *Journal of the American Medical Association* (*JAMA*) intravenous injections of amobarbital (Sodium Amytal) in a number of psychiatric conditions, including depression: "The depression is certainly less profound and the course of the illness is materially shortened, with the use of the drug." In schizophrenia, "normal lucid intervals" of 4 to 14 hours had been achieved. Later that year in the *Wisconsin Medical Journal*, Bleckwenn added for depression, "[The patients] are more active, more talkative, have less constrained and less awkward attitudes" (p. 694). Over time, this procedure became known as the "amytal interview." Bleckwenn was said to have originated the term "truth serum," although it is now widely disbelieved that amobarbital serves any such function.* (In this 1930 article in *JAMA*, Bleckwenn also

* Bleckwenn mentioned in passing in his *JAMA* article, under the rubric "schizophrenia," that amobarbital had been of value in the relief of "catatonic excitement"; later, he said

proposed amobarbital for the relief of **catatonia**, where it functioned better than as an antidepressant.)

In 1931, Erich Lindemann (1900–1974) at the Psychopathic Hospital in Iowa City, Iowa, called attention in the *Proceedings of the Society for Experimental Biology and Medicine* specifically to the ability of intravenous Sodium Amytal to induce "a feeling of serenity and well-being, a desire to communicate and to speak about problems or personal matters usually not spoken of to strangers. There was also the feeling of being unable to guard against saying things which one does not want to and an inability to refuse to answer questions even if they refer to very intimate matters" (p. 865). Therapeutically, the drug made catatonic patients who had been mute for months again communicative, and silent, guilt-stricken depressed patients willing to talk about their feelings.

Meanwhile, in 1936 John Stephen Horsley (lic. MRCS Eng., LRCP, 1932 [MRCS = Member of the Royal College of Surgeons; LRCP = Licentiate of the Royal College of Physicians]), a staff psychiatrist at Dorset Mental Hospital in England, described in the *Journal of Mental Science* intravenous injections of another barbiturate, pentobarbital sodium (Nembutal), to achieve what he called "narco-analysis"—"a practical substitute for the economically unavailable, if desirable, method of psychoanalysis."

In 1945, Roy R. Grinker (sen.) (1900–1993) and John Paul Spiegel (1911–?) of Chicago, first in their book *War Neuroses in North Africa* (1943) then in *Men Under Stress* (1945), suggested "narcosynthesis" using intravenous sodium pentothal as a way of performing the "uncovering of anxieties and conflicts and the production of adequate abreactions" in the brief time available to military medicine. The technique: "The patient is given the drug until his counting aloud ceases and he begins to take deep, stertorous breaths." The interview begins at that point. "The best method is to start the patient talking and let him continue uninterrupted in spite of associations leading him far from the subject of war" (*Men Under Stress*, pp. 389–390). "Synthesis" meant the "recapture by the ego of alienated ideas and emotions" and "the synthesis of related feelings that have been separated by the process of dissocation" (p. 393).

Narcotherapy represents one of the first important American contributions to the international narrative of psychiatry (if one exempts the diagnosis "**neurasthenia**" [from George M. Beard, an electrotherapist, 1839–1883] and the "rest cure" treatment [from **Silas Weir Mitchell**, a neurologist]).

The restorative effects of barbiturates in schizophrenia (1948). A team of researchers led by neurophysiologist Seymour Kety (1915–2000) and including Carl Frederic Schmidt (1893–1988), Fritz Freyhan (1912–1982), and Kenneth E. Appel (1896–1979)—all at the Pennsylvania School of Medicine with the exception of Freyhan

---

that it "awakened" catatonic patients, an observation that had considerable impact on the treatment of psychosis. **Max Fink** recalls, "One of the delights of being a medical student in 1942–1945 and then as a resident at Bellevue 1949–1951 was the opportunity to use amobarbital for catatonic patients. We were given syringe, needles, tourniquet, water and allowed (encouraged) to give IV injections when so ordered."

(who was a psychiatrist at the Delaware State Hospital)—set out to study changes in the cerebral blood flow of schizophrenics produced by various therapies, including barbiturates. They found rather serendipitously that Sodium Amytal and pentothal produced a significant but temporary lessening of symptoms in schizophrenia. Of this publication in 1948 in the *American Journal of Psychiatry* Kety later said, "[Here] I saw the temporary but remarkable restoration in the thinking and affect of some schizophrenics under the influence of sodium amytal narcosis. I was impressed that a drug could produce such dramatic effects, which suggested that biochemical processes . . . were responsible for the psychotic symptoms" (Shepherd, *Psychiatrists on Psychiatry*, p. 85). On the basis of this research, in 1951 Robert Felix made Kety the first scientific director of the **National Institute of Mental Health**.

The barbiturates as Delay's "psycholeptics" (1949). In a paper in the *Proceedings of the Royal Society of Medicine*, **Jean Delay** called the sodium barbiturates "psycholeptic" because they produced a lowering of intrapsychic tensions "and are depressants of psychological tonus." By contrast, the amphetamine methamphetamine (Methedrine), at the time used therapeutically, was a "psychogogue" because it increased "intrapsychic tension."

Charles Shagass's "sedation threshold" (1954). In 1954 in *Electroencephalography and Clinical Neurophysiology*, Charles Shagass (1920–), a psychiatrist–electrophysiologist at **McGill University**, showed quantitatively that the presence of the "sedation threshold" with the barbiturates differs in different kinds of illnesses. (Schizophrenic and anxious patients require larger amounts of amobarbital than do patients with major depression and organic brain disease.) This was an early exercise in using psychopharmacology as a diagnostic torch.

The Weinstein–Kahn amobarbital test for organic brain disease (1955). As a result of the Grinker–Spiegel reports (*see* above), military doctors became accustomed to using amobarbital freely. In 1955, Edwin Alexander Weinstein (1909–1998),* a Washington, D.C., neurologist and psychiatrist who consulted widely in area military hospitals, and Robert L. Kahn (1918–), a psychologist at Mount Sinai Hospital in New York, proposed in their "denial hypothesis" of behavior that the administration of amobarbital in patients with organic brain disease would, in inquiries about orientation, elicit denial and minimization of illness but have no such effect in psychiatric patients with normal brain function. *See* their *Denial of Illness* (1955).

The barbiturates revived in the treatment of catatonic mutism (1992). Many years after the above discoveries, W. Vaughn McCall (1958–) in the Department of Psychiatry at Duke University and co-investigators conducted a randomized controlled trial of amobarbital versus placebo in catatonic mutism: They found it fairly effective, placebo not at all. They chose amobarbital over a **benzodiazepine** because they felt it had maintained its historic reputation as the "gold standard" (*see* their article in the *American Journal of Psychiatry*, 1992).

---

* Weinstein is also remembered for a medical biography of President Woodrow Wilson (1981); in 1968 he moved to New York, becoming professor of neurology at Mt. Sinai Medical School.

BATTIE, WILLIAM (1703–1776). One of the founders of the concept of the therapeutic asylum, Battie was born in a small town in the county of Devon, the son of a vicar. He read medicine at Cambridge (A.M. in 1730) then, obtaining a license to practice from the university, practiced medicine in Cambridge while lecturing on anatomy at the university. In 1737, he took his M.D. degree at Cambridge, moving in the same year to London, where he soon became a fellow of the College of Physicians. He was instrumental in founding St. Luke's Hospital for Lunaticks in 1750, becoming its chief physician, and simultaneously owned and supervised several private asylums. Publication in 1758 of his *Treatise on Madness*, the first manual to be based on actual cases rather than theoretical considerations, made him one of the most prominent "mad-doctors" of the day. Battie was, along with **Chiarugi** and **Pinel**, among the earliest of physicians to conceive of insane asylums as having a therapeutic role and to see in psychiatry a distinctive kind of medical specialty. In the judgment of psychiatry historians Richard Hunter and Ida Macalpine, "Battie . . . initiated a new era in psychiatry. . . . As the first physician of repute with a scientific background and distinguished social position who made insanity his whole time work he raised the 'Mad Business' to a respectable medical specialty" (*Three Hundred Years of Psychiatry*, p. 404).

BEERS, CLIFFORD (1876–1943). The founder of the "mental hygiene" movement, Beers grew up in New Haven, Connecticut, his family in the produce business. While Beers was a student at Yale University, in 1894 a beloved brother became stricken with epilepsy. Beers found that his mind dwelled upon the fear of developing the illness himself. As he said in his autobiography, *A Mind That Found Itself* (1908), "This was the thought that soon got possession of my mind. The more I considered it and him, the more nervous I became; and the more nervous, the more convinced that my own breakdown was only a matter of time" (pp. 7–8). Indeed, by the time Beers graduated in 1897 he was, as he said, "a sick man." He went in and out of several private institutions before his final recovery; in 1908, the same year in which he published his book, he founded the Connecticut Society for Mental Hygiene, and the following year (1909) he organized the National Committee for Mental Hygiene, later called the National Association for Mental Health, of which he was general secretary until 1939. The mission of the National Association for Mental Health was to prevent mental illness, to remove the stigma from the condition, and to promote the training of professionals and research in the field. As writer Albert Deutsch (1905–1961) later said in his influential work, *The Mentally Ill: A History of Their Care and Treatment from Colonial Times* (1937)—a book sponsored by the American Foundation for Mental Hygiene—"*A Mind That Found Itself* created a profound impression in professional and lay circles. Its rallying cry was heard and heeded. Men and women from all walks of life flocked to the banner flung aloft by the young reformer" (p. 309). Indeed, by 1966 the book had had 38 printings. The term "mental hygiene," already in widespread use in Europe, was suggested by **Adolf Meyer**, a charter member of Beers' National Committee for Mental Hygiene. In 1931, Beers became cofounder of an International Committee for Mental Hygiene, of which he served as general secretary until 1939.

A key concept for the mental hygiene movement was "mental health," by which they understood any quantitative variation from the norm. Psychiatric illness, by contrast—a clinician's concept—involved qualitative distinctions among kinds of diseases. With the emphasis of the mental hygiene movement on outpatient facilities, one might see in the work of Beers the beginnings of social psychiatry.

BEHAVIORAL THERAPY. *See* COGNITIVE-BEHAVIORAL THERAPY.

BENZODIAZEPINES, A CLASS OF ANTIANXIETY DRUGS (from 1960). Stimulated by the success of such drugs as **chlorpromazine** in the mid-1950s, the branch of the Hoffmann La Roche company in Nutley, New Jersey, asked chemist Leo Sternbach (1908–) to lead the search for other innovative compounds. Born in Abbazia on the Istrian Peninsula, then part of Austria, Sternbach had been working for Roche in Basel when the Second World War began, and the company sent him and other Jewish scientists to their American branch for safety. In Nutley, as a group chief in organic chemistry, in 1955 he created the chemical class of benzodiazepines, the first of which, chlordiazepoxide—a so-called 1,4 benzo because of nitrogen atoms at positions 1 and 4 on the diazepine ring—was patented in 1959 and marketed as Librium in 1960. The "benzos," or "BZDs," were a highly successful drug class because they acted effectively on anxiety, mixed anxiety–depression, and other conditions while at the same time being comparatively safe. Although they were later taxed with addictiveness, it remains unclear how addictive they were compared to other related classes of psychoactive compounds.

In 1963, Roche launched the benzodiazepine that was to become by the late 1960s the then most successful drug in pharmaceutical history: Valium (generic name, diazepam). Diazepam was ultimately marketed worldwide under some 87 different brand names and figured as "mother's little helper" in a song by Mick Jagger of the Rolling Stones. By 1971, Librium and Valium accounted for $200 million of Roche's $280 million in sales in the United States, and *Fortune* magazine was calling the two drugs "the greatest commercial successes in the history of prescription drugs." By 1977, about 8000 tons of benzodiazepines were being consumed annually in the United States.

Among other popular benzodiazepines, on the basis of year patented (year of marketing refers to the United States), were the following:

- 1963: flurazepam (marketed by Roche as Dalmane in 1970)
- 1963: lorazepam (marketed by Wyeth as Ativan in 1977)
- 1963: flunitrazepam (marketed by Roche as Roipnol in Italy in 1976; not licensed in the United States)
- 1964: clonazepam (marketed by Roche as Clonopin in 1975)
- 1965: temazepam (marketed by Sandoz as Restoril in 1981)
- 1965: oxazepam (marketed by Wyeth as Serax in 1965)
- 1970: triazolam (marketed by Upjohn as Halcion in 1982)
- 1970: alprazolam (marketed by Upjohn as Xanax in 1981)

In April 1977, Richard F. Squires (1933–), a scientist at A/S Ferrosan Research Laboratories in Soeborg, Denmark, aided by Claus Braestrup (1945–), then a Ph.D. student on work-study at Ferrosan, announced in *Nature* that they had evidence for the existence of a single binding site on brain membranes (a receptor) for diazepam. This initial discovery of a benzodiazepine receptor was followed later that year, in November, by a similar find of Hanns Möhler (1940–), a biochemist at Roche in Basel and lecturer in nearby Freiburg University, and Toshikazu Okada, a pharmacologist at Nippon-Roche Research Center, Kamakura City, Japan (*see* their report in *Science*). Locating a specific site of action for the benzos helped to explain the mechanism of action of these drugs.

By the 1990s, there were more than a hundred different benzodiazepines on world markets. In retrospect, the benzodiazepines were one of the safest and most efficacious drug classes in the history of psychopharmacology. They virtually drove the **barbiturates** from the field as the hypnotics and sedatives of choice.

BERGER, HANS (1873–1941). The inventor of electroencephalography (EEG), Berger was born in Coburg in northern Germany, his father the chief physician of the local hospital. In 1897, he wrote his state exam in medicine in Jena (pronounced YAY-na), the last of the medical schools at which he had studied, remaining thereafter. He finished his Habilitation in 1901 and by 1919 had become Otto Binswanger's (1852–1929) successor as professor of psychiatry. He was dismissed in 1938, retreated to a small sanatorium in Bad Blankenburg, and committed suicide in 1941 in an episode of depression. It had been Berger's hope that the "psychic energy" of the brain would permit him to measure its activity with a string galvanometer, although the idea aroused the derision of his colleagues. In fact, he could record through the intact skull electrical changes that take place in cerebral activity. His classic description of EEG, "On the Electroencephalogram in Man," appeared in 1929 in the *Archive of Psychiatry and Nervous Diseases* (*Archiv für Psychiatrie und Nervenkrankheiten*), followed thereafter by a long series of articles on the interpretation and administration of EEG. The "third communication" in 1931 in the *Archiv für Psychiatrie* was about changes in EEG induced by drugs and laid the basis for the science of pharmaco-EEG. His student Kurt Kolle (1898–1975) judged Berger, next to **Emil Kraepelin** and **Ernst Kretschmer**, to be among the three most famous German psychiatrists in the world. EEG represents the first procedure to "objectivize" the mind, the goal of the intensely biologically oriented Berger. In practical terms, Berger was the first to measure the electrical activity of the brain.

BETHLEM HOSPITAL/"BEDLAM" (from 1247). Bethlem hospital was the only asylum in England until the foundation of Norwich asylum in 1724, then St. Luke's Hospital in London in 1751. It therefore, as Richard Hunter and Ida Macalpine observe, "occupies a unique place in the history of the insane in the British Isles" (*Three Hundred Years*, p. 306). Founded in 1247 as the Hospital of St. Mary of Bethlem in the Bishopsgate district of London, the hospital served initially as a base for the Crusaders' sallies into the Holy Land; only over time did it assume the role of hospice for the poor and asylum for the insane. The City of London acquired control over its administration in 1547 and put it under a board of governors; a little more than a century later, in 1676, the hospital opened new quarters in the Moorfields district.

By the mid-sixteenth century, it had sufficiently acquired the role of a specialist hospital for the insane that the corruption of its name, "Bedlam," became a generic term for craziness. As recent British historians of psychiatry have pointed out, tales of abuse and neglect at Bethlem have vastly been overdrawn.

In 1815, the hospital moved again, this time to St. George's Fields in the district of Southwark, where it remained until its removal in 1930 to Monk's Orchard in suburban Kent (at which time the Southwark building, minus the dormitory wings, became the Imperial War Museum). In the 1850s, under its first nonresident superintendent, Sir William Charles Hood (in office 1852–1862; life dates 1824–1870), it was transformed from a receptacle for the poor and mad to a mental hospital for private patients. Dating from 1823, when Scottish-born psychiatrist Alexander Morison (1779–1866) began lecturing there, Bethlem played a minor role in training medical students and post-graduate registrars (residents); yet, it was never really integrated into the University of London, and after a big reorganization of graduate education beginning in 1944, Bethlem was excluded from training to the benefit of the **Maudsley Hospital**. Under the threatened loss of prestige of this downgrade, in 1948 Bethlem and the Maudsley merged, and the hospital's centuries-long distinctiveness came to an end.

Some of the signal names in the history of British psychiatry have been associated with the Bethlem, notably the Monro dynasty of "physicians," or medical supervisors, who presided over Bethlem for four generations beginning with James Monro (dates, 1680–1752) in 1728; John Monro (life dates, 1715–1791) was in office in the period 1751–1791 and is remembered for a highly publicized controversy with **William Battie**; Thomas Monro (life dates, 1759–1833), in office 1787–1816, was dismissed after a scandal involving the longtime chaining of a patient named William Norris (c. 1760–1815); and Edward Thomas Monro (life dates, 1790–1856), in office 1816–1855, who was the last of the "physicians" and who left under something of a cloud. Among the hospital's "apothecaries," or medical officers, might be mentioned John Haslam (life dates, 1764–1844), author of *Observations on Madness and Melancholy* (1809)—the detailed cases of which are among the earliest reported in psychiatry*—who served from 1795 to 1816. (The last of the Monros involved with psychiatry was Henry Monro [1817–1891], who was not associated with Bethlem but rather was an early advocate of biological theories and a physician at St. Luke's Hospital.)

BIOLOGICAL PSYCHIATRY, BEGINNING OF IN UNITED STATES (1946). In 1946 at the Fairmont Hotel in San Francisco, two California neurologists—Johannes M. Nielsen (1890–1969, professor of neurology at the University of Southern California) and his student George N. Thompson (1909–?), chief psychiatrist at the Los Angeles General Hospital)—organized a meeting of a select group of investigators interested in "the biological basis of behavior"; from this meeting emerged the Society of Biological Psychiatry. Among those chartering the new society were Percival Bailey (1892–1973), a Chicago neurologist who had studied in Paris and was among other things attending neuropsychiatrist at Presbyterian Hospital; Karl M. Bowman (1888–1973), on staff at the Langley Porter clinic in San Francisco and professor of psychiatry at the University of California; Stanley Cobb (1887–1968), professor of neuropathology at Harvard University and psychiatrist-in-chief at the Massachusetts General Hospital; Roland P. Mackay (1900–1968), attending neurologist at the Neuropsychiatric Institute in

* An earlier edition entitled *Observations on Insanity* was published in 1798, but the second edition was so extensively revised as to constitute a new book.

Chicago; Harry C. Solomon (1889–1982), medical director of the Boston Psychopathic Hospital; and Samuel Bernard Wortis (1904–1969), professor and chair of psychiatry and neurology at New York University School of Medicine. This was the elite of the U.S. neuroscience establishment. In 1947, Nielsen and Thompson published the first textbook of biological psychiatry in the United States, *The Engrammes of Psychiatry*.

BIPOLAR DISORDER. *See* **MANIC-DEPRESSIVE ILLNESS.**

BLEULER, EUGEN (1857–1939). Known for his interest in the psychology of schizophrenia and for his coinage of the term schizophrenia, Bleuler was born in Zollikon, near Zurich, into a farming family. During his undergraduate studies in medicine, he decided to become a psychiatrist, and after passing the state exam in medicine in 1881, he became an assistant physician at the university psychiatric clinic Waldau in Berne. He then studied abroad—in London and with **Jean-Martin Charcot** in Paris and Bernhard von Gudden (1824–1886) in Munich—before becoming an assistant of **Auguste Forel's** at the **Burghölzli psychiatric clinic.** In 1886, at age 29, he became director of the Cantonal Chronic Care Asylum in Rheinau, and then in 1898 he became Ordinarius professor of psychiatry in Zurich. He was emerited in 1927. In addition to his brief flirtation with psychoanalysis and friendship with Freud, Bleuler is known for his work on affectivity in 1906 (*Affektivität, Suggestibilität, Paranoia*) and for his careful clinical research on schizophrenia in 1908 and 1911. (*See* **SCHIZOPHRENIA: EMERGENCE: Bleuler** [1908, 1911].) In 1910, he coined the term autism. Bleuler's other major contribution was his *Textbook of Psychiatry* (*Lehrbuch der Psychiatrie*, 1916), widely used in Europe.

In retrospect, Bleuler shifted the emphasis in schizophrenia from course and outcome to the cross-sectional study of symptoms, essentially broadening the concept of the disease and giving it a more generous prognosis.

BODY IMAGE: DISTURBANCES OF. These are of interest in psychiatry because the image that the mind gives a person of his or her body is of importance in one's perception of trouble.

Reil's theory of cenesthesia (body feeling) (1803). Leipzig psychiatrist Johann C. Reil saw psychiatric illness as a disorder of sensations arising in the mind, as well as of sensations that the mind created in the body (Gemeingefühl). As he wrote in his *Rhapsodies on the Application of the Psychic Method of Cure in Mental Disorders* (*Rhapsodien über die Anwendung der psychischen Curmethode auf Geisteszerrüttungen*) in 1803, "When unpleasant feelings arise in the wake of mental sensations, do these feelings exist because of excitable mind images [erregte Vorstellungen] or because of abnormal activity in the brain fibers? At least it is this brain route that gives unpleasant feelings their painful consequences for the body's cenesthesia (Gemeingefühl)" (p. 159). Reil pointed out that the power of suggestion lent to the mind the ability to cause all kinds of physical symptoms of illness. (*See* **GERMAN "ROMANTIC" PSYCHIATRY: Reil.**)

Phantom-limb (1871). **Silas Weir Mitchell,** the Philadelphia neurologist who had been a surgeon in the Union army during the U.S. Civil War, noted that many patients with severed limbs continued to "feel" the amputated part as though it were still present. "When a limb has been cut off the sufferer does not lose the consciousness of its existence. . . . [Amputees] retain a sense of its existence so vivid as to be more definite and intrusive than is that of its truly living fellow-member. A person in this condition is haunted, as it were, by a . . . phantom of so much of himself as has been lopped away—an unseen ghost of the lost part. . . . There is something almost tragical, something ghastly, in the notion of these thousands of spirit limbs haunting as many good soldiers, and every now and then tormenting them with the disappointments which arise when, the memory being off guard for a moment, the keen sense of the limb's presence betrays the man into some effort, the failure of which of a sudden reminds him of his loss" (pp. 565–566). Mitchell said that, "Sometimes the ghostly members are in a perpetual state of automatic activity, and the fingers open and shut or twist across one another, especially when there is about to be a change of weather" (p. 568). His 1871 article in *Lippincott's Magazine of Popular Literature and Science* is an early example of understanding breakdowns between actual somatic states and the mind's appreciation of them.

Anorexia nervosa (later understood as a disorder of body image) (1873). Although reports of young women refusing food for psychogenic reasons were long familiar, only in 1873 did **Ernest-Charles Lasègue** coin the diagnostic term "hysterical anorexia" (l'anorexie hystérique) in a paper in the *Archives générales de médecine.* Laségue described the onset: "[The female patient] experiences at first some malaise following her meals: vague sensations of fullness, of pain, gastralgia post prandum or else occurring at the beginning of the meal." The refusing of food continues under various pretexts of pain and such. "After several weeks, it is no longer a supposedly transitory dislike of eating; it is a refusal of food that continues indefinitely. The illness has begun" (p. 388). Later that year, in a lecture, William Gull (1816–1890), a consulting physician to Guy's Hospital in London, called this kind of food refusal "Anorexia hysterica (Apepsia Hysterica)." As the paper was published in 1874 in the *Transactions of the Clinical Society of London,* it bore the title "Anorexia nervosa." Neither clinician considered that a disorder of body image was involved, but the diagnosis itself had entered the medical marketplace.

See **DYSMORPHOPHOBIA** (1891). A belief in the ugliness of one's looks.

Henry Head's study of the body image in the brain (1918). Head (1861–1940), a neurologist at London Hospital, had learned a good deal about the representation of the body in the brain from the head trauma of the First World War. In the journal *Brain* (1918), he explained that some aspects of the body, such as the axis of a limb, were not represented topographically in the brain but functionally: "It is the functions, rather than the anatomical relationships, of any one part of the body that are represented [in the cortex]" (quotation from his collected articles, *Studies in Neurology* [1920], p. 736).

Schilder: body image as a social and biological phenomenon (1935). Shortly after **Paul Schilder** arrived in the United States in 1928—first at Johns Hopkins University then moving to Bellevue Hospital in New York—he developed an interest in body image and its determinants. After a series of articles, especially one published in the psychoanalytic journal *Imago* in 1933 on "Body Image and Social Psychology" ("Das Körperbild und die Sozialpsychologie"), in 1935 he wrote a book on *The Image and Appearance of the Human Body* in which he determined that body image changed throughout the life cycle in accordance with the body's underlying physiology and with people's emotional lives and relations with others, that it represented an expression of the total personality, and that all life experiences influenced it. Individuals internalize the sensations of organic disease, which in turn influences their images of their bodies.

Anorexia nervosa as a disorder of body image (1966). From the beginning of her academic career in the United States, Hilde Bruch (1904–1984), who had fled Nazi Germany in 1933, was interested in disorders of body image. In her days as a pediatrician, she had studied overweight children (*see* her 1940 article on "Obesity in Childhood" in *Psychosomatic Medicine*). Then, after her formal shift to psychiatry, which she taught at Columbia University beginning in 1943, she focused on body image in the overweight (*The Importance of Overweight*; 1957); in a landmark article published in 1962 in *Psychosomatic Medicine*, she said: "The first symptom [in anorexia nervosa] is a disturbance in body image of delusional proportions" (p. 188). After the appearance in 1973 of her influential work, *Eating Disorders: Obesity, Anorexia Nervosa and the Person Within*, the standard interpretation in the eating disorders field came to see anorexia as a problem not of appetite but of body image.

DSM-III highlights disturbances of body image in anorexia nervosa (1980). The third edition of the ***Diagnostic and Statistical Manual*** of the American Psychiatric Association emphasized that, among the essential features of the disorder, were "intense fear of becoming obese" and "disturbance of body image, e.g. claiming to 'feel fat' even when emaciated."

BORDERLINE PERSONALITY DISORDER. Borderline personality disorder (BPD) is important because it became a highly popular diagnosis after the 1980s, applied almost exclusively to young women who previously would have been called "hysterical."

Beginning of "borderline personality disorder" (1938). New York psychoanalyst Adolph Stern (1879–1958) described in the *Psychoanalytic Quarterly* "a large group of patients [who] fit frankly neither into the psychotic nor into the psychoneurotic group. . . . This border line group of patients is extremely difficult to handle effectively by any psychotherapeutic method" (p. 467). Highly narcissistic and insecure, these patients "are constantly being deeply insulted and injured by trifling remarks made by people with whom they come into contact, and occasionally develop mild paranoid ideas" (p. 471). His description involved 10 characteristics that might or might not be present and was quite nonspecific.

"Borderline personality" becomes specified (1967–1968). In 1967, Menninger Foundation psychoanalyst Otto F. Kernberg (1928–) specified in the *Journal of the American Psychoanalytic Association* the psychopathology of what he called "borderline personality organization," which he believed to be a stable character structure and not "a transitory state fluctuating between neurosis and psychosis." He offered a list of operational criteria, any two or three of which would suffice to make the diagnosis. They included anxiety, "polysymptomatic neurosis," and "manifest sexual deviation." Giving rise to this pattern of personality organization were various "aspects of ego weakness," including inability to tolerate anxiety, to control impulses, or to sublimate one's drives in other ways.

In 1968, Chicago neurologist and psychoanalyst Roy R. Grinker, Senior (1900–1993) and colleagues attempted to characterize borderline patients in a quantitative analysis. They admitted to hospital a number of young adults with uncertain psychiatric diagnoses, performed a long battery of tests on them, and observed them closely for 2 weeks. After a factor analysis of the data, the investigators concluded that borderline patients had defects in their affective relations centering about angry explosions, inconsistent self-identity, and depressions characterized by loneliness rather than guilt. They subdivided these patients into four categories, including those who are impulsively angry, those whose personal relations with others vacillate, those who show little spontaneity and prefer to withdraw, and those who have anxiety mixed with a "child-like, clinging depression." Grinker's monograph *The Borderline Syndrome* (1968) put BPD on the map.

Borderline personality disorder: Gunderson defines (from 1978). In an article in 1978 in the *American Journal of Psychiatry*, John G. Gunderson (1942–) and Jonathan E. Kolb (1943–), both at **McLean Hospital**, defined BPD as involving low achievement, impulsivity, manipulative suicidal gestures, heightened affectivity, mild psychotic experiences, high socialization (intolerance of being alone), and disturbed close relationships. Later, Gunderson served on the advisory committee of ***DSM-III-R*** for personality disorders and in 1984 wrote the influential manual *Borderline Personality Disorder*.

Borderline personality disorder enters *DSM-III* (1980). The definition in the *Manual* reflected recent scholarship, characterizing BPD by "instability in a variety of areas, including interpersonal behavior, mood, and self-image. . . . Frequently there is impulsive and unpredictable behavior that is potentially physically self-damaging. . . . There may be problems tolerating being alone, and chronic feelings of emptiness or boredom" (p. 321).

BORDERLINE STATES (from 1909). The term "borderline" has found various usages in the recent history of psychiatry. (*See* **BORDERLINE PERSONALITY DISORDER.**) Carl Pelman (1838–1916), a longtime asylum superintendent who in 1908 had just become professor of psychiatry in Bonn, introduced the term as the title of his rather rambling account of *Psychic Borderline States* (*Psychische Grenzzustände:* 1909); by it he meant virtually everything in psychiatry outside of mainline psychosis, including sexual deviance, alcoholism, pathological lying, the homeless, and so forth.

In 1924, Robert Wälder spoke of "border-line psychosis" as a psychoanalytic concept. (*See* **FREUDIAN INTERPRETATIONS OF PSYCHOSIS: "border-line" psychosis** [1924].)

In 1938, Adolph Stern (1879–1958) described a certain form of personality disorder (one unresponsive to psychoanalysis) as "borderline personality disorder," a term that underwent several permutations before ending in the personality disorders section of the ***DSM*** series. (*See* **BORDERLINE PERSONALITY DISORDER** [1938].)

In 1949, Paul Hoch (1902–1964) and Phillip Polatin (1905–1980) at the New York State Psychiatric Institute used "borderline" to describe "pseudoneurotic schizophrenia," a form of schizophrenia without delusions or hallucinations. (*See* **SCHIZOPHRENIA: RECENT CONCEPTS: pseudoneurotic schizophrenia** [1949]).

BOWLBY, JOHN (1907–1990). Known for his "attachment theory" of maternal–infant bonding, Bowlby was born into a patrician medical family—his father, Sir Anthony Bowlby, was president of the Royal College of Surgeons—and discovered an interest in psychoanalysis during his years at Cambridge (1925–1928). Following graduation, he first observed the importance of separation while working at a school for emotionally maladjusted children. From 1929 to 1933, he read medicine at University College Medical School, then trained in psychiatry at the **Maudsley Hospital** between 1933 and 1936, during which time he was a student-candidate at the British Psychoanalytic Society, analyzed by Joan Riviere (1883–1962), and supervised by **Melanie Klein**. In 1936, he came on staff at the London Child Guidance Clinic and began the study of the relationship of early life events to the formation of neurosis in adults, his first publication on the subject appearing in the *International Journal of Psychoanalysis* in 1940. After the Second World War, in 1946 he became head of the children's department of the Tavistock Clinic, where he remained until his death.

In his three-volume trilogy on *Attachment and Loss*, Bowlby revised classical psychoanalytic theory by arguing that neurosis stemmed from real-life experiences of the mother and child with attachment and dependency rather than from unconscious fantasies. He said that the bond between infant and mother was not merely derived from primeval appetites for food and sex, but served an evolutionary function—protecting the child from predators, and could be elicited experimentally among primates. Volume one in the triology discussed *Attachment* (1969); volume two explored *Separation: Anxiety and Anger* (1973); and volume three was given over to *Loss: Sadness and Depression* (1980). These became classic works in developmental psychology and influenced much research on "maternal–infant bonding," and the importance of the mother (or a similar caregiver) in the playroom of the child.

BRIEF PSYCHOTHERAPY. *See* **FREUDIAN PSYCHOTHERAPY: TECHNIQUE: Stekel's "brief" psychoanalytic technique** (1919); **Sifneos's "short-term psychotherapy"** (1972); **PSYCHOTHERAPY: "interpersonal psychotherapy of depression"** (from 1967).

BULIMIA. In an economy of scarcity, where the population is chronically undernourished, frenzied episodes of overeating wax and wane like the moon. Thus, the symptom of bulimia, which according to its Greek roots means hungry enough to eat an ox ("bous" = ox; "limos" = hunger), goes back to the Ancients. Yet the syndrome of what Gerald F. M. Russell (1928–) of the **Maudsley Hospital** called "bulimia nervosa" in a 1979 article in *Psychological Medicine* seems of relatively recent date. Russell argued that bulimia nervosa grew out of anorexia nervosa, a demonstrably recent illness. In bulimia nervosa, episodes of gorging alternate with periods of anorexia, and the patients maintain a normal weight through induced vomiting and laxatives. Russell's bulimia nervosa became simple "bulimia" in ***DSM-III*** in 1980, an eating disorder that was insisted to be separate from anorexia nervosa (anorexia being a body-image disorder; bulimia an inability to control food cravings) in the pages of the *Manual*. (*See* **BODY IMAGE, DISTURBANCES OF: anorexia nervosa**.) By ***DSM-III-R*** in 1987, the term "bulimia nervosa" was accepted in the *Manual* and gone was the belief that it was separate from anorexia nervosa. In 1994, the disease-designers of ***DSM-IV*** shifted bulimia and anorexia entirely from the childhood–adolescence part of the *Manual* to a newly created section on "eating disorders." Here, a bulimic subtype of anorexia nervosa was accepted, yet bulimia nervosa remained an independent diagnosis as well, with "purging" and "nonpurging" subtypes.

BURGHÖLZLI, THE UNIVERSITY PSYCHIATRIC CLINIC OF ZURICH (1870 and after). In 1863, **Wilhelm Griesinger**, who had come to Zurich in 1860 as professor of medicine and director of the university medical clinic, organized in the old city asylum a "psychiatric clinic" and began lecturing to the medical students. Appointed director of the asylum, he left for Berlin 2 years later. In 1869, psychiatry teaching in Zurich was elevated to a professorship, the chair holder simultaneously being head of the new university hospital ("clinic"), which was erected in 1870 and called the "Burghölzli" (known as the "Bli").

Among Griesinger's successors were a number of well-known psychiatrists. Between 1869 and 1872, Bernhard von Gudden (1824–1886), who pioneered research in neuroanatomy and physiology, occupied the chair. He drowned together with his patient, the mentally ill King Ludwig II of Bavaria (1845–1886), in Lake Starnberg near Munich under tenebrous circumstances. In the brief period 1873–1874, Gustav Huguenin (1838–1907) was the chair holder, succeeded in 1875–1879 by **Eduard Hitzig** (1838–1907). Between 1879 and 1898, **Auguste Forel** (1848–1931) was professor of psychiatry; and in the years 1898–1927, **Eugen Bleuler** (1857–1939) held the chair and left one of the greatest marks of anyone upon the discipline of psychiatry. Bleuler was followed by Hans Wolfgang Maier (1882–1945) in the years 1927–1941, after which in the period 1942–1969, Eugen Bleuler's son Manfred (1903–1994) became the professor of psychiatry. Manfred Bleuler was known for research on psychopathology and—stimulated by his year of study in 1929 in Boston under Stanley Cobb (1887–1968) where he saw some of neurosurgeon Harvey Cushing's (1869–1939) patients with pituitary tumors—on the endocrinological aspects of schizophrenia. Manfred Bleuler's book *Endocrinological Psychiatry* (*Endokrinologische Psychiatrie*) was published in 1954. Bleuler was also known for his work on long-term outcomes in schizophrenia, many of which turned out to be surprisingly positive: *Die schizophrenen Geistessörungen im Lichte langjähriger Kranken- und Familiengeschichten* (1972) (translated into English in 1978 as *The Schizophrenic Disorders: Long-term Patient and Family Studies*). After Bleuler, the clinic was divided.

C

CARDIAZOL SHOCK THERAPY. *See* CONVULSIVE THERAPY: CHEMICAL.

CATATONIA. Catatonia is motor abnormalities in association with severe disorders of mood and thought. Catatonic excitement means an increase in spontaneous and purposeless movements; it is a feature of manic illness among other disorders. Catatonic stupor is a decrease in reactivity to the environment with a reduction of movements and is a feature of depressive illness among others. Catatonia can also be seen as an independent disease.

The term "catatonia" was coined by **Karl Ludwig Kahlbaum** in an 1874 monograph (*Die Katatonie, oder das Spannungsirresein*), but he had used it in public lectures since 1868. The phenomenon had, however, been long familiar in psychiatry and was recognized as part of the immobile apathy traditionally called melancholia attonita (attonita = thunderstruck).

Emil Kraepelin at first accepted Kahlbaum's view that catatonia was an independent illness. He said in the fourth edition (1893) of his textbook, *Psychiatry* (*Psychiatrie*), that Kahlbaum's own classification was overly diverse in terms of cause, clinical picture, and prognosis. "Nonetheless on the basis of clinical experience I feel justified in selecting out a certain group of cases from the category 'catatonia' as a distinctive disease. We are talking here about the acute or subacute forms of distinctive kinds of excitement, that then pass into stupor or dementia with confused delusions and sporadic hallucinations" (pp. 444–445). Here, he made catatonia a form of the "psychic processes of degeneration" alongside dementia praecox.

Yet, in the sixth edition in 1899, Kraepelin changed his mind: catatonia was a subform of dementia praecox. Among the clinical manifestations of dementia praecox, he said, were the hebephrenic forms, the paranoid forms, and the catatonic forms. As he noted in the eighth edition of his textbook in 1913, the last edition he was to complete himself, "On the basis of course, namely of outcome, and apparently on the basis of autopsy findings, there remain no distinctive differences [between catatonia and dementia praecox]; thus we are justified in seeing Kahlbaum's catatonia chiefly as a distinctive kind of course of dementia praecox" (vol. III, 6th ed. [2], p. 809).

For **Eugen Bleuler** as well, catatonia was one of the subdivisions of "the schizophrenias" (alongside the paranoid, hebephrenic, and schizophrenia-simplex subdivisions). As he said in his *Textbook of Psychiatry* (*Lehrbuch der Psychiatrie*) in 1916, "Following acute catatonic attacks a tolerable condition may again recur; the cases that begin furtively all have a bad prognosis without any remissions that are worth mentioning" (A. A. Brill's 1924 English translation of the fourth German edition, p. 417). Kraepelin and Bleuler had thus hijacked Kahlbaum's catatonia and buried it in schizophrenia (where it has been ever since).

In 1930, William J. Bleckwenn (1895–1965), assistant director of the Wisconsin Psychiatric Institute, noted in the *Journal of the American Medical Association* (*JAMA*) that intravenous injections of amobarbital relieved catatonia. Under the category "schizophrenia," he wrote, "The catatonic patient has shown some extremely interesting and rather striking responses." "Periods of from four to fourteen hours of a 'normal lucid interval' have been a constant result of the treatment" (p. 1169). These observations took catatonia out of the concept of "psychological defenses"; some observers view Bleckwenn's procedure as the real beginning of **psychopharmacology**.

As for the recent history of catatonia, ***DSM-III*** continued the Kraepelinian tradition of seeing catatonia as a kind of schizophrenia. In 1980, the existence of a "catatonic type" of schizophrenia, marked by "stupor, negativism, rigidity, excitement, or posturing," was noted in the *Manual* (p. 190). ***DSM-IV*** in 1994 extended the possibility of catatonic symptoms to mood disorders, adding the term as a "specifier": "when the clinical picture is characterized by marked psychomotor disturbance that may involve motoric immobility, excessive motor activity, extreme negativism, mutism" (p. 382).

In the 1970s, interest in catatonia as independent of schizophrenia began to revive with the report in 1973 of James R. Morrison, then at the University of Iowa, in the *Archives of General Psychiatry* that catatonia occurred in about 10% of a series of 2500 patients admitted to the inpatient service of the Iowa State Psychopathic Hospital during the years 1920–1971 with a diagnosis of schizophrenia. He found that catatonia was also quite common in mood disorders: "It would appear that approximately one quarter of patients who have been diagnosed as catatonia, excited type, in fact may suffer from an affective disorder" (p. 41). In 1976 in the *Archives of General Psychiatry*, Richard Abrams (1937–) and Michael Alan Taylor (1940–), using data collected while they were at New York College of Medicine (Metropolitan Hospital), showed that two thirds of a series of consecutive inpatients with signs of catatonia in fact had a mood disorder, usually mania.

In 2003, Taylor, now at the University of Michigan, and **Max Fink** recommended in the *American Journal of Psychiatry* that catatonia be considered an independent syndrome in its own right: "[It] is found in about 10 percent of acutely ill psychiatric inpatients and is more commonly observed in persons with mood disorder than in those with schizophrenia. It is found in many conditions and presents mainly as retarded-stuporous or excited-delirious forms" (p. 1233). This contradicts the commonly held view that catatonia is "rare." (Interested readers will find an overview in Fink and Taylor, *Catatonia: A Clinician's Guide to Diagnosis and Treatment* [2003].) (On periodic catatonia *see* **PSYCHOSIS: EMERGENCE** [1932].)

CATECHOLAMINE HYPOTHESIS OF DEPRESSION (1965). In the most frequently cited article ever published in the *American Journal of Psychiatry*, Harvard psychiatrist Joseph Schildkraut (1934–) argued that depression was an illness linked to the catecholamine **neurotransmitters** (those having a "catechol" portion, such as dopamine and norepinephrine; these and the "indolamines" such as serotonin are collectively referred to as "monoamines").* Schildkraut had graduated with an M.D. from Harvard in 1959,

* It is widely forgotten that in 1959 psychiatrist Abram Hoffer (1917–), director of psychiatric research in the Department of Public Health in Saskatchewan, noted at a conference at McGill University on depression: "The evidence suggests that the catecholamines must play a vital and perhaps villanous role in the causation of depression," and adduced the biochemical evidence on which this hypothesis was based (*Canadian Psychiatric Association Journal*, suppl., pp. S118–S119).

trained in psychiatry at the Massachusetts Mental Health Center, then between 1963 and 1967 went down to the **National Institute of Mental Health** (NIMH) to study neuropsychopharmacology (returning then to "Mass Mental," where he spent the rest of his career). At NIMH, Schildkraut's awareness of several circumstances began to crystallize into the belief that disordered neurochemistry was the cause of depression: Already at Mass Mental he had been impressed at the response of depressed patients to the monoamine oxidase inhibitor phenelzine (Parke-Davis's Nardil). (*See* **IPRONIAZID; NEUROTRANSMITTER.**) This pointed the gun at the monoamines as implicated in depression: if one could inhibit the enzyme that broke them down, the patients got better. Then, in an experiment he determined that phenelzine acted on norepinephrine (a monoamine), and discovered at NIMH that the tricyclic antidepressant **imipramine** did so as well. It was thus clear from this and other evidence, he reasoned, that norepinephrine played a key role in depression. "There is good evidence," he concluded, "to support the thesis that the antidepressant effects of both the monoamine oxidase inhibitors and the imipramine-like drugs are mediated through the catecholamines, and that, by different biochemical mechanisms of action, both of these classes of drugs increase the active catecholamines at adrenergic receptor sites." "The catecholamine hypothesis currently seems to be the strongest and most useful pathophysiological hypothesis of affective disorders" (pp. 516, 517). This represented the "catecholamine" theory of depression that would dominate drug discovery research and academic psychopharmacology for years to come. An exclusive role for norepinephrine in mood disorders, however, is no longer credited. (*See* **SELECTIVE SEROTONIN REUPTAKE INHIBITORS.**) Yet, the hypothesis sparked much research. Psychiatric historian David Healy refers to Schildkraut's 1965 article as "the 1960s equivalent to Freud's *Interpretation of Dreams*."

CHARCOT, JEAN-MARTIN (1825–1893). Often incorrectly identified as a psychiatrist, Charcot was an internist and neurologist whose contributions to psychiatry were largely limited to his doctrine of hysteria. Born in Paris into the family of a wagonmaker, Charcot began his internship in the Paris hospitals in 1848, a protegé of the internist Pierre François Olive Rayer (1793–1867). After his M.D. thesis on gout in 1853, he soon became a ward chief (médecin des hôpitaux) in charge of a service at Lourcine hospital. Passing his Agrégation in 1860 on the second try—the Agrégation is a major exam that qualifies one to teach at university level—and now eligible for a teaching post, in 1862 he chose that vast warehouse of elderly, invalid, ailing, and insane women, the **Salpêtrière hospice**, where he became chief physician of the infirmary. He evidently selected the hospice because it gave him an opportunity to follow patients over the long term and then to link the postmortem findings to signs and symptoms seen antemortem. In this manner, in the 1860s he made a number of important discoveries in neurology, including—from 1868 on—differentiating multiple sclerosis from Parkinson's disease. For these accomplishments in internal and neurological medicine, Charcot became much celebrated.

As Charcot received the chair of clinical pathology in 1872, he was already involved with **hysteria**, a condition that had come to interest him in the early 1860s. His interest intensified in 1870 as he received a ward of "hysterics" as part of his service. Hysteria meant roughly pseudoepilepsy in those days, but Charcot considerably expanded the definition to include what he called hysteria minor (la pétite hystérie) and hysteria major (la grande hystérie). Both were constitutional (inborn) lifelong diseases that affected mainly but not just women. Hysteria minor was characterized by various "stigmata," such as constricted peripheral vision and hypnotizability; hysteria major involved various "phases" of behavior through which the patient would supposedly migrate. In retrospect, almost all of this was artifactual behavior induced in the patients by the physicians' expectations. Yet, Charcot had become so renowned that his flights of fancy were accepted by his medical colleagues as the iron laws of hysteria. At the height of his career, as the president of France in 1882 created a clinical chair for him in nervous diseases, Charcot's hysteria had become a psychiatric doctrine that widely appeared in international textbooks. After his death in 1893, the house of cards fell in, and Charcot's hysteria vanished from the scene. His views were published in the late 1880s in his *Tuesday Lectures at the Salpêtrière* (*Leçons du mardi à la Salpêtrière*).

CHIARUGI, VINCENZO (pronounced KEY-ah-ROO-jee) (1759–1820). The director of one of the first therapeutic asylums, Chiarugi was born in Empoli in Tuscany, his father a physician. He graduated with an M.D. from the University of Pisa in 1779, and in 1785, at the initiative of the Grand Duke Pietro Leopoldo (1747–1792), he became involved in the renovation of the ancient Bonifazio Hospital, which in 1788 opened its doors exclusively to psychiatry patients (instead of remaining a standard "hospice" of the day, mingling together the criminal, the poor, the halt, the elderly, and the insane). In accordance with the principles of the Enlightenment then much in vogue in northern Italy, Chiarugi designed ways of making the experience of institutionalization actually therapeutic instead of merely custodial. He spelled these out in his 1789 book, *Administrative Guide to the S. Maria Nuova and Bonifazio Hospitals* (*Regolamento dei Regi Spedali di S. Maria Nuova e di Bonifazio*), which gave details on gardens, divided the patients into wards on the basis of degree of illness, and insured for them proper meals and humane treatment. In 1793–1794, he wrote a psychiatry textbook in three volumes, *On Insanity* (*Della pazzia*), which was devoted for the most part to the "causes" of insanity and to classifying the major varieties. In a brief section on treatments, Chiarugi also specified some of his therapeutic ideas: for psychological sedation it was necessary to keep the patients in calm, quiet environments. "The sweet songs of gentle, moving music in many cases will represent the first-line treatment" (I, pp. 211–212). As for stimulating treatments, the patients should do moderate athletic workouts in the asylum and at home. In the treatment of melancholy, Chiarugi found it "absolutely necessary that . . . [the physician] finds his way into the patient's heart, gaining his confidence and trust." Chiarugi referred to this approach as "the psychological treatment" (la cura morale) (II, pp. 67, 75). After the publication of his text, Chiarugi lost interest in research in psychiatry as such and devoted himself to dermatology—pellagra and venereal disease represented huge sources of psychiatric illness—resigning the superintendentship of Bonifazio in 1817.

CHLORPROMAZINE AND THE PHENOTHIAZINE ANTIPSYCHOTICS (from 1952). Prehistory: In 1883, August Bernthsen (1855–1931), a postdoctoral student in chemistry at Heidelberg, synthesized a hydrocarbon molecule with two benzol rings connected to each other by a sulfur and a nitrogen atom. Writing in the *Reports of the German*

Chemical Society (*Berichte der Deutschen Chemischen Gesellschaft*), Bernthsen called it "thiodiphenylamine" and later scholars rebaptized it as "phenothiazine." Only in 1934 was this base developed as an insecticide.

Then in 1944, a research group headed by Paul Charpentier at the Rhône-Poulenc research labs in Vitry-sur-Seine, searching for new antihelminthics, hit on the idea of hooking an amino group to a hydrocarbon chain that they dangled from the base of the phenothiazine. The following year, in 1945, others at Rhône-Poulenc started screening Charpentier's compounds as possible antihistamines, and out of this back-and-forth came a drug called promethazine (RP 3277), which had as a side effect pronounced sleepiness. This led the researchers to think the drug might have central (brain) effects—and indeed it did: an antihistamine with strong sedative qualities, it is still widely available for sale today as Phenergan.

In the late 1940s, a French naval surgeon named Henri Laborit (1914–1995) obtained some promethazine and used it in a "lytic cocktail" with other drugs to slow down the autonomic nervous system and reduce shock in surgery. Stimulated by these successes, Charpentier synthesized still more compounds from the phenothiazine nucleus and in December of 1950 sent one, RP 4560, to Simone Courvoisier for pharmacological testing; it was a compound that he had developed not as an antihistamine but with high hopes for central effect.

RP 4560 was chlorpromazine, the single most important drug in the history of psychiatry: As it was launched for trials in 1952 (upon the recommendation of Laborit), first at the Val-de-Grâce military hospital, then by **Jean Delay** and **Pierre Deniker** at **Ste.-Anne mental hospital,** it tamed the symptoms of psychosis without unduly sedating the patients. In 1953, in an article in *Presse médicale* that was widely ignored outside of France because it had no statistics, Jean Sigwald (born 1903, lic. med. qualified 1932) and Daniel Bouttier (lic. 1948) at the Brousse Psychiatric Hospital reported "chloropromazine" [sic] effective in a wide variety of outpatient conditions. They emphasized especially its antidepressant qualities.

No one connected with this story ever won a Nobel Prize. Yet in 1957, Deniker and Laborit received Lasker Awards (along with **Heinz Lehmann**) for their part in this story. They had touched off a pharmacological revolution, demonstrating that a major psychiatric illness could be improved, not with psychotherapy but with chemotherapy, and that the seat of such illnesses must therefore be in the brain rather than in the mind.

Outside of France, chlorpromazine was tested first in Switzerland. In 1953, John Eugen Staehelin (1891–1969), director of the Basel university psychiatric clinic, and Paul Kielholz (1916–1990), then an assistant psychiatrist (later Staehelin's successor), reported in the *Swiss Medical Weekly* (*Schweizer Medizinische Wochenschrift*) on the usefulness of the drug in "psychic disturbances" where the "vegetative tone" was down, and in those where a "reduction" of the patient's emotional drives was desirable, in order to make him or her more accessible to psychotherapy. Despite the opaque language, however, it is clear they were administering it to patients with major psychiatric illnesses.

Rhône-Poulenc took out a U.S. patent in 1953, selling the license for the drug to Smith Kline & French Laboratories in Philadelphia. Trials by **Heinz Lehmann** in Canada and by Willis H. Bower (1916–2000) at **McLean Hospital**, the latter trial published in 1954 in the *New England Journal of Medicine*, proved especially influential. Smith Kline marketed the drug in 1954 as Thorazine; Rhône-Poulenc brought it out elsewhere as Largactil. Interestingly, in the early days chlorpromazine was tried for indications going far beyond psychosis: it was marketed for pain, high-grade anxiety, nausea, hyperactivity in children, and menopausal distress, among many other conditions (and it does have a pharmacological effect in pain and nausea, at least). Only later, in the Drug Efficacy Study Implementation (DESI) of the U.S. Food and Drug Administration during the years between 1968 and 1972 were the indications for chlorpromazine limited essentially to psychosis.

Because of the great commercial success of chlorpromazine, other phenothiazines followed in short order. None was ever therapeutically superior to chlorpromazine—the gold standard in antipsychotic therapy—yet had differing side-effect profiles. In order of year of U.S. patent, the main phenothiazine antipsychotics were as follows:

- 1956: perphenazine (Schering launched as Trilafon in 1957).
- 1957: prochlorperazine (Smith Kline & French launched as Compazine in 1956 [*sic*]); this ceased relatively soon to be used as a psychiatric drug and was indicated instead for gastrointestinal upset.
- 1958: thioridazine (Sandoz launched as Mellaril in 1959).
- 1959: trifluoperazine (first described 1957; Smith Kline & French launched as Stelazine in 1958).
- 1960: fluphenazine (White Laboratories launched as Permitil in 1959; Squibb launched as Prolixin in 1960).

A page was turned in the history of antipsychotic therapy in 1967 when E. R. Squibb & Sons brought out Prolixin Enanthate, a twice-a-month injectable form of fluphenazine. This was the first of the so-called "depot" antipsychotics, long-acting injectable doses that made possible the community treatment of schizophrenic patients, who no longer had to take medications daily in a supervised setting. In 1973, Squibb launched Prolixin Decanoate, an injectable form administered once every 3 weeks.

The early days of phenothiazine therapy were marked by the administration of very high doses. It was not unheard of in the United States for patients on chlorpromazine to receive up to 3000 mg a day, at a time when 150 mg per day was considered in Europe to be a healthy dose. The big decline in dosages began with the publication of the book *The Action of Neuroleptic Drugs* (1965) by Hans-Joachim Haase (1922–), professor of psychiatry in Düsseldorf, and by Paul Janssen (1926–2003), director of research of a pharmaceutical company in Beerse, Belgium, named after his family. The authors built upon a discovery that Haase had made in 1955 about the shrinking size of handwriting under neuroleptic treatment: In 1965, they said that when the patient's handwriting starts to get smaller, the therapeutic dose ("neuroleptic threshold") has been reached: it became clear that the threshold was reached at much smaller doses.

Another body blow to large doses came in 1991 as Stephen R. Marder (1945–) and associates at the West Los Angeles Veterans Administration Medical Center emphasized in *Schizophrenia Research* that in order to limit the symptoms of **extrapyramidal syndromes** (EPS) such as **tardive dyskinesia** (TD), "the lowest effective dose" should not be exceeded. Then in 1994, Paula Bollini (otherwise at the International Organization for Migration in Geneva) and co-workers at the Technology Assessment Group of the Harvard School of Public Health, in a "meta-analysis" (pooling of data) of 22 published trials that appeared in *Psychological Medicine,* offered a definitive demonstration of the harmfulness of high doses: at doses above 375 mg-equivalents of chlorpromazine, patients stopped getting better, but the rate of side effects increased significantly.

Leo Hollister (1920–2000), a veteran U.S. psychopharmacologist, said that in his lifetime he had been present at three medical miracles: one was penicillin and he had witnessed the spectacle of patients with bacterial endocarditis, "an otherwise fatal illness," saved with the drug; the second was seeing patients wheelchair-bound with rheumatoid arthritis get up and walk around the ward after treatment with corticosteroids; the third was chlorpromazine (Healy, *Psychopharmacologists,* II, p. 235).

CLAUDE, HENRI-CHARLES-JULES (1869–1945). Professor of mental diseases at the University of Paris from 1922 to his retirement in 1939, Claude was born in Paris, concentrated in internal medicine and neurology (much influenced by **Jean-Martin Charcot**), and by 1903 had acquired the rank of ward chief (médecin des hôpitaux). The following year, he passed the Agrégation exam and became the assistant of Fulgence Raymond (1844–1910), who had the chair of nervous diseases at the **Salpêtrière hospice** (the former Charcot chair). Here, Claude encouraged Raymond to organize an outpatient service for nonpsychotic illnesses ("les petits mentaux," as they were familiarily known). In 1922, Claude was appointed professor of mental diseases in the chair situated at **Ste.-Anne mental hospital** (in the French system, these chairs are located at certain hospitals), where he remained until his retirement in 1939. At Ste.-Anne, he sought immediately to make the teaching of psychiatry more interesting for medical students, giving them the feeling that psychiatry was a part of medicine rather than, as **Jean Delay** put it in his obituary of Claude, "appearing to them as an inaccessible domaine of purely speculative interest and walled off by a hermetic vocabulary" (*L'Encéphale,* 1950, p. 389).

Claude is known for having introduced such physical therapies as the malarial fever cure (*see* **NEUROSYPHILIS; WAGNER VON JAUREGG**), **insulin** coma, and metrazol convulsion (*see* **CONVULSIVE THERAPY: CHEMICAL**) into France; he is also associated with a rather unsuccessful effort, called organo-dynamic thinking, to synthesize psychiatry with the basic anatomical–clinical method of doing research in medicine (a method that much influenced his student **Henri Ey**). Not uncongenial to **Sigmund Freud's** doctrines, Claude had among his residents such prominent later figures in French psychoanalysis as **Jacques Lacan**, Raymond de Saussure (1894–1971), and Rudolph Loewenstein (1898–1976). Claude encouraged the formation in 1925 of the pro-psychoanalytic Groupe de l'Évolution psychiatrique. **Pierre Pichot** calls Ste.-Anne under Claude "one of the most lively centres of French psychiatry between the wars" (*History of Psychiatry,* p. 104).

Despite Claude's neurobiological orientation, much reinforced by the epidemic of encephalitis of 1917, he was a great benefactor of the psychoanalytic movement—as Pierre Morel points out in his biographical dictionary of French psychiatry. In 1923, Claude asked René Laforgue (1894–1962) to organize a psychoanalytic consultation service at Ste.-Anne, where the founders of the future Paris Psychoanalytic Society later met. Three years later, he started a lecture series on psychoanalysis in the psychiatric clinic of the hospital. A number of later psychoanalysts, such as Lacan, passed through Claude's clinic as assistant physicians. Yet, in his memoirs, Henri Baruk (1897–1999) has left an unforgettable image of Claude as petty and vain and quite uncomfortable with clinical psychiatry (*People Like Us* [*Des hommes comme nous*], 1976, pp. 28–33).

CLÉRAMBAULT'S SYNDROME. *See* **EROTOMANIA; FRENCH CHRONIC DELUSIONAL STATES: mental automatism** (1920).

COGNITIVE-BEHAVIORAL THERAPY (CBT). Behavioral techniques concern activities that may be modified by reflex action without much cogitation on the part of the subject. As "operant conditioning" was conceived by Burrhus Frederick Skinner (1904–1990)—notably in his book *Science and Human Behavior* (1953)—actions lead either to a reward or to the prevention of a painful stimulus, thus changing behavior by reinforcement or discouragement ("extinction"). Cognitive techniques address such intellectual functions as the reality testing of "automatic thoughts" and involve more the kind of rational persuasion that Paul Dubois conceived (*see* **PSYCHOTHERAPY: Dubois's "rational psychotherapy"** [1904]). CBT thus draws on two sources: a rich tradition of behavioral therapy going back to Ivan Petrovich Pavlov (1849–1936) and the Russian school of physiologists (that will not be further considered in this *Dictionary*; however, *see* **EYSENCK**); it draws as well on more recent efforts to identify errors in cognition as the root problem in such illnesses as depression.

This more recent tradition begins with the South African psychiatrist Joseph Wolpe (1915–), a lecturer at the University of Witwatersrand, who in 1954 in the *AMA Archives of Neurology and Psychiatry* described "reciprocal inhibition" as the basis of the effect of psychotherapy (he amplified these ideas in his 1958 book, *Psychotherapy by Reciprocal Inhibition*): The anxiety response is inhibited if a stimulus the opposite of anxiety is evoked in an anxiety-producing setting. Applying this theory to humans with phobias, he found that prolonged exposure to the feared setting produced "systematic desensitization." Wolpe was very much a behaviorist and attempted, for example, to convert homosexuals into heterosexuals with behavior therapy techniques. (*See also* **HOMOSEXUALITY AND PSYCHIATRY** on psychoanalytic attempts to effect this kind of "reparative" therapy.) Yet, his work begins the CBT stream.

Building on these findings, in 1963 Aaron Beck (1921–), then associate professor of psychiatry at the University of Pennsylvania, argued in the *Archives of General Psychiatry* that depression arose in part as a result of "cognitive distortions" involving such themes as "low self-evaluation, ideas of self-deprivation, exaggeration of problems and difficulties, self-criticisms and self-commands, and wishes to escape or die" (p. 333). As Beck elaborated his ideas about depression and cognition in his book *Depression: Clinical, Experimental and Theoretical Aspects* (1967), the triad of cognitive patterns forcing the individual to "view himself, his world, and his future in an idiosyncratic way" were (1) construing experiences negatively, (2) viewing himself negatively, and (3) viewing the future negatively (p. 255). Cognitive, or insight, psychotherapy, said Beck, focused on neutralizing "automatic thoughts, validating basic truths, and using induced fantasies to modify mood." In an article published in *Behavior Therapy* in 1970, he spelled out the relationship of cognitive therapy to behavior therapy. His seminal book was *Cognitive Therapy of Depression* (1979).

Cognitive therapy was launched in a medical environment still dominated by psychoanalysis. One colleague informed Beck that cognitive therapy was "like treating malaria with an electric fan." Yet, in clinical trials, cognitive therapy demonstrated roughly the same efficacy in nonhospital depression as did psychopharmacology. In 1994, Beck founded in Bala Cynwyd, Pennsylvania, the Beck Institute for Cognitive Therapy and Research to help train therapists.

Establishing the effectiveness of "exposure" therapy in the treatment of obsessive-compulsive disorder (1973). It was Janet who in *Principles of Psychotherapy* (*La médecine psychologique*) in 1923 initially established that continually ordering a patient to repeat a given compulsive action, or exposure, diminished the patient's need to do so. Calling them "treatments by suggestion," Janet said that the patients "know very well that they are incapable of performing certain acts voluntarily or else that they will retard their execution by a mass of scruples . . . and they themselves desire to be made to execute certain acts in a forced or automatic way. 'Have you absolutely decided to feed me with the tube if I do not eat?' 'Exactly.' 'In that case I am forced and it is you who take the responsibility; I prefer that.' And she eats as she should" (Eng. Trans., p. 198).

Yet the observation was not taken up. In 1973, psychiatrist Isaac M. Marks (1935–) at the Institute of Psychiatry of the **Maudsley Hospital** in London determined that "exposure in vivo," continuously subjecting patients who had rituals and phobias to a stimulus that evokes their symptoms, produced a lasting diminution of the symptoms themselves. He published the exposure principle first in 1973 in the *Canadian Psychiatric Association Journal*, advocating "continued exposure to the phobic situation until anxiety and avoidance responses are extinguished" (p. 11). Eight years later, in 1981, he wrote in an article in the *American Journal of Psychiatry* that on the basis of controlled studies, self-exposure was at least as effective as therapist-accompanied exposure: "For a ritualizer the evoking stimulus might be the discomfort brought on by the perception of dirt, disarray, or uncertainty. Such a stimulus evokes the response of compulsive washing, tidying up, or checking. . . . The compulsive tidier . . . might be asked to untidy his or her possessions. . . . In time, the resultant evoking stimulus of discomfort will be tolerated without evoking rituals or avoidance" (p. 585).

COMMUNITY PSYCHIATRY. (*See* **BEERS, CLIFFORD;** also **PSYCHOTHERAPY: group psychotherapy; "therapeutic community"** [both 1939].) The premise of community psychiatry is that patients with serious illnesses are best treated in the community rather than in closed mental hospitals. Although this preference had been adumbrated throughout the nineteenth and early twentieth centuries, only in the 1940s does it start to swell into a movement. Particular landmarks in the unfolding of the community approach are given below.

The Mental Health Treatment Act of Great Britain (1930). The act provided for voluntary treatment in mental hospitals so that patients might be less resistant to admission if they could leave at will; the act also authorized outpatient clinics based in asylums and general hospitals; indeed, the act discarded the term "asylum" in favor of "mental hospital."

"Day hospitals" (from 1946). As notions of "therapeutic community" expanded after the Second World War, it became apparent that the community needed a site where discharged patients in particular could be treated during the day without being formally admitted to a psychiatric bed. D. Ewen Cameron (1901–1967), head of psychiatry at **McGill University**, created the first day hospital in the world in 1946 at the Allan Memorial Institute in Montreal. In 1948, psychotherapist Joshua Bierer (1901–1984) established the first in England, a "social club" at the Social Psychiatry Centre in London that he had set up 2 years previously. A number of other such day hospitals then followed in Great Britain, so that by 1959 more than 38 existed. The movement incorporated Bierer's philosophy that, "Treatment must include the whole social environment of the patient and all his social relationships. He must be treated not only as a person but as part of a community," as he wrote in the *Lancet* in 1959 (p. 901).

The Community Mental Health Centers Act in the United States (1963). Stimulated by the report *Action for Mental Health* in 1961 (*see* **PSYCHOTHERAPY: "therapeutic community"**), in 1963 Congress passed an act designed, as Robert Felix, head of the **National Institute of Mental Health**, put it, "to reduce substantially, within a decade or two, the numbers of patients who received only custodial care—or no care at all—when they could be helped by the application of . . . the modern methods of dealing with . . . mental illnesses." Yet the program was never adequately funded, and many centers became diverted toward psychotherapy for middle-class people with adjustment disorders rather than looking after recently discharged patients with serious illnesses. In the words of psychiatry historian Gerald N. Grob, "Within a decade after the passage of the act of 1963, it had become clear that CMHCs, whatever their original purposes, had neither replaced mental hospitals nor provided alternative services for the severely mentally ill" (*From Asylum to Community*, p. 256).

The promotion of "community mental health services" by the Regional Office for Europe in Copenhagen of the World Health Organization (from 1970). The efforts of the World Health Organization (WHO) Regional Office for Europe had a large impact on community psychiatry in Europe, particularly from the viewpoint of (1) implementing community care programs based on the principles of "continuity of care" (up and down the ladder of referral from mental hospital to community), (2) creating "integrated care" (meaning a number of different mental-health disciplines and institutions collaborating smoothly), and (3) augmenting the resources given to mental health. As a WHO report in 1971 noted, "The trend towards caring for the mentally ill in the community wherever possible and recognition of the need to consider the patient in the context of his social environment are modern phenomena. This approach is the antithesis of custodial care in large isolated institutes and of an exclusively medical approach which seeks to treat mental illness in the same terms as a physical disease" (WHO, *Trends in Psychiatric Care: Day Hospitals and Units in General Hospitals*, p. 18).

The advent of the "depot" antipsychotics (from 1973). A major obstacle to community psychiatry had been the reluctance of many discharged schizophrenic patients to continue taking their antipsychotic medications because of the movement disorders known as **"extrapyramidal side effects"** that often accompany chronic use of antipsychotics. (*See also* **PARKINSONISM: NEUROLEPTIC-INDUCED; TARDIVE**

DYSKINESIA.) Once these patients discontinue their medications, they relapse easily and become resistant to the ministrations of community care. Thus, the Squibb company's introduction in 1973 of long-acting fluphenazine, marketed as Prolixin Decanoate, an injectible form of the drug—dissolved in oil, allowing for slow release—that acts for up to a month (instead of having to be taken daily), had a big impact on community psychiatry. As a World Rehabilitation Fund report commented in 1986, "Easily accessible depo-neuroleptic clinics dispense these medications to patients living in the community and patients appear less resistant to medication maintenance."

COMPULSIVE BEHAVIOR. *See* **OBSESSIVE-COMPULSIVE DISORDER.**

CONDUCT DISORDER. The medicalizing of persistent antisocial behavior on the part of children goes back to **Cesare Lombroso** and the degeneration theorists of the nineteenth century. (*See* **CRIMINALITY AND PSYCHIATRY; PSYCHIATRIC GENETICS: degeneration theory** [1857].) Lombroso believed that criminals were born, and demonstrated from youth onward signs of "moral insanity" (he called them "pazzi morali"). Moreover, youthful antisocials were in many cases, he said, afflicted with epilepsy, and their outbursts could be seen as ictal in nature. In the second edition of 1878 of *The Criminal Male* (*L'uomo delinquente*), Lombroso pointed to "The complete identity and analogy between the morally insane man and the born-criminal." As Lombroso wrote in 1902 in the *New Anthology of Sciences* (*Nuova Antologia di Scienze*) of one youthful criminal who became a notorious brigand in adult life, "He was a born criminal, above all because . . . he was subject to epileptic episodes, an illness that is . . . at the bottom of born criminality. . . . It manifested itself acutely between ages of 12 and 15, at the time in which he became incorrigible and cruel toward his father."

Even after the driven determinism of degeneration theory had passed from the scene, the concept of innate criminality remained in the literature of forensic and adolescent psychiatry. In the eighth edition of his textbook (1915), **Emil Kraepelin** raised "the question of the born criminal."

From the 1920s onward, psychoanalysts saw conduct disorder, or juvenile delinquency, as a problem of individual character pathology. Here, a key contribution stemmed from Viennese educator and psychoanalyst August Aichhorn (1878–1949); namely, his 1925 classic work, *Verwahrloste Jugend: Die Psychoanalyse in der Fürsorgeerziehung* (translated into English in 1935 as *Wayward Youth*—the German subtitle meant "psychoanalysis in foster institutional care"). Freud wrote the preface. Aichhorn said, "It has been well established that much delinquent behavior arises on the basis of neurosis, meaning that neurotic changes in ego-structure occur in connection with delinquency" (p. 29).

As well, Chicago psychoanalyst Franz Alexander (1891–1964) suggested the concept of "acting out" in a 1930 article on "the neurotic character" in the *International Journal of Psychoanalysis*: "The asocial tendencies, which the neurotic represses and confines to substitutive gratification . . . are all given free rein by the true criminal without the presence of inner conflict." Whereas some neurotics "acted out" their impulses in such forms as masturbation, others did so in life (pp. 296, 304). (Alexander was not writing expressly of adolescents with conduct disorder, yet the notion of "acting out" subsequently was applied not to adult murderers but wayward teenagers.)

Simultaneously, a sociological perspective on delinquency flourished, initiated by sociologists Clifford Robe Shaw (1895–1957) and Henry Donald McKay (1899–1980), both at the Institute for Juvenile Research in Chicago. In 1929, President Herbert Hoover had created the National Commission on Law Observance and Enforcement, known popularly as the Wickersham Commission after its chairperson, New York lawyer George W. Wickersham, in response to public concern about gang wars in Chicago among other matters. In 1931, Shaw and McKay, in their *Social Factors in Juvenile Delinquency* (volume two of the *Report on the Causes of Crime*, published by the National Commission), noted that, "The community fails to function effectively as an agency of social control in these areas of high rates of delinquents" (p. 387). In 1942, Shaw and McKay brought out *Juvenile Delinquency and Urban Areas*, an opening gong in the sociology of delinquency.

After the Second World War, conduct disorder and juvenile delinquency became widely considered as socially caused. In 1946, Lester Eugene Hewitt of the Child Guidance Institute of the University of Michigan and Richard L. Jenkins (1903–?), a Chicago child psychiatrist, argued in *Fundamental Patterns of Maladjustment* that youthful antisocial behavior was the result of "particular environmental situations" rather than either psychodynamics or biology. Psychiatrists took leading roles in the 1950s in the huge wave of concern about "juvenile delinquency," distinguishing bewtween "individual delinquency," for which there would be psychoanalytic explanations, and "sociologic delinquency," attributable to ethnic subcultural behavior.

In 1966, sociologist Lee Nelken Robins (1922–) of Washington University in **St. Louis** reported a follow-up study of 500 children brought to child guidance clinics in St. Louis and then tracked down 30 years later: In her book *Deviant Children Grown Up: A Sociological and Psychiatric Study of Sociopathic Personality*, she found that conduct-disordered children often became sociopathic adults.

As for official postwar diagnosis in American psychiatry, ***DSM-II*** in 1968 had no particular label for the conduct-disturbed, noting only an "adjustment reaction of adolescence: irritability and depression associated with school failure and manifested by temper outbursts, brooding and discouragement" (p. 49).

"Conduct disorder" as a diagnosis for willful and misbehaved adolescents, mainly boys, entered ***DSM*** in the third edition in 1980, having as its essential feature, "a repetitive and persistent pattern of conduct in which either the basic rights of others or major age-appropriate societal norms or rules are violated." The disorder was subdivided on the basis of how socialized and aggressive the children and adolescents were. "Conduct disorder" was, in the *DSM* typology, the childhood version of "antisocial behavior" in adults, and nestled alongside "oppositional disorder," the latter being "a pattern of disobedient, negativistic, and provocative opposition to authority figures." The *Manual* also struck a genetic note that became more accentuated in successive editions: "Familial pattern: the disorder is more common in children of adults with antisocial personality disorder and alcohol dependence than in the general population." ***DSM-III-R*** (1987) and ***DSM-IV*** (1994) made no essential changes to the overall concept.

CONOLLY, JOHN (1794–1866). Born in Lincolnshire, England, into a family of Irish origin, Conolly first served in a county militia, going into medicine as he was unable to make ends meet. He graduated with an M.D. at Edinburgh, then drifted about as a family physician and lecturer in medicine at University College London. He returned to the Midlands in 1830 and served as an inspector to county asylums, all the while becoming a cofounder of the Provincial Medical and Surgical Association, which turned into the British Medical Association. In 1839, Conolly became superintendent of the Middlesex Asylum at Hanwell, just outside of London.

After his arrival at Hanwell, Conolly accelerated a revolutionary change underway in English asylum medicine by abolishing the use of mechanical restraints. It is not that he originated the practice of treating asylum patients with kindness and "nonrestraint"—the concept goes back to the system originated at the Quaker private asylum at York, the Retreat, by its founder **William Tuke**. (*See also* **"MORAL TREATMENT"**.) Several other psychiatrists had already implemented nonrestraint in the British Isles. Yet Conolly's prestige meant that his 1856 book, *The Treatment of the Insane without Mechanical Restraints*, became widely followed at home and abroad, and efforts to preserve the dignity of asylum patients and to offer more humane care became common in the asylum world after Conolly's success became known. In his book he noted that "The mere abolition of fetters and restraints constitutes only a part of what is properly called the non-restraint system." Rather it was a "complete system" for managing patients involving reassurance "by a few kind words that no ill-treatment is any longer to be feared," that the patient is given clean and comfortable clothing, that he or she eats with proper tableware on a clean table, and that the patient's "irritable brain" is given quiet and repose in his own bedroom, or, for violent patients, in a "padded room" (pp. 35–43). "The old system," Conolly said, "placed all violent or troublesome patients in the position of dangerous animals. The new system regards them as afflicted persons, whose brain and nerves are diseased, and who are to be restored to health, and comfort, and reason" (p. 53).

"CONVERSION" DISORDER INTRODUCED (1795). The term "conversion" had occasionally been used in humoral medicine in the sense of the complication of a disease or the side effect of a treatment. In 1795, John Ferriar (1763–1815), physician to the Manchester Infirmary and Lunatic Hospital, wrote, "Many cases of conversion produce insanity; this disorder supervenes on the imprudent suppression of eruptions; on the extinction of continued fevers." He remarked upon a case in which a woman became manic as a result of the suppression of her menses. "She continued insane during seven years, and was restored to her senses by an uterine haemorrhage" (*Medical Histories and Reflections*, 2nd ed., vol. II, p. 120). Elsewhere, Ferriar also described "hysterical conversion," in which the body produces alarming symptoms without real underlying disease. (*See* **FREUDIAN DOCTRINE OF HYSTERIA** [1892 and after].)

CONVULSIVE THERAPY: CHEMICAL (METRAZOL) (1934). Budapest neuropathologist Ladislaus von Meduna (1896–1964) introduced the modern practice of convulsive therapy by chemical means. Meduna, a graduate of the Semmelweis Medical University in 1922, had trained as a neuropathologist at the Budapest Interacademic Institute for Neurological Research, then in 1926 followed his chief Prof. Károly Schaffer (1864–1939)—who educated an entire generation of Hungarian psychiatrists in histology (the equivalent of biochemistry today)—to the university department of psychiatry; Meduna was also a ward chief at the state asylum at Budapest-Lipótmezö. Meduna had noticed under the microscope that glia cells (the connective tissue of the brain) in schizophrenic patients looked quite different from those in epilepsy patients, and because epilepsy and schizophrenia rarely occurred in the same patient, Meduna hypothesized a kind of opposition between the two illnesses. It followed, he thought, that if epileptiform fits could be induced in schizophrenics, it might ameliorate the disease. He began by using camphor as the epileptogenic drug. (There had been previous attempts in medicine to induce fits with camphor, although these were unknown to Meduna at the time.) Shortly thereafter, Meduna switched to the more soluble and faster-acting pentylenetetrazol as the convulsion-inducing drug, which had been marketed as a mild cerebral and cardiac stimulant under the brand names Cardiazol in Europe and Metrazol in the United States.

In 1935, in the *Journal of Combined Psychiatry and Neurology* (*Zeitschrift für die gesamte Neurologie und Psychiatrie*), he reported on the first 26 patients, some of whom had received camphor, others Cardiazol. Of the 26, 10 experienced substantial improvement; this was at the time when the therapeutics of schizophrenia were virtually nonexistent. In 1937, he provided a comprehensive view of his treatment in *The Convulsive Therapy of Schizophrenia* (*Die Konvulsionstherapie der Schizophrenie*). Meduna's treatment was soon overtaken by **electroconvulsive therapy (ECT)** because the latter was easier to use, better tolerated by the patients, and had equal efficacy. Also, outpatients often disliked Metrazol therapy because of the problem of delayed convulsions: They would return home and experience yet another convulsion there. Yet, Cardiazol (Metrazol) is important as the first of the convulsive therapies.

Meduna emigrated to the United States in 1939, becoming professor of psychiatry first at Loyola University, then at the University of Illinois medical school, both of which are in Chicago. In Chicago, he occupied himself with the understanding of oneirephrenia, a form of schizophrenia characterized by clouding of consciousness (*see* his monograph in 1950; *see also* **Willi Mayer-Gross's** 1924 monograph); he also became involved with the possible carbon-dioxide treatment of neurosis, writing a monograph on the subject in 1955; it was a method that failed to catch on.

First to report on Metrazol in the United States was Hungarian-born psychiatrist Emerick Friedman (1910–?), who read a paper on it at a staff conference of the Buffalo City Hospital in May 1937.

CONVULSIVE THERAPY: ELECTRICAL. *See* **ELECTROCONVULSIVE THERAPY (ECT).**

COTARD'S SYNDROME (the delusion of negativity [le délire de négation]) (1880). In 1880, Jules Cotard (1840–1889) presented to the Société médico-psychologique in Paris (the French Psychiatric Society) a paper on patients, such as those at the private nervous clinic in suburban Vanves where he worked, who customarily deny the existence of anything to which their attention is directed. "You ask them their name? They don't have a name. Their age? They don't have an age. Where they were born? They were never born. . . . If they have a headache or a stomach ache? They don't have a head, don't have a stomach." In line with the differentiation of psychosis that **Ernest-Charles Lasègue** and his successors had begun in 1852 (*see* **PARANOIA; PSYCHOSIS: EMERGENCE**), Cotard suggested that this was a "special form of psychosis [une évolution délirante spéciale] that seems to me to apply to quite a large number of melancholic patients who are not persecuted, particularly to those with anxiety, and it is based above all on the very chronic negative dispositions that these patients have" (p. 153). The syndrome is found in schizophrenia, psychotic depression, and frequently in the dementias of the elderly. The paper was published in 1882 in the *Archives de neurologie*.

CRICHTON-BROWNE, JAMES (1840–1938). A pioneer of the study of mental illness in Britain, he was born in Edinburgh, the son of William A. F. Browne (1805–1885), superintendent of the Crichton Royal Institute at Dumfries (the foremost asylum in Scotland) and of Magdalene Howden, a Shakespearian scholar. (Crichton-Browne received "Crichton" as his second Christian name in honor of James Crichton, the benefactor of the Dumfries asylum, and he later added it to his surname.) He read medicine at Edinburgh University, qualifying as a surgeon in 1861 and earning an M.D. with a thesis on hallucinations in 1862. After serving on the medical staff of several provincial asylums, in 1866 he became medical director of the large West Riding asylum at Wakefield, also lecturing in psychiatry at Leeds University. He began the annual *West Riding Lunatic Asylum Medical Reports*, which included notable scientific articles. (Crichton-Browne also co-edited the journal *Brain* from 1878 to 1885.) He left the West Riding asylum in 1875 and removed to London to become a "Visitor in Lunacy," or mental-hospital inspector, and continued in that function until he retired in 1922. In London, he also became one of the first British psychiatrists to have an extensive private practice.

Crichton-Browne is known for having introduced the scientific study of psychiatry to British asylums, and his most distinguished visiting fellow was probably neurophysiologist David Ferrier (1843–1928), who did research at Wakefield in the early 1870s. In the late 1920s and early 1930s, Crichton-Browne published a series of amusing popular books containing observations about life and medicine, such as *Victorian Jottings* (1926) and *What the Doctor Thought* (1930), many of which retain their charm. "Crichton-Browne's true faith was the brain," write his biographers Michael Neve and Trevor Turner, quoting him: "The brain-cell is an altar before which spiritual unions take place, a tabernacle in which the holy of holies is enshrined" (*Medical History*, 1995, p. 417).

CRIMINALITY AND PSYCHIATRY. In his novel *East of Eden* (1952), John Steinbeck wrote of the character Cathy Ames:

> It is my belief that Cathy Ames was born with the tendencies, or lack of them, which drove and forced her all of her life. Some balance wheel was misweighted, some gear out of ratio. She was not like other people, never was from birth. And just as a cripple may learn to utilize his lack so that he becomes more effective in a limited field than the uncrippled, so did Cathy, using her difference, make a painful and bewildering stir in the world. (Viking ed., 1970, pp. 72–73)

The term "psychopath" was anticipated by English philosopher Jeremy Bentham (1748–1832) in his 1817 work on hedonism, *A Table of the Springs of Action: Shewing the Several Species of Pleasures and Pains*: "Psychological dynamics . . . has for its basis psychological pathology. Pleasure and exemption from pain fail to be considered everywhere in the character of ends: pleasure and pain here in the character of means" (*Collected Works*, p. 87). Some writers have seen **James C. Prichard's** diagnosis "moral insanity" in his *Treatise on Insanity* (1835) as the first practical incorporation of the concept of psychopathy, yet the term as Prichard uses it is too vague to qualify for that distinction.

The "Central European" criminal psychopath. Viennese psychiatrist Ernst von Feuchtersleben (1806–1849), in his 1845 *Textbook of Medical Psychology* (*Lehrbuch der ärztlichen Seelenkunde*), popularized the term "psychopathy" in the narrower sense of a disordered personality rather than an urge to avoid pain: "We call psychopathies or disorders of the personality [Psychopathieen oder Persönlichkeits-Krankheiten] . . . those composite conditions, in which the reciprocal relationship between the psychic and the physical is diseased in a number of ways, so that the empirical personality of the individual appears disordered [getrübt]" (pp. 262–263).

As early as **Morel's** writing on mental disorders in 1860, the psychopath is seen as a criminal. Morel said of "degenerate persons" (he did not use the term "psychopath"): "From the intellectual and moral viewpoint, hereditary influences of a pernicious nature . . . become converted early into unhealthy tendencies such as drunkenness, suicide, and vagabondage" (p. 580). Among European writers under the influence of Morel's degeneration theory, criminals became increasingly "born criminals."

In 1888, Julius Ludwig August Koch (1841–1908), director of the state asylum at Zwiefalten in Württemberg, introduced in his *Brief Guide to Psychiatry* (*Kurzgefasster Leitfaden der Psychiatrie*; 1888) the concept of what he called "psychopathic inferiorities" (psychopathische Minderwertigkeiten). Of those with "inborn psychopathic degeneration," he said: "These creatures appear quite frequently in the ranks of the evil-doers [Bösewichte]" (p. 45).

It was via the writings of **Cesare Lombroso** and **Eugen Bleuler** that this kind of psychopath influenced generations of scholarship on criminality and character disorder. Eugen Bleuler's 1896 book on *The Born Criminal* (*Der geborene Verbrecher*), together with Lombroso's earlier writings on *Criminal Man* (1876) and *Criminal Woman* (1893), created the dark figures who stalked through life driven as much by their genes as by poverty and social conditions.

In 1929, right-wing Munich psychiatrist Johannes Lange (1891–1938) buttressed these views by adumbrating the genetics of criminality in a book entitled *Crime and Destiny: Studies of Criminal Twins* (*Verbrechen als Schicksal: Studien an kriminellen Zwillingen;* translated into English in 1930). Lange said, "The biologist, and even more the doctor who has to deal with the individual criminal, cannot help again and again seeing fate in crime, stronger than the free-will of the individual. The natural tendencies one is born with, the surrounding world he grows up in, these are essentially destiny" (p. 21 of English translation). As Willi **Mayer-Gross** and co-authors commented in their 1954 textbook, *Clinical Psychiatry*, "The effect of Lange's work, which attracted very great attention at the time, was to suggest that . . . the make-up of personality was determined almost exclusively by hereditary factors; and that social behaviour itself was the almost inevitable product of the personality" (p. 99).

Yet, Lange's findings received some confirmation in the work of another pioneer of psychiatric genetics, Aaron J. Rosanoff (1878–1943), at the time in private practice in

Los Angeles, in an article in 1934 on "Criminality and Delinquency in Twins" in the *Journal of Criminal Law and Criminology*. Rosanoff wrote, "Our material indicates that in two-thirds of the cases of adult criminality in monozygotic twins, when one is criminal the other is likewise criminal" (p. 932). He amplified his views in a 1941 book on the same subject (in 1939 he became director of the Department of Institutions in California). These eugenist views of criminality and psychopathy fueled sterilization laws in a number of countries.

The psychoanalytic psychopath. Psychoanalytic writing produced a milder version of psychopathy in which the psychopath was made not born. The 1925 work of Viennese educator and psychoanalyst August Aichhorn (1878–1949), *Verwahrloste Jugend* (translated into English in 1935 as *Wayward Youth*), accented libidinal misadventures: "Given certain disturbances in the libido organization . . . the child remains asocial. . . . This means that he has not repudiated completely his instinctual wishes but has suppressed them so that they lurk in the background awaiting an opportunity to break through to satisfaction. This state we call 'latent delinquency'; it can become 'manifest' on provocation" (p. 4 of English translation). Franz Alexander's (1891–1964) research (begun in Berlin, continued in Chicago) on the "neurotic character," notably as found in the *International Journal of Psychoanalysis* in 1930, asserted that misbehaving psychopaths were basically "acting out."

The Anglo-American criminal psychopath. The doctrine of social causation inspired much Anglo-Saxon research on psychopathy, beginning with Edinburgh psychiatry professor Sir David Henderson's (1884–1965) 1939 book, *Psychopathic States*. Henderson saw psychopathy more as a result of social emargination than heredity: "There is so much more security and courage and happiness when we form part of the herd, but the psychopath does not correspond to the herd type, he has not the instinct of fellowship with his fellow-men. Such a state leads almost inevitably to fatalism and despair, the reaction to which may be either aggressive or submissive" (p. 133). Henderson believed such individuals could be rehabilitated.

An American milestone was Hervey Cleckley's *The Mask of Sanity: An Attempt to Clarify Some Issues About the So-Called Psychopathic Personality* (1941). Cleckley (1914–1984), professor of psychiatry at the Medical College of Georgia in Augusta, indicted the psychopath's upbringing, not his genetics. Comparing the family dynamics of psychopathy to those Leo Kanner had described for **autism**, Cleckley said, "There is . . . reason for me to feel that degrees of central coolness . . . have played a part in the early environment of some patients who, when we see them twenty years later, react as psychopaths" (p. 475). (Cleckley is also remembered as co-author of *The Three Faces of Eve* [1957], which sparked an epidemic of "**multiple personality disorder.**" The title of prison psychologist Robert M. Lindner's (1914–1956) portrait, *Rebel Without a Cause: The Story of a Criminal Psychopath* (1944), echoes on in the James Dean movie of 1955. Lindner called psychopathic personality "a Pandora's box," and said that the multitude of terms for it evidenced its half-understood nature: "constitutional psychopathic inferiority, moral imbecility, semantic dementia, moral insanity, sociopathy, anethopathy, moral mania, egopathy, tropopathy, etc." (p. 3).

Different entirely from the European psychopath was the one that stepped forth from William Maxwell McCord (1930–1992) and Joan Fish McCord's (1930–2004) book, *Psychopathy and Delinquency* (1956)—he was an instructor in social psychology at Harvard; she a member of the Laboratory of Human Development there. The McCords' juvenile psychopath was asocial, "driven by primitive desires," highly impulsive, aggressive, and felt little guilt. Above all, he had "a warped capacity for love" (pp. 6–14). The authors recommended an innovative sort of "milieu therapy." (*See* **PSYCHOTHERAPY** on the origins of milieu therapy.)

In 1952, in the first edition of the *DSM* series, ***DSM "One,"*** the psychopathic personality became "sociopathic personality disturbance: antisocial reaction"; in subsequent ***DSM*** editions as well, "psychopath" ceased to be an independent diagnosis, although the term remained in use within psychiatry.

In the 1970s and after, under the influence of behavioral genetics, the classical Central European approach to psychopathy experienced something of a rebirth. In 1976, **Samuel Guze** in *Criminality and Psychiatric Disorder* wrote that "at least some cases of sociopathy may arise from 'abnormal' or 'altered' brain function." "It is not yet possible to unravel the tangled skein of evidence concerning heredity and environment in sociopathy, but it is difficult to ignore completely the indications of a biological contribution to its etiology" (p. 142). Almost 30 years after those lines were penned, In his *Biology and Crime* (2001), David C. Rowe (ca. 1950–2003) of the Interdisciplinary Program in Genetics at the University of Arizona was able to ask, "is there a gene for crime"? (*See also* **CONDUCT DISORDER; PERSONALITY DISORDERS; PSYCHIATRIC GENETICS.**)

CROW, TIMOTHY JOHN (1938–). A prominent English biological psychiatrist, Crow read medicine at London Hospital Medical College and trained in psychiatry at the **Maudsley Hospital**, receiving his diploma in psychological medicine (D.P.M.) in 1966. After lecturing at Aberdeen and Manchester, in 1974 Crow became head of the division of psychiatry of the clinical research centre at Northwick Park Hospital. In 1995, he became scientific director of the Prince of Wales Centre for Research into Schizophrenia and Depression, and in 1998 professor of psychiatry at Oxford. He is associated with a **positive vs. negative** typology in 1980 of schizophrenia, with brain biology studied in **neuroimaging** in 1976, and with understanding the substantial role of heredity in the genesis of schizophrenia.

CULLEN, WILLIAM (1710–1790). The great Enlightenment systematizer of illnesses, especially psychiatric, Cullen was born in Hamilton, Scotland, into the family of an estate official of the Duke of Hamilton. After years of study and itinerant work as a medical practitioner, he graduated with an M.D. from Glasgow University in 1740. He began lecturing at Glasgow in 1744—mostly in chemistry rather than medicine—becoming in 1751 professor of medicine there. In 1755, he came to Edinburgh University as the professor of chemistry, then from 1766 until his death professed the institutes of medicine and the practice of physic. Although he had little experience with psychiatric ailments, in his *First Lines of the Practice of Physic*, published in Edinburgh in 1777 and in following years, he laid out a new classification of psychiatric and neurological disorders that replaced the old concept of the humors with a modern notion of the "neuroses," based on clinical observation and a theory of pathology. One of the four orders of neuroses were the Vesaniae, or "disorders of the intellectual functions." The Vesaniae were then subdivided into (1) amentia, meaning "imbecility of the judgment";

(2) melancholia, meaning "partial insanity"; (3) mania, meaning "universal insanity"; and oneirodynia, meaning "inflamed or disturbed imagination during sleep." Given that Edinburgh was then the premier academic center in Britain and Cullen its most renowned professor, his classification became highly influential in detaching psychiatric nosology from a millennia-old tradition of humors and steering it toward a nosology based on the principle of cutting nature at the joints.

D

DEEP-SLEEP THERAPY AND BARBITURATES (1922). (*See also* **BARBITURATES.**) In 1920, Zurich-**Burghölzli** psychiatrist Jakob Klaesi (1883–1980) began using a combination of two of Roche's barbiturates for deep-sleep therapy. The idea of putting patients into a therapeutic stupor was not original with Klaesi and had been previously attempted with other barbiturates and with bromine. But Klaesi's sleep therapy with the combination product Somnifen, which he described in 1922 in the *Journal of Combined Neurology and Psychiatry* (*Zeitschrift für die gesamte Neurologie und Psychiatrie*), became widely known, and barbiturate sleep-therapy represented an occasionally used remedy for psychotic illness in the 1930s and 1940s. Deep-sleep therapy joined **insulin coma therapy**, **electroconvulsive therapy**, and chemical convulsive therapy (*see* **CONVULSIVE THERAPY: CHEMICAL**) as one of the innovative "physical," or somatic, therapies. It ceased to be used after the introduction of **chlorpromazine** and other antipsychotic drugs in the early 1950s.

DEGENERATION. *See* **PSYCHIATRIC GENETICS: degeneration theory** (1857).

DELAY, JEAN-LOUIS-PAUL (1907–1987). A pioneer of psychopharmacology in France, Delay was born into a surgeon's family in Bayonne in southwest France, and his career was marked with brilliance at practically every step. At 22, he was an intern of the Paris hospitals, by 1937 rising to ward chief (médecin des hôpitaux); in 1939, he passed the Agrégation exam, and in 1942 earned a Ph.D. in arts and science; in 1946, he was appointed to the chair of mental diseases (maladies mentales) at the **Ste.-Anne mental hospital**. On the basis of a two-volume biography of French novelist André Gide, Delay was appointed in 1959 to the Académie française. In psychiatry, he had a profoundly biological orientation—indeed so biological that it irritated him to see patients, which he almost never did except in his private practice.

Beginning in 1939, he helped to introduce electroencephalography in France. Yet aside from his 1942 Ph.D. thesis on memory (considerably influenced by **Pierre Janet**, whose pupil Delay was), Delay is mainly known for advances in psychopharmacology, or for encouraging his students such as **Pierre Deniker** (1917–1998) and **Pierre Pichot** (1918–) to make them. (Whether Delay contributed or not, his name went onto every paper.) In 1949, in research published in the *Proceedings of the Royal Society of Medicine*, Delay introduced narcoanalysis with Sodium Amytal in France (*see* **BARBITURATES: narcotherapy**), contrasting the therapeutic effects of barbiturates in manic-depressive illness, acute neuroses, and schizophrenia, compared to those of methamphetamine. (Delay called it "chemical psychoanalysis.") Although credit for discovering the psychiatric efficacy of **reserpine** is usually accorded to **Nathan Kline**, Delay and Deniker were in print on the subject only months after him (in the Congress of French Psychiatry [*Congrès des aliénistes et neurologistes de langue Française*], 1954, pp. 836–841).

Delay is associated above all with the discovery of the therapeutic efficacy of the antipsychotic drug **chlorpromazine** (CPZ). Although it was not Delay's team that discovered initially the drug's value, they did in fact conduct the first systematic clinical trial and reported in the summer of 1952 that they had made a find of capital importance. When in the upheavals of 1968 a group of students messed up his office, Delay was so shocked that he never again returned to it. In 1952, at a French-language psychiatry conference in Paris, Delay and Deniker coined the term "neuroleptic" (known in North America as "antipsychotic," a term **Heinz Lehmann** proposed in the *Canadian Medical Association Journal* in 1961).

DELIRIUM. Defined as acute brain failure, delirium means a reduced clarity of awareness of the environment caused by a medical condition or a substance. An important symptom of delirium* is loss of orientation: not really knowing where one is, what day it is, or who one is. It is primarily a clouded state of consciousness but may be associated with a narrowing or lowering of consciousness as well, in addition to visual hallucinations. The term was evidently introduced into medicine by the Roman writer Celsus (25 B.C.–A.D. 50) in the first century after Christ. Yet, for many years its use remained ambiguous and was often made co-terminous with madness, psychosis, or dementia. Nonetheless, in an era when infectious illnesses with high fevers were so common, delirium also acquired a core meaning of organically caused confusion and disorientation.

According to Zbigniew J. Lipowski (1924–1997), a major student of delirium, the term is first used in English in the sixteenth century, where medical writers differentiate it from mania and melancholia—general terms for madness—as neither was associated with fever. The seventeenth-century physician Thomas Willis (1621–1675), in his *Two Discourses Concerning the Soul of Brutes* (published in 1672 and translated into English in 1683), said that delirium was not a disease in its own right but a symptom of various physical illnesses. In his account, Willis focused on disorientation and psychosis. In 1794, Erasmus Darwin (1731–1802; grandfather of Charles Darwin), in his *Zoonomia, or the Laws of Organic Life,* proposed that delirium was a sign of impaired consciousness—essentially the modern definition—and likened it to dreaming.

In France, the term "délire" has tended to mean delusional disorder more than delirium, although it was a French sanatorium psychiatrist, Alexandre-Jacques-François Brierre de Boismont (1797–1881), who in 1845 introduced the phrase "acute delirium" (délire aigu) in the *Mémoires* of the Academy of Medicine. In 1851, Louis-Jean-François Delasiauve (1804–1893), who had just taken over the service of mental retardation and epilepsy at Bicêtre Hospital in Paris, proposed in the *Annales de médecine* the term "stupidity," or "mental confusion," for delirium: "Hallucinations and irrational fears are a consequence of stupidity, as are the shadows into which intelligence falls." Delasiauve

* The "three Ds" help distinguish these concepts: in acute organic illness there is *d*elirium, a consciousness disturbance; in a subacute disorder, such as **alcoholism**, there is *d*ysmnesia, a disturbance of memory; in dementia, a chronic organic brain change, there is a *d*eterioration of personality (Alzheimer's disease [*see* **DEMENTIA**] is not primarily a disorder of memory, as is popularly thought).

assigned the mental confusion of alcoholism or narcotics to "stupidity" (Semelaigne, *Pionniers de la Psychatrie Française*, I, 306). (In English, "mental confusion" is disorder of thought, whereas delirium is a disorder of consciousness.)

In Germany, psychiatry professor Karl Bonhoeffer (1868–1948), then in Breslau, later in Berlin, made a fundamental contribution to delirium in 1909 by distinguishing in the *Central Journal for Nervous Diseases and Psychiatry* (*Zentralblatt für Nervenheilkunde und Psychiatrie*) between the "endogenous psychoses," including depression (*see* **DEPRESSION: EMERGENCE: exogenous vs. endogenous**), and the "exogenous psychoses" arising acutely from somatic disorders outside the brain. "Among such exogenous forms of reaction might be mentioned the deliria [die Delirien], and the occasional hallucinoses that occur in their context"; he went on to enumerate several others (p. 499). Yet, this insistence that delirium was a specific exogenous psychiatric reaction to organic illness sufficed to focus the entire field of psychiatry on exogenous versus endogenous sources of illness.

The definition of delirium as a disturbance in levels of consciousness, a result of brain changes measured by electroencephalography (EEG), was begun in 1944 by John Romano (1908–1994) and **George L. Engel**, then in the departments of psychiatry and medicine at the University of Cincinnati (later they went to Rochester). In an article in *Medical Clinics of North America* in 1944 on "Physiologic and Psychologic Considerations of Delirium," they demonstrated that different levels of disturbance in brain function, as seen in EEG slowing, correspond to different levels of delirium. They wrote, "The close correlation between the electrical activity of the cortex and the basic disturbance in delirium, i.e. the alteration in the level of consciousness, provides convincing evidence that the psychologic symptoms are . . . the result of disturbances in higher cortical function" (p. 635).

DELIRIUM TREMENS. Delirium tremens (DTs) is a special form of delirium caused by withdrawal of alcohol from the brain and often accompanied by a coarse tremor, vivid hallucinations, and agitated behavior. It was first described in the *Talmud* in the fourth and fifth centuries after Christ. Thomas Sutton (1767?–1835) coined the term in 1813 in his *Tracts on Delirium Tremens* and differentiated it from meningitis ("phrenitis") by discovering that DTs responded to opium. "It has been remarked," he said, "that the parties attacked with delirium tremens have been given to drinking; and I feel firmly persuaded, that all cases of this disease are connected with indulgences of that nature" (Hunter and Macalpine, p. 682).

DELUSION, DELUSIONAL DISORDER. *See* **FRENCH CHRONIC DELUSIONAL STATES** (from 1909); **PARANOIA; PARAPHRENIA; PSYCHOSIS: EMERGENCE; SCHIZOPHRENIA: EMERGENCE.**

DEMENTIA. Dementia, in the sense of a temporary or permanent loss of brain function that could affect people of all ages, has always been familiar to physicians. The elderly in particular have often been implicated in global deficits in personality, intelligence, and emotion. Medicine once knew many phrases for this, including "melancholia." As Robert Burton (1577–1640), an Oxford cleric, wrote in 1621 in his *Anatomy of Melancholy*: "After 70 years . . . all is trouble and sorrow. [The elderly] are overcome with melancholy in an instant. Or if they do continue in such courses, they dote at last (an old man is twice a boy) and are not able to manage their estates through common infirmities incident in their age. Full of ache, sorrow, and grief, children again, dizzards [fools], they carle [are gruff and snarling] many times as they sit, and talk to themselves" (p. 183). Some landmarks in the narrowing of brain pathology to our current concept of dementia as cognitive dysfunction and personality deterioration in the elderly are as follows:

Cullen's "amentia" (1777). In *First Lines of the Practice of Physic*, published in 1777 and in following years, Edinburgh's **William Cullen** described "amentia" as a subclass of the "Vesaniae," or disorders of judgment. One variety of amentia was "amentia senilis, from decay of perception and memory, in old age." In 1785, **Philippe Pinel** translated the fourth edition (1784) of Cullen's work into French, rendering amentia as "dementia." That represents the definitive appearance of the term on the medical stage, although it had been used occasionally before.

Esquirol's "senile dementia" (1814). (*See* **DEPRESSION: EMERGENCE: differential diagnosis of depression from dementia** [1814].) **Étienne Esquirol** was among the first to differentiate dementia from the form of depression that he called lypemania. In his essay "On dementia" in the *Dictionary of Science and Medicine* (*Dictionnaire des sciences médicales*), he wrote that "in an illness that is frequently the end point of a large number of other illnesses, [dementia] is, so to say, the constitutional state of old age" (vol. 2, p. 237). "Senile dementia" was differentiated from the "chronic" and "acute" varieties in representing "the result of the process of aging. As the individual is imperceptibly pushed toward old age, he loses his sensibility together with the free exercise of his faculties of reasoning, yet before reaching the final stage of decrepitude. Senile dementia installs itself slowly. It begins with the weakening of memory, especially that of recent events" (p. 262).

Bayle's "chronic arachnitis": the first organic dementia identified (1822). *See* **PSYCHOSIS: EMERGENCE; UNITARY PSYCHOSIS.**

Krafft-Ebing differentiates reversible "dementia" in younger patients from "senile" dementia (1872, 1879). Although a number of authors had been differentiating dementia from mental illness, or "vesanic dementia" from senile dementia, in 1872 **Richard von Krafft-Ebing** in his textbook drew a clear line between "primary treatable dementia," which he also called "stupidity" (Stupidität), and "Dementia senilis." Stupidity-style dementia was a "psychoneurosis" chracterized by the slowing or indeed the suspension of psychic functioning with emotional flattening (Stimmungsmangel). Stupor, hallucinations, and delusions were complications. Although stupidity was conditioned by a heavy constitutional predisposition, it was, unlike mental retardation, acquired in adult life. As causes, Krafft-Ebing hypothesized either brain "exhaustion" or "masturbatory excesses." Krafft-Ebing introduced the concept of "stupidity" in the 1872 edition, then expanded on it in subsequent editions. As he noted of "stupidity: primary treatable dementia" in the second edition in 1879, "Those affected by it are usually youthful, primarily male individuals under 30." Yet the prognosis, in contrast to that of senile dementia, was favorable: "Only in seldom cases does the functional exhaustion [of the brain] pass into irreparable dementia" (vol. II, pp. 47, 49). Here, Krafft was adumbrating a distinction between favorable-outcome psychosis and senile dementia.

Korsakoff separates amnesia from dementia (Korsakoff's psychosis) (1887). Sergei S. Korsakoff (1853–1900) was at the time of his discovery a staff psychiatrist at a clinic for nervous disease in Moscow; in retrospect, he counts as one of the founders of Russian psychiatry. Writing in a Russian psychiatry journal, the *Arkh. Psikhiat. Nevrol.*, in 1887, Korsakoff identified an amnestic syndrome, often involving neuritis, occurring in alcoholics that he called "cerebropathia psychica toxaemica" (today, "Korsakoff's syndrome" or "Korsakoff's psychosis"). "The disorder of memory manifests itself in an extraordinarily peculiar amnesia, in which the memory of recent events, those which just happened, is chiefly disturbed, whereas the remote past is remembered fairly well" (p. 398 of English translation in *Neurology* in 1955). In 1904, psychiatry professor Karl Bonhoeffer (1868–1948), then at **Heidelberg**, differentiated toxic (as in alcoholism) Korsakoff memory loss from senile memory loss in an article published in the *Allgemeine Zeitschrift für Psychiatrie*. He said that loss of recent memory was the distinguishing characteristic of the syndrome. Later, it was established that Korsakoff's patients were suffering from Wernicke's disease, a pattern of brain lesions caused by thiamine deficiency (secondary usually to alcoholism). (*See* **WERNICKE–KORSAKOFF SYNDROME**.)

Beginning the differentiation of the organic dementias: the dementia of neurosyphilis (1894). In his laboratory at the Frankfurt asylum, **Alois Alzheimer** began his careful delineation of dementia caused by "progressive paralysis," or "general paralysis of the insane" (later, neurosyphilis). His 1894 article in the *Neurological Central Journal* (*Neurologisches Centralblatt*) marked the beginning of his work in this area, which culminated in a 1902 contribution in the *General Journal of Psychiatry* (*Allgemeine Zeitschrift für Psychiatrie*).

Alzheimer's presenile dementia (1906, 1910). In November 1906, **Alois Alzheimer** reported at a meeting the case of a 51-year-old woman who was fully psychotic, lacking in short-term memory, and had localized neurological signs and progressive dementia. At autopsy, he identified various pathological brain changes, some of which were already known in the literature, namely brain atrophy, arteriosclerosis, and senile plaques. A fourth finding, neurofibrillary tangles, Alzheimer himself had already described. Plaques and tangles had not been previously noted in dementia cases in younger patients. Alzheimer's paper for that meeting was summarized in the *General Journal of Psychiatry* (*Allgemeine Zeitschrift für Psychiatrie*) in 1907; in no way did he claim that he had identified a new disease, but rather that this case represented "such a divergent pattern that it is not to be classified among any of the known diseases; anatomically there are findings that deviate from all of the disease processes presently known." He said that in recent years there had been an increasing number of such cases, and that "at some point we should be able to delineate them clinically in a more precise manner." The title of the article was "On a Distinctive Illness of the Cerebral Cortex" ("Über eine eigenartige Erkrankung der Hirnrinde"). (There was no discussion following the presentation.) Alzheimer did not use the term "presenile dementia." (Indeed, an early use of the expression "presenile dementia" occurs in 1898 in Jena psychiatry professor Otto Binswanger's [1852–1929] brief research note without postmortem histology in the *Munich Medical Weekly* [*Münchener Medizinische Wochenschrift*].)

In the eighth edition of his textbook in 1910, **Kraepelin** argued that these cases of early psychosis that progressed rapidly to dementia probably represented a separate category of illness sui generis. He noted that in the three cases that had come to autopsy, Alzheimer had discovered identical pathology. Kraepelin made these patients part of the larger group of "presenile insanity" (praeseniles Irresein) and said, "The area of the presenile psychoses is currently perhaps the most baffling in psychiatry" (*Psychiatrie*, 8th ed., II(1), p. 534).

"Pick's" disease (1892 and after). As early as 1892, Arnold Pick (1851–1924), professor of psychiatry at the German university in Prague, began reporting cases of cerebral atrophy resulting in dementia with focal symptoms, meaning symptoms localizable to a certain area of the brain; these were of interest at the time because Carl Wernicke believed that the symptoms of senile dementia were always nonfocal. (*See* **WERNICKE–KLEIST–LEONHARD PATHWAY**.) Pick articulated these views in 1892 in the *Prague Medical Weekly* (*Prager Medicinische Wochenschrift*) in the article "On the Relationship of Senile Brain Atrophy to Aphasia" ("Über die Beziehungen der senilen Hirnatrophie zur Aphasie"). This case is often cited as the locus classicus for "Pick's disease." Yet, it is not. A 60-year-old man whose case Pick reported in 1906 did have severe frontal- and temporal-lobe wasting at autopsy (in the *Monthly Review of Psychiatry and Neurology* (*Monatsschrift für Psychiatrie und Neurologie*), the kind of pathology that was evident in the disease later named after him and that is really the first reported case of "Pick's disease."

In 1906, it occurred to no one that Pick was describing a new disease, as this kind of neuropathological work was becoming common in the literature. Yet in 1926, Hugo Spatz (1888–1969), head of neuropathology in the Munich Psychiatric Clinic, together with a co-worker, in the *Journal of Combined Neurology and Psychiatry* (*Zeitschrift für die gesamte Neurologie und Psychiatrie*), wrote that the regional wasting of neurons in the frontal and temporal zones represented a specific disease for which they proposed the name "Pick's Disease." The authors acknowledged that this coinage was not exactly what Pick, who had just died, would have had in mind because he was interested in local, not regional, lesions. Throughout Pick's histopathological work ran an important general point: that there were a variety of dementias, each corresponding to a different pattern of local changes in the brain.

"Lewy-body" dementia (1912). In 1912, in volume 2 of Max Lewandowsky's (1876–1918) textbook, *Practical Neurology for Physicians* (*Praktische Neurologie für Ärzte*), Friedrich (Fritz) Heinrich Lewy (1885–1950), who had just graduated in medicine in Berlin in 1910, described intracytoplasmic inclusions, later called "Lewy bodies," in the brain stem in Parkinsonism. These inclusions were later discovered to be characteristic of a common form of dementia, called "senile dementia of the Lewy body type," involving fluctuating cognitive impairment and psychosis or depression. Lewy subsequently became an important neurologist and psychiatrist and emigrated to the United States in 1934. (In 1962 neuropathologist John S. Woodard [1923–] at the Camarillo State Hospital in Camarillo, California, proposed Lewy-body mental illness in late-adulthood as a separate disease. He argued in the *Journal of Neuropathology and Experimental Neurology* that, "The cases seemed to represent a discrete clinicopathologic entity in relation to mental disease," and were characterized by paranoid or affective disorders in addition to "unprovoked violence and assaultiveness" [pp. 448–449].)

Bleuler's "organic syndrome" (1916). In his *Textbook of Psychiatry* (*Lehrbuch der Psychiatrie*), **Eugen Bleuler** argued that a range of diffuse disturbances of the cerebral cortex, referred to as "organic syndrome," could cause a "weakening of intelligence," especially affecting memory. "The various intellectual abilities do not disappear uniformly . . . and practiced abilities escape the general deterioration the longest. The senile bookkeeper can be markedly demented in all other directions and yet surpass many a healthy person in addition" (p. 232). As examples of the organic brain syndrome, Bleuler mentioned the "senile psychoses," of which there were three: arteriosclerotic insanity, simple brain atrophy ("dementia senilis") and "presbyophrenia" (pp. 276–277 of the English translation, 1924). The feature common to the three was "the diffuse reduction of the brain substance and symptomatologically the complex of the 'organic psychic' symptoms." Bleuler's "organic syndrome" greatly influenced European thinking on dementia.

Alzheimer's disease and senile dementia are the same disease (1948). Although German histopathologists had long believed that Alzheimer's pre-senile dementia and the dementia of senescence represented a single pathological process, Robert Denis Newton, a London Harley-Street psychiatrist (1904–1985), clearly articulated this notion in 1948 for a psychiatric readership in the *Journal of Mental Science* (later *British Journal of Psychiatry*). Alzheimer's disease thus soared from a pathological curiosity affecting a small number of individuals in mid-life to the commonest disease of the elderly. "There can be no justifiable grounds for speaking of Alzheimer's disease and senile dementia as separate entities," he wrote. "The term Alzheimer's dementia is suggested to describe this organic syndrome" (pp. 235, 248).

Martin Roth says dementia is only one of several psychogeriatric outcomes (1955). In his paper "The Natural History of Mental Disorder in Old Age," published in the *Journal of Mental Science* in 1955, Martin Roth (1917–), at Graylingwell Hospital in Chichester, England, laid the basis of modern psychogeriatric classification by subdividing the mental disorders of later life into five groups: "affective psychosis," "late paraphrenia," "arteriosclerotic psychosis," "acute confusion," and, finally, "senile psychosis," the only member of the group that was unrecoverable. As psychogeriatrician Jeremia Heinik at Ichilov Hospital in Tel-Aviv, Israel, remarks, Roth's classification "shed a spirit of optimism in a field considered to deal only with irreversibility (e.g. dementia)." (On Martin Roth, *see also* **PARAPHRENIA.**)

Separating benign and progressive memory dysfunction (1958). Psychiatrist Vojtech Adalbert Kral (1903–1988), of the Gerontological Unit at **McGill University**, distinguished in the *Journal of Gerontology* between the "impaired recall of specific remote memories" and "progressive impairment of recent memory . . . leading to a senile amnestic syndrome" (p. 175). The following year, in *Geriatrics*, he and psychologist Blossom Temkin Wigdor (1924–) administered the oral androgen Halotestin to one group of elderly patients with "mild" memory dysfunction and to another with senile amnestic syndrome. The former group responded well, the latter did not, indicating that memory loss in dementia is qualitatively different from the normal forgetfulness of the elderly.

Based on this research, benign senescent forgetfulness (BSF) became considered physiological, meaning a normal accompaniment of aging, whereas mild cognitive impairment (MCI) was thought of as a preliminary stage of Alzheimer's disease.

Associating the degree of dementia with the amount of pathological change in the brain (1967). Martin Roth (1917–) and co-workers in Newcastle upon Tyne in England demonstrated in the *Proceedings of the Royal Society of Medicine* in 1967 that the quantitative degree of dementia was associated with the extent of neuritic plaques in the cerebral gray matter. The severely demented probably represent a separate group, the authors said. Yet otherwise: "There is a highly significant correlation between mean plaque counts and scores given for dementia and performance in psychological tests. The findings suggest that psychological and pathological indices are closely related to one another" (p. 258). (On Martin Roth, *see* **PARAPHRENIA.**)

Alzheimer's disease is not just an acceleration of the natural aging process but an acquired age-linked disease (1977). Rejecting Martin Roth's argument (*see* **above**), Raymond Adams (1911–), a neurology professor at Harvard, and Maurice Victor (1920–), professor of neurology at Case Western University in Cleveland, argued in their *Principles of Neurology* that the disease was a pathological eruption into old age, not an accelerated extension of it. They pointed out, among other arguments, that "*Homo sapiens* is the only animal species in which Alzheimer fibrillary changes and senile plaques are found in the aging brain. . . . It seems to us unbiologic that human aging should differ from that of all other animal species" (quotation from 2nd ed., 1981, p. 421).

Linking familial Alzheimer's disease to a specific chromosomal locus (1987). An international team of researchers led by Peter H. St George-Hyslop (1953–), then at the Neurogenetics Laboratory of Massachusetts General Hospital (later at the University of Toronto), suggested in an article in *Science* in February 1987 that a defective gene on chromosome 21 might be the cause of Alzheimer's disease. The authors said of the significance of this discovery, "The existence of DNA markers linked to the FAD [familial Alzheimer's disease] gene raises the possibility that they might be of use for presymptomatic or prenatal diagnosis of FAD in appropriate families" (p. 889).

Linking early-onset Alzheimer's disease to a specific chromosomal locus (1992). In an article in *Nature Genetics*, Mike Mullan and co-workers at the psychiatry center of the University of South Florida in Tampa, together with a group based in the departments of biochemistry and neurology at St. Mary's Hospital Medical School in London, found evidence in 10 "early-onset" families that the precursor protein gene in Alzheimer's disease was situated on the middle long-arm of chromosome 14. This suggested that a significant subset of Alzheimer's cases—the early-onset type—were genetically caused.

DENIKER, PIERRE-GEORGES (1917–1998). Pioneer of psychopharmacology, Deniker was born into a French diplomatic family. After finishing his medical studies in 1945 and his internship in 1946–1949, he became an assistant physician (chef de clinique) until 1952 in the Paris Faculty of Medicine, also serving from 1949 on as a staff psychiatrist under **Jean Delay** in the Paris psychiatric hospitals. In 1961, having passed the Agrégation, he became a professor (professeur agrégé) in the faculty of medicine; from 1971 until his retirement in 1985 he was head of the newly created (after Delay's retirement) university department of mental health and therapeutics of the **Ste.-Anne mental hospital**. The work of Delay and Deniker in 1952 on **chlorpromazine** had great importance for the development of psychiatry as a discipline, turning it from a profession based on an empirical approach to syndromes (in the United States based on psychotherapy) to one based on the prescription of medication.

In 1954, Delay and Deniker made, simultaneously with **Nathan Kline** in the United States, the discovery of **reserpine**'s usefulness as a psychotropic drug. In 1952, Delay and Deniker described "neuroleptics" (known in the United States as antipsychotics) as an independent drug class for psychosis; in 1955, they convened a landmark scientific colloquium in Paris, the first international psychopharmacology meeting, to discuss these new drugs. In 1957, Deniker received a Lasker Award. In a series of books and papers during the years—especially in his textbook of psychopharmacology (*Méthodes chimiothérapiques en psychiatrie*) cowritten with Delay in 1961—Deniker laid much of the conceptual basis of the discipline of psychopharmacology. Deniker and his colleagues also emphasized the efficacy of low doses of antipsychotic drugs at a time when the international community was moving toward steadily higher doses and caused wonder that all the unpleasant side effects of the high doses were not being seen in the Paris hospitals.

DEPENDENCE (DRUG). *See* **ALCOHOLISM; SUBSTANCE ABUSE.**

DEPERSONALIZATION. The term "depersonalization," meaning the feeling that one's being and thoughts are unreal, was coined by French philosopher Ludovic Dugas (1857–?) in the *Revue philosophique* in 1898: "I should define as alienation of the personality or depersonalization the state in which the ego [le moi] feels its actions escaping control and becoming foreign" (p. 502). Even though the phenomenon itself had previously been described in the medical literature, **Pierre Janet** and Fulgence Raymond (1844–1910), the latter being Charcot's successor, in their monograph in 1903 on *Les obsessions et la psychasthénie*, applied the term to several patients, of whom they reported: "She feels that she has lost her personhood, that she is no longer anything. It seems to her that it is not she who is seeing, is not she who is hearing, is not she who is eating. It seems to her that her arms and legs work on their own, without her. . . . Basically it is as if she was dead, at most as if her legs continued to live; but she herself is deceased, or in any event absent" (*Les obsessions*, I, p. 41).

For **Karl Jaspers**, in his *General Psychopathology* of 1913, depersonalization belonged to the disorders of "consciousness of personhood" (Persönlichkeitsbewusstsein), in which Jaspers stressed the feeling of automatic thoughts and actions (der Automatismus der Willensvorgänge)—close to some of the "first-rank" symptoms of schizophrenia numerated by his friend **Kurt Schneider** (*see also* **SCHIZOPHRENIA: EMERGENCE**). Depersonalization thus became shifted from a neurotic to a psychotic symptom, and during the years was mentioned frequently by the asylum psychiatrists who saw severe mental illnesses as well as by psychoanalysts who saw neurotic patients. The term entered the ***DSM*** series with the second edition in 1968 as one of the "neuroses": "depersonalization neurosis." The patient is "dominated by a feeling of unreality and of estrangement from the self, body, or surroundings" (p. 41). (The latter sentiment is often called "derealization.") In ***DSM-III*** in 1980, depersonalization joined the "dissociative disorders" and remained there essentially unchanged in subsequent editions.

In 2003 Daphne Simeon (1958–) and co-workers at the Mt. Sinai School of Medicine in New York characterized depersonalization disorder in the *Journal of Clinical Psychiatry* as typically beginning between 16 and 25 and running a chronic course: "Chronic depersonalization is in part developmentally driven and the adolescent years are a vulnerable period for the formation of a 'real' and 'well-grounded' self-experience" (p. 995).

DEPRESSION AND MOOD DISORDERS: EMERGENCE. The word "depression" has a number of meanings, depending on the discipline. Within neurophysiology, it refers to a decrease in the brain's electrical activity causing, for example, "cortical depression." For the pharmacologist, depression means drug actions that decrease the activity of the central nervous system, such as barbiturates and anesthetics. In psychology, depression stands for any decrease in performance, such as in psychomotor activity or intellectual agility. As for psychiatry, depression can mean a normal human emotion, a symbol of mood that may become pathological if it is retained too long or too deeply; a depressive syndrome that may, or may not, include a depressed mood; or a reactive depression precipitated by certain life events. First described as **melancholia**, a term of such amplitude reverberates across the history of psychiatry. There follow some important concepts in the emergence of the diagnosis of depression. (For more current events, *see* **DEPRESSION AND MOOD DISORDERS: RECENT CONCEPTS**.)

Traditional depressive-equivalents. Before the mid-nineteenth century, several diagnostic terms in medicine were historically equivalent to depression, such as "vapours" and "hysteric fits." In 1707, London physician John Purcell (1674?–1730) said of patients with "vapours," "Those who have laboured long under this distemper are oppressed with a dreadful anguish of mind and a deep melancholy, always reflecting on what can perplex, terrify, and disorder them most, so that at last they think their recovery impossible. . . . They decline all diversions." "Melancholy in hysterical people is easily cured in the beginning, but when it has taken deep root, and the patients avoid and shun company, then . . . it is to be feared they will endeavour to make themselves away" (*A Treatise of Vapours or Hysterick Fits*, 2nd ed., pp. 13–14, 170). Such terms clearly include many other symptoms than those conventionally reckoned to depression, yet they do embrace depression.

By mid-eighteenth century, spleen and "hyp" [-ochondria] had become fashionable diagnoses. As society physician George Cheyne (1671–1743), then practicing in the spa town of Bath, explained to novelist Samuel Richardson (1689–1761) in a letter in 1742, "We call the hyp every distemper attended with lowness of spirits, whether it be flatulence from indigestion . . . head-pains, or a universal relaxed state of the nerves, with numbness, weakness, startings, tremblings, etc., so that the hyp is only a short expression for any kind of nervous disorder with whatever symptoms" (Mullett, ed., *Letters*, p. 108).

In 1786, James M. Adair (1728–1802), who had a tony practice for nerve patients in Bath, suggested that both spleen and hyp had been ascribed to the recent nervous illness of Queen Anne, who "was frequently subject to depression of spirits, for which, after the courtly physicians had given it a name, they proceeded to prescribe Rawleigh's confection and pearl cordial. This circumstance was sufficient to transfer both the disease and the remedy to all who had the least pretensions to rank" (*Medical Cautions for the Consideration of Invalids*, p. 13).

"Depression" as a term (pre-1850). Although **melancholia** was the preferred expression for dysphoria and insanity, the term "depression," from the Latin "de" (down) and "premere" (to press), nonetheless appeared in medical writing as early as the seventeenth century in the context of mood disorder, or emotional disorder. In 1765, Edinburgh physician Robert Whytt (1714–1766), one of the founders of neurophysiology, in his *Observations on the Nature, Causes, and Cure of those Diseases which Have Been Commonly Called Nervous, Hypochondriac or Hysteric*, described "depression of mind" associated with hypochondriasis and dysphoria (p. 312). He added: "When low spirits proceed from a suppression of the menses or haemorrhoids, if these evacuations cannot be restored, some others must be substituted in their place: but nothing has such sudden good effects as bleeding" (p. 519).

"Depression of mind may be induced by causes that are forgotten," noted American psychiatrist **Benjamin Rush** in 1812 in his *Medical Inquiries and Observations upon the Diseases of Mind* (quote from 3rd ed., 1827, p. 44).

In 1818, Johann Christian August Heinroth, an asylum psychiatrist in Leipzig (1773–1843) (*see* **GERMAN "ROMANTIC" PSYCHIATRY**), in his *Textbook of the Disturbances of Mental Life* (*Lehrbuch der Störungen des Seelenlebens*), became one of the first psychiatric writers to use the terms "depression" and "exaltation" in an account of mood disorders. "The principle and the stimulus of evil affect men in two ways, just as poison works in two opposite manners: positively or negatively, stupefyingly or paralyzingly. A life affected by the first kind is distinguished by exaltation and that affected by the second, by depression" (Mora's English translation, I, 125).

Karl Wigand Maximilian Jacobi (1775–1858), director of the Siegburg asylum in Germany, often used the term "depression" in its modern sense in his descriptions of clinical cases. In his 1844 text on *The Main Forms of Mental Illness* (*Die Hauptformen der Seelenstörungen*), Jacobi described one patient who alternated "episodes of raucous and boisterous excitement" with delirium and "depression" (I, p. 121).

Differential diagnosis of depression from dementia (1814). **Étienne Esquirol** was among the first to differentiate dementia from the form of depression that he termed lypemania. In his essay "On dementia" in the *Dictionary of Science and Medicine* (*Dictionnaire des sciences médicales*), he illustrated the difference: "The anger [of the demented] lasts only a moment. It has nothing of the tenacity of those with mania and above all of those with lypemania [melancholic depression]" (pp. 221–222).

Lypemania (1820). (*See also* **PSYCHOSIS: EMERGENCE: Esquirol's monomania**.) Although **Esquirol** earlier introduced the term "lypemania" as a virtual synonym for melancholia, it was only in 1820, in an essay "On Lypemania or Melancholia" ("De la lypémanie ou mélancholie"), that he fully characterized the disorder and differentiated it from other illnesses. He considered lypemania primarily an affective, or emotional, form of melancholia and scorned the term "melancholia" itself as associated with discredited humoral theories involving "bile." Esquirol's lypemania represents the first occasion in which a prominent psychiatrist presented melancholic depression as a disturbance of affect rather than a form of "insanity."

Dysthymia (1844). Carl Friedrich Flemming (1799–1880), chief physician at a newly opened asylum in Sachsenberg bei Schwerin in Germany, proposed "dysthymia atra" as a replacement for melancholia, which had become a heterogeneous kind of grab bag of symptoms. (Atra means black in Greek, and atrabile was a classical Greek term for melancholy.) It consisted of "sadness, fear and anxiety, mistrust, and irritability (Übelwollen)" (*General Journal of Psychiatry* [*Allgemeine Zeitschrift für Psychiatrie*], p. 114). Flemming considered "dysthymias" to be "emotional disorders" (Gefühlskrankheiten). Yet, Flemming's own ardor for his new concept was tepid, and he had abandoned it in favor of "mood depression" (Gemüths-depression) by the time he wrote his big textbook in 1859, *Pathology and Treatment of the Psychoses* (*Pathologie und Therapie der Psychosen*) (p. 66).

Circular insanity (1851). *See* **MANIC-DEPRESSIVE ILLNESS: circular insanity** (1851).

Hypochondria as a subform of depression (1860). Although hypochondria had been associated with melancholia since the Ancients, what was previously understood by melancholia had little to do with depression and much with undifferentiated madness. In the early nineteenth century, a whole generation of psychiatrists began to use "depression" and "melancholia" in the modern sense: hence the relationship of depression to hypochondria became of renewed interest. Unlike public-asylum psychiatrists, who rarely saw such conditions as hypochondria, those in the private sector did. **Vienna** psychiatrist Max Leidesdorf (1819–1889) had extensive experience with private psychiatric clinics, where the threshold of illness was lower. In 1860, in addition to lecturing at the university, he had just joined the staff of a prestigious private clinic in Vienna's Ober-Döbling suburb when he brought out his psychiatric textbook, *Pathology and Therapy of Psychic Illnesses* (*Pathologie und Therapie der psychischen Krankheiten*). In the section on "conditions of psychic depression," he distinguished among hypochondria, which was the milder stage, and melancholia, the more severe stage. In hypochondria, "the patients' feelings turn entirely about their health, the condition of which occupies their whole attention." The difference between hypochondria and melancholia, said Leidesdorf, was that "the hypochondriac seeks medical advice and assistance constantly; he makes contact and has confidence, albeit tenuous and short-lived. The melancholic does not seek medical advice, and occupies himself with plans for his suicide" (p. 154 of the second edition, in 1865, entitled *Textbook of Psychiatric Illnesses* [*Lehrbuch der psychischen Krankheiten*]).

Dysthymia (revived) (1863). **Karl Kahlbaum** distinguished systematically between underlying diseases, which might produce affective disorders, and the actual symptoms of melancholia, which he called dysthymia. He made this discrimination in a larger work on nosology called *The Classification of Psychic Illnesses* (*Die Gruppirung der psychischen Krankheiten*). Kahlbaum thus nailed down a distinction begun by Flemming and others (**PSYCHOSIS: EMERGENCE: distinction . . .** [1844]) between primary disease and momentary illness presentation. Some scholars feel that Kahlbaum's dysthymia is significant as "the hour of birth of endogenous depression" (Schmidt-Degenhart, p. 65). In the book, Kahlbaum also distinguished between psychotic melancholy (a Vesania, as he borrowed **William Cullen**'s term for the class) and nonpsychotic dysthymia (a kind of partial insanity for which he coined the term "Vecordia": vecordy was a seventeenth-century English expression for madness). (Elsewhere, Kahlbaum also chiseled out pieces of what would later be called schizophrenia, thus narrowing dysthymia to its modern meaning of emotional disorder, rather than a synonym for "madness.") (*See* **SCHIZOPHRENIA: EMERGENCE: Vesania typica** [1863]; **catatonia** [1874].) Also among the Vecordia was "paranoia," a "disturbance of intelligence" (not **paranoia** in the sense of delusional disorder, which latter he called "diastrephia"). It is noteworthy that for dysthymia and paranoia, as "partial mental diseases," the personality remains intact, unlike the Vesaniae (p. 90).

Periodical melancholia (1875 and following years). Although Falret and Baillarger had by 1854 described the periodic alternation of depression and mania (*see* **MANIC-DEPRESSIVE ILLNESS**), it was not until the work in 1875 of Russian emigré physician and New York electrotherapist William Basil Neftel (1830–1906) that recurrent unipolar depression was characterized. (*See* his article "On Periodical Melancholia," in the *Medical Record* in 1875.) Apparently unaware of Neftel's article, in 1878 Ludwig Kirn (1839–1899), a student of Christian F. W. Roller (1802–1878) and a staff psychiatrist at the Illenau asylum, in his book *The Periodic Psychoses* (*Die periodischen Psychosen*) gave a sharply defined picture of all the periodic affective disorders, including the circular psychoses; thus, Kirn provided a kind of collective label for these recurrent illnesses.

In 1886, Danish physician Carl Georg Lange (1834–1900), professor of pathological anatomy at the University of Copenhagen and considered Denmark's "first neurologist," described "periodic psychic depression" as an independent illness with sudden onset, retardation, and numerous bodily changes such as loss of appetite and physical collapse. This constituted "an energetic declaration," in Danish psychiatrist Hans Jacob Schou's words (H. J. Schou lived from 1886 to 1952 and was the father of Mogens Schou—*see* **LITHIUM**), that endogenous depression had a possibly physical cause (Lange found elevated uric acid in the patients' urine). (The work was published in Danish; *see* the German translation of the second Danish edition, *Periodische Depressionszustände* [1896]. *See also* Schou's 1927 summary of it in the *Acta psych. et neurol.* An English translation [2001], edited by Johan A. Schioldann, is also available.)

In 1898, Ewald Hecker (1843–1909), chief physician of a private nerve sanatorium in Wiesbaden, Germany, voiced the suspicion that most of these cases of periodic depression really corresponded to **Karl Kahlbaum's** cyclothymia (*see* **MANIC-DEPRESSIVE ILLNESS** [1882]) ("Cyclothymia: a Circular Mood Disorder" ["Die Cyclothymie, eine circuläre Gemüthserkrankung"], *Journal of General Practice* [*Zeitschrift für praktische Ärzte*], p. 7).

Anxiety as a fundamental part of depression (1880). Although clinicians had always noted that depression and anxiety tended to occur together, among the first psychiatry writers to characterize depression as including anxiety was Christian Roller (?–1897), the son of Christian F. W. Roller (1802–1878), who practiced in a private asylum in Strasbourg. Writing in the *General Journal of Psychiatry* (*Allgemeine Zeitschrift für Psychiatrie*), Roller said that, "If anything is typical of the large group of mental disorders that we are inclined to group together under the name of melancholia, it is anxiety" (p. 197). Subsequent generations of psychiatrists debated whether anxiety and depression were really the same disorder or two separate disorders.

See **HYPOMANIA AND MANIA** (1881).

Cyclothymia (1882). *See* **MANIC-DEPRESSIVE ILLNESS.**

See **PARANOIA** (1883) as a late complication of melancholia.

Exogenous vs. endogenous (1893, 1909). In his 1893 textbook on nervous diseases, Paul Julius Möbius (1853–1907), a neurologist in Leipzig, initiated the distinction between "exogenous" nervous diseases, meaning illnesses having a specific and definable cause, and endogenous nervous diseases, "for which the only essential precondition [is] a certain inborn predisposition; once this is present, the disease may be caused by a variety of factors" (*Outline of the Doctrine of Nervous Diseases* (*Abriss der Lehre von den Nervenkrankheiten*; p. 140). Möbius, who prided himself on having devised a system of practical use, said, "From the practical viewpoint, it must be emphasized that we are almost powerless against all endogenous illnesses. . . . Once the illness is manifest, direct influencing of it is impossible" (p. 141).

The distinction was not widely noted until the terms were again picked up in 1909 by Karl Bonhoeffer (1868–1948), then psychiatry professor in Breslau, who distinguished between exogenous causes of affective disorders (meaning organic causes coming from outside, such as alcoholism, poisoning, or peripheral organ disease) and endogenous (meaning inborn, intrinsic, or constitutional). In affective disorders, he considered some kinds of mania (such as febrile) to be exogenous, whereas manic-depressive illness and pure depression were endogenous. In his article in the *Central Journal for Nervous Diseases and Psychiatry* (*Zentralblatt für Nervenheilkunde und Psychiatrie*), Bonhoeffer did not confine himself to affective disorders. (Note: In Bonhoeffer's parlance, exogenous is restricted to biological causes; it does not mean "reactive.")

See **ANHEDONIA** (1896 and later).

Involutional melancholia (1896). In the 1896 edition (fifth edition) of his influential textbook, *Psychiatry*, **Emil Kraepelin** distinguished between forms of melancholia that were acquired, such as the melancholia of middle and old age (the result of "involution," which required no predisposition), and all the other forms of mania, depression, and circular insanity, which were constitutional, or inborn, in nature. (In this edition, Kraepelin started using the term "depression" rather than "melancholia" for all the others.) Kraepelin, however, abandoned the notion of involutional melancholia in the eighth edition (1913) of his book, after familiarizing himself with Georges L. Dreyfus's (1879–1957) finding (in *Melancholy* [*Die Melancholie*], 1907) that almost all cases of involutional melancholia in fact displayed the features of manic-depressive illness. The concept of involutional melancholia itself, however, went on to a hearty life outside of Kraepelin's textbooks and was put to rest only by the demonstration in the 1970s that depression in the elderly responded in the same way to medication as in other age groups.

Manic-depressive illness (das manisch-depressive Irresein) (1899). *See* **MANIC-DEPRESSIVE ILLNESS: Kraepelin** (1899).

"Depression" becomes preferred to "melancholia" (ca. 1904). After **Emil Kraepelin** abandoned melancholy for depression in the fifth edition (1896) of his text, he lent his great prestige to this change. Then, in the United States, **Adolf Meyer**, professor of psychiatry at Johns Hopkins University, gave the decisive push. In 1904, he told a meeting of the New York Neurological Society that, in the words of the stenographer, "On the whole, he was desirous of eliminating the term melancholia, which implied a knowledge of something that we did not possess. . . . If, instead of melancholia, we applied the term depression to the whole class, it would designate in an unassuming way exactly what was meant" (*Journal of Nervous and Mental Diseases*, 1905, p. 114).

Neurotic depression (1911). The Berlin psychoanalyst and psychiatrist Karl Abraham (1877–1925) initiated the use of this concept in the psychoanalytic literature, writing in the *Central Journal of Psychoanalysis* (*Zentralblatt der Psychoanalyse*): "The neurotic becomes overwhelmed with anxiety when his drive aims at a satisfaction that his repression forbids him from achieving. Depression eventuates when, unsuccessful and unsatisfied, he abandons his sexual goal." Abraham noted that the literature contained "strikingly little about the psychology of neurotic depression" (p. 303).

Vital depression as an aspect of endogenous depression (vs. reactive depression) (1920). Building on the work of philosopher Max Scheler (1874–1928) about the layering of the psyche, in 1920 **Kurt Schneider** (1887–1967), then an academic psychiatrist in Cologne, distinguished between endogenous and reactive depression. The term "endogenous" he would have borrowed from the eighth edition in 1913 of Kraepelin's textbook (*see* **SCHIZOPHRENIA: EMERGENCE: Kraepelin**), where Kraepelin had used it as a qualifier for dementia praecox (schizophrenia). Endogenous depression in Schneider's view represented a disturbance of the body's "vital" feelings, situated in a very physical plane of vitality. Schneider summarized Scheler's views about this vital feeling of life (Lebensgefühl) as follows: "[It] participates in the body's entire feeling of corporization (Gesamtausdehnungscharakter des Leibes), without being localized in any particular part." "In such a feeling we grasp life itself, and in this feeling something is imparted to us: ascent, decline, health, illness, [and] danger." Endogenous depressions, therefore, were unprovoked, or autonomous ("motivlose"), disorders of these vital feelings; reactive depressions were disorders of the mental plane (seelische Gefühle) as such, often caused by external problems. Endogenous depressions were characterized by disturbances of the body's physical functions, such as diurnal variation (feeling worse in the morning), weight, and menstruation. For Schneider, vital depression and endogenous depression were synonymous. "Reactive depressions," by contrast, produced sadness (Traurigkeit) at the level of "emotional feelings" (Empfindungsgefühle), rather than unmotivated dysphoria (motivlose Verstimmung) at the vital level. Yet, vital depressions could occur in reaction to external events. For Schneider, the difference between "reactive" and "vital" was that they occurred at different "emotional layers," not that one was caused by events, the other uncaused. Schneider's article, in 1920 in the *Journal of Combined Neurology and Psychiatry* (*Zeitschrift für die gesamte Neurologie und Psychiatrie*) had great influence on subsequent generations of psychiatrists in Europe, and the term "endogenous depression" remained part of the standard vocabulary of mood disorders until the appearance of ***DSM-III*** in 1980.

Vital depression itself later became understood as physical symptoms in depression, or psychosomatic issues in depression. (*See* the work of Maarten H. Cohen-Stuart (1922–), at the Delta Hospital of Rotterdam, in *Psychiatria, Neurologia, Neurochirurgia*, 1965).

Benign stupor (1921). In an effort to get away from the straightjacket of the **Kraepelinian** system and its two great disease entities—dementia praecox and manic-depressive illness—New York psychiatrist August Hoch (1868–1919), who was born in Basel but emigrated to the United States in 1887, proposed "benign stupor" as a disease entity resembling manic-depressive illness and having a favorable outcome, as contrasted with "malignant stupor," a kind of catatonic stupor characteristic of dementia praecox. (Stupor means being unreactive to and unaware of one's surroundings.) Hoch, was Swiss-born **Meyer**'s successor as director of what was then called the Psychiatric Institute of the New York State Hospitals. He was among the first Americans beside

Meyer and Neftel—all had come from the Central European nosological tradition—to contribute to the international narrative of depression or schizophrenia. His book *Benign Stupor* was published posthumously in 1921, 2 years after his death.

Psychogenic depression (1926). Although earlier authors had alluded to nonconstitutional forms of "acquired neurasthenia," it was **Emil Kraepelin's** student Johannes Lange (1891–1938) at the German Psychiatric Research Institute (Deutsche Forschungsanstalt für Psychiatrie) in Munich who fleshed out the concept of "psychogenic forms of depression" ("psychogene Depressionszustände") as opposed to melancholic depressions in a 1926 article in the *Journal of Combined Neurology and Psychiatry* (*Zeitschrift für die gesamte Neurologie und Psychiatrie*). Psychogenic depressions, he said, were reactive in nature (unlike melancholy), were not characterized by retardation, and improved as the patients' situation changed. All of the somatic events of melancholy such as diurnal variation, stubborn constipation, and the feeling that the entire body was somehow involved were absent in psychogenic depression, where fatigue, irritability, and an inability to get going at work were, as well as sadness, the main symptoms.

Depressive neurosis (1927). **Sándor Radó** differentiated depressive neurosis from melancholia, saying at a meeting in 1927, "The most striking feature [of depression] is the fall in self-esteem and self-satisfaction. The depressive neurotic . . . attempts to conceal this disturbance; in melancholia it finds clamorous expression in the patients' self-accusations and self-aspersions, which we call 'the delusion of moral inferiority' " (*International Journal of Psychoanalysis*, 1928, p. 421).

British debate about "two depressions" vs. "one" (1920s). As the German concepts of endogenous depression vs. reactive filtered into Britain, they ignited a debate. In 1929, Ronald Dick ("R. D.") Gillespie (1897–1945), who 3 years previously had just become physician for psychological medicine at Guy's Hospital in London, wrote an article in *Guy's Hospital Reports* about depressed patients he had seen earlier on a studentship at Cassel Hospital in Penshurst. He divided them into two main groups: the "reactive" depressions, who displayed a host of "psychoneurotic" features, were quite anxious, and worried a lot about their health; and the "autonomous" depressions, who did not clear up at good news, tended to express ideas of unworthiness, and did not blame the environment for their problems: their dark mood seemed to come more out of the blue and less from their previous personalities. Thus, from Gillespie's work, the dichotomy "reactive-autonomous" arose.

Meanwhile, in 1926 Edward Mapother (1881–1940), who had recently become the first medical superintendent of the **Maudsley Hospital** in London, had weighed in with quite different views. He agreed with Kraepelin that there was just one disorder, manic-depressive psychosis, and apparent types of depression were just differences in degree. "Kraepelin, if anyone, has the right to settle what conditions the term 'manic-depressive psychosis' shall connote. . . . I entirely agree with his . . . views in this matter" (*British Medical Journal*, p. 872).

As the big authorities at these two different London power centers—Guy's and the Maudsley—dueled, in 1934 **Aubrey Lewis** (an assistant physician at the Maudsley) published his contribution: it was a paper on "melancholia" that he had written in 1931 on the basis of cases collected in 1928–1929, just after he had come to the Maudsley as a resident ("registrar"). Enormously self-confident for such a junior scholar,

Lewis announced that subtyping was very difficult because of "the interaction of organism and environment" (p. 370). "Gillespie even gives a table showing the differences, so that the general practitioner and the student can carry out the diagnostic exercise readily. But it has been made sufficiently apparent in the various sections of this study that these criteria fail" (p. 374). For Lewis, too, there was just one depression.

DEPRESSION AND MOOD DISORDERS: RECENT CONCEPTS. Starting in the middle third of the twentieth century, the diagnosis of depression increased many-fold. Though some of this increase was owing to the systematic marketing of the diagnosis by pharmaceutical companies, other elements of the increase involved refocusing the psychiatric nosology as such. Classic diagnoses such as "hysteria," "neurasthenia," and "nervousness" started to go out of style. Psychoanalysis popularized "neurotic depression" or "depressive neurosis" as workaday diagnoses, and the great relabeling of psychiatric diagnoses that occurred with ***DSM-III*** in 1980 elevated "major depression" to prominence. By the end of the twentieth century, "depression" had come to represent more than half of all psychiatric diagnoses made in clinical practice.

"Vegetative" depression (1949). There was a tradition of associating affective disorders with autonomic disturbances that went back to Max Rosenfeld's (1871–1956) 1906 article in the *Central Journal for Nervous Diseases* (*Centralblatt für Nervenheilkunde*). Rudolf Lemke (1906–1957), professor of psychiatry at Jena University in East Germany, alluded to it in 1949, proposing in the newly founded journal *Psychiatrie, Neurologie und Medizinische Psychologie* the diagnosis "vegetative depression," characterized by an anxious-depressed mood and autonomic symptoms. It differed from such diagnoses as "vegetative dystonia" (*see* **HYSTERIA: "vegetative dystonia"** [1934]) in that the patients were at risk of suicide.

Lopez Ibor's "anxious thymopathy" (timopatia ansiosa) (1950). Departing from the **Kraepelinian** tradition of seeing anxiety as part of manic-depressive disorder, in 1950 Juan J. Lopez Ibor (1907–1991), a member of the department of psychiatry of the University of Madrid and a former student of **Karl Jaspers** and **Kurt Schneider**, argued that anxiety and anguish represented an autonomous disease of an entirely "endogenous" nature; anxious thymopathy possessed deeply somatic roots and was not at all psychogenic. It came from the "vital" level of the body; in his book *La Angustia Vital* (*Patologia General Psicosomatica*), published in 1950, he proposed the term "vital anguish" (la angustia vital) for the whole complex. (Thymo- is derived from the Greek, meaning mind or will; in modern parlance, however, "thymopathy" refers to diseases of the thymus.*) He believed it to be part of a "circular" disorder ("el circulo timopatico") and said it might overlap in some patients with endogenous depression, giving rise to "idiopathic anxious depression."

---

* As Eugen Bleuler wrote in 1916 in his *Textbook of Psychiatry* (in the English translation [1924] by New York psychoanalyst Abraham Arden Brill [1874–1948]—an early translator of Freud's work as well), "Since the affective dispositions fluctuate greatly in different people, they also most readily cross the borderline of the 'normal.' The so-called psychopaths are really nearly all exclusively or mainly thymopaths" (translation of the fourth German ed. of *Lehrbuch der Psychiatrie*, 1923, p. 117).

Kraepelin's manic-depressive illness seems to consist of separate diseases: bipolar and unipolar disorders (1957). *See* **MANIC-DEPRESSIVE ILLNESS** (1957).

Atypical depression (1959). **William Sargant's** group in the department of psychological medicine at St. Thomas's Hospital in London found that a certain subset of depressive patients responded readily to the drug **iproniazid** (Marsilid), an inhibitor of brain monoamine oxidase. The subset was characterized by patients who did not have the classic picture of endogenous depression, with self-reproaches and early-morning worsening, but rather were highly anxious, phobic, and greatly fatigued. Sargant's "registrars" (the British term for resident) Eric Douglas West (M.B. 1951) and Peter John Dally (M.B. 1953) published on this in the *British Medical Journal* in 1959, then Sargant himself co-wrote several subsequent follow-up articles, saying for example in 1960 in *Psychosomatics* that, "[These patients] may . . . have become bad tempered, irritable, hyperreactive and aggressive, quite unlike so many of the more endogenously depressed patients" (p. 15). Sargant's work represents one of the first attempts to identify a subclass of depression patients differentially responsive to a given drug. Marsilid was subsequently withdrawn from the market as toxic.

Tellenbach's "melancholic type" (1961). Hubert Tellenbach (1914–), associate professor and head of the department of clinical psychopathology at Heidelberg, postulated in his book *Melancholie* (1961) that a certain "melancholic type" of character exists that predisposes individuals to clinical melancholy. Its main characteristic is a highly developed sense of orderliness (Ordentlichkeit) that leads to "exceptionally high demands regarding one's own achievements." Said Tellenbach: "The melancholic individual wants to achieve much, and to do so regularly. But he wants to maintain his achievements at a level that is simultaneously a ceiling." Thus, the melancholic is interested only in the "possible," while anything "that might appear impossible is never even aspired to. That is probably the reason that melancholic types almost never achieve a high social position" (pp. 53–54). Although the diagnosis was never taken up in American psychiatry, it has remained influential in Central Europe.

Vital depression vs. personal depression (1965). Herman van Praag (1929–) and co-workers, then at the Dijkzigt Hospital in Rotterdam, contrasted these two forms of depression as the equivalents of endogenous vs. reactive depression, with the difference that the latter set of terms implied causation of some kind (constitutional vs. external events), whereas Van Praag considered the causes of depression to be unknowable. The defining characteristic of vital depression was its "motiveless" nature, or inexplicable onset, coming out of the blue. Also, the patient may not necessarily feel sad, but rather physically dragged down. "One might speak of a continuous hangover, or, with **Schneider** (*Clinical Pathology* [*Klinische Pathologie*], 1959), of a depressio sine depressione." The article appeared in *Psychiatria, Neurologia, Neurochirurgia*, a Dutch medical journal (quote, p. 331). Van Praag was first to devise a scale for measuring vital depression.

"Primary vs. secondary" depression (1969). Drawing on the work of Robert Woodruff (1934–) and colleagues, **St. Louis school** members **Eli Robins** and **Samuel Guze** proposed in 1969, at a large **National Institute of Mental Health** conference on "the psychobiology of the depressive illnesses," the division of affective disorders (depression and mania) into primary and secondary forms; "primary" meaning patients with no previous history of psychiatric illness and "secondary" patients who had "a preexisting, diagnosable psychiatric illness, other than a previous primary affective disorder" (p. 292 of the proceedings of the conference, edited by Thomas A. Williams and others, published in 1972). The authors found this classification superior to the other conventional classifications of affective disorders: endogenous vs. reactive, and neurotic vs. psychotic.

Psychotic depression as an independent entity (1975 and after). There was a European tradition of treating all serious depressions as "psychotic." The study of psychotic depression goes back at least to **Kahlbaum**'s work on catatonia in 1874, when he described patients with catatonia who were depressed and psychotic. (*See* **SCHIZOPHRENIA: EMERGENCE: catatonia** [1874].) During the years, the observation was commonly made that depressed patients who displayed symptoms such as catatonia and delusions did less well than other kinds of depressed patients. Yet, in the absence of specific treatments or a common family history for such patients, little was made of the finding. Also, these depressions responded equally well to electroconvulsive therapy, so it did not really matter what the subgroups were.

Then, starting in 1975, it began to become apparent that a subgroup clearly existed—with psychotic delusional symptoms—that did poorly on standard antidepressants, as Alexander Glassman (1934–) and associates at the New York State Psychiatric Institute, linked to Columbia University, reported in the *American Journal of Psychiatry*; these patients also responded much better to ECT, as David Avery (1946–) and Aldo Lubrano (1950–) at the Palo Alto Veterans Administration Hospital found in a reanalysis of an earlier Italian study that had compared ECT to the tricyclic antidepressant **imipramine** (*American Journal of Psychiatry*, 1979).

In 1992, Alan F. Schatzberg (1944–) and Anthony J. Rothschild (1953–), at the time in the department of psychiatry of Harvard Medical School, asked in an article in the *American Journal of Psychiatry*, "Psychotic (Delusional) Major Depression: Should It Be Included as a Distinct Syndrome in *DSM-IV*?" They answered yes. "[The data] point to both the rationale and the need for designating psychotic major depression as a distinct syndrome in *DSM-IV*" (p. 743). ("Severe with psychotic features" continued, however, in the *Manual* to be just a specifier for "major depressive episode.")

The concept of psychotic "depression" would cause misgivings in researchers who believe that catatonia, a brutal slowing, is not the same as the retardation of depression. Thus, a psychotic depression that included catatonia caused some international eyebrow-raising. Under the leadership of **Max Fink**, the treatment of psychotic depression with ECT became well defined. (*See* Georgios Petrides [1957–] and Max Fink, *Journal of ECT*, 2001.)

See **"FEIGHNER DIAGNOSTIC CRITERIA"** (1972)

The introduction of "major depression" (1978). Continuing the work of the **St. Louis school** (*see also* **"FEIGHNER"** [1972]), in 1978 **Robert L. Spitzer** and psychologist Jean Endicott (1936–) of the New York State Psychiatric Institute and department of psychiatry of Columbia University, together with **Eli Robins**, extended their nosology—which they were now calling the Research Diagnostic Criteria (RDC)—to 25 principal diagnostic categories, including "major depressive disorder" (which had 11 subtypes) and "minor depressive disorder with significant anxiety." This article in the *Archives of General Psychiatry* became part of the intellectual scaffolding of ***DSM-III***.

Atypical depression (revived) 1979. In searching for treatment-specific depression subtypes, a group of researchers led by Frederic Quitkin (1937–) and Michael

Liebowitz (1945–) and including **Donald Klein** and Arthur Rifkin (1937–), of the department of psychiatry of Columbia University and the New York State Psychiatric Institute, identified a subset of patients whom they believed especially responsive to monoamine oxidase inhibiting drugs (monamine oxidase inhibitors, or MAOIs) (*see* **IPRONIAZID**). The patients, who were given the diagnosis "atypical depression" (with reference to the earlier English work of **William Sargant**), had the following characteristics: some degree of dysphoria on the basis of Research Diagnostic Criteria, plus "mood reactivity" (patient gets better when things change), plus two or more of the following symptoms: overeating, gaining weight, oversleeping, sensation of leaden fatigue, taking rejection poorly. In 1979, Quitkin and colleagues began to publish on this in the *Archives of General Psychiatry*; Liebowitz and colleagues wrote another key article in the *Journal of Clinical Psychology* in 1984. Atypical depression was accepted as an official psychiatric diagnosis ("atypical features specifier") in ***DSM-IV*** (1994).

DSM-III enshrines "major depression" and revives "dysthymia" (1980). In 1980, the Task Force on Nomenclature and Statistics of the American Psychiatric Association, led by **Robert Spitzer**, published the third edition of its ***Diagnostic and Statistical Manual of Mental Disorders***. Among the many disorders to be reconfigured were the depression diagnoses ("affective disorders"), but in a manner sharply different from the Research Diagnostic Criteria of 1978 (*see* above). ***DSM-III*** created three new disease labels in the mood area: (1) "major depression" (anticipated in 1978), which was a mixture of psychotic and nonpsychotic depressive conditions; (2) "dysthymic disorder" (a term coined by Flemming in 1844; *see* **DEPRESSION: EMERGENCE**), which was a new label for what had been known as "neurotic depression"; and (3) "adjustment disorder with depressed mood" for minor depressions supposedly treatable with psychotherapy alone (as the correspondence of the drafters indicates). Manic-depressive illness, for which the *DSM* drafters adopted Karl Kleist's label "bipolar disorder" (*see* **WERNICKE–KLEIST–LEONHARD PATHWAY**) remained intact. *DSM* adopted the **Kahlbaum** label "cyclothymic disorder" for less serious manic-depressive illness (*see* **MANIC-DEPRESSIVE ILLNESS** [1882]). As in the Feighner article (*see* **"FEIGHNER DIAGNOSTIC CRITERIA"** [1972]), "operational criteria" were stipulated for the granting of each of these diagnoses. Thus, to meet the criteria for major depressive episode, the patient had to have a dysphoric mood for a certain period of time plus four of a list of eight other criteria that included such symptoms as poor appetite, insomnia, and loss of pleasure in formerly pleasurable activities. (The drafters did not use the term "anhedonia.") Subsequent editions of ***DSM*** did not change significantly the nature of the affective diagnoses.

The new *DSM* diagnosis of "major depressive disorder," with its checklist of heterogeneous symptom pictures and absence of reference to the patient's past history, was not without critics. As Bernard James ("Barney") Carroll (1940–), then professor of psychiatry at Duke University, said in 1982 at a conference in Berlin on *The Origins of Depression* that Jules Angst (1926–) of Zurich had convened, the concept of major depressive disorder was far too nonspecific. Also, "These criteria are deficient in another important respect—they give a flat, two-dimensional view of the patient's illness because they ignore features that earlier clinicians placed much weight upon—family history, for example, previous episodes, responses to previous treatments, and a history of hypomanic or manic phases" (p. 166). Nonetheless, "major depression" went on to become the single most important diagnosis in psychiatry.

Double depression (1982) Martin B. Keller (1946–), then in the department of psychiatry of the Massachusetts General Hospital, and Robert W. Shapiro (1938–1980), whose name was added posthumously, characterized double depression as the overlapping of two Research Diagnostic Criteria depression categories (*see* above): a patient having, at the same time, major depressive disorder superimposed on an underlying chronic depression ("dysthymic disorder"). The article, in the *American Journal of Psychiatry,* thus aired publicly an overlapping that ***DSM*** insiders had discussed throughout the drafting. Keller and Shapiro argued that the prognosis for patients with double depression was worse than for those with major depression alone.

"Seasonal affective disorder" (SAD) (1984). The existence of a certain kind of depression that routinely worsens in the winter months was proposed and named in 1984 by Norman E. Rosenthal—himself a sufferer—and co-workers at the **National Institute of Mental Health** in the *Archives of General Psychiatry*. Bright light was said to have "a marked antidepressant effect" upon SAD. The concept was incorporated in ***DSM-III-R*** in 1987 as a "specifier" for major depression (*see* above) and for bipolar disorder (*see* **MANIC-DEPRESSIVE ILLNESS**), defined as "a regular cyclic relationship between onset of the mood episodes and a particular 60-day period of the year," especially the time from early October to late November. Despite international misgiving about the diagnosis, it reappeared in ***DSM-IV*** (1994).

Recurrent, brief depression (1985). In the context of a longitudinal study of a cohort of young adults in Zurich, Jules Angst (1926–), chair of the research department of the Psychiatric University Hospital in Zurich (**Burghölzli**), realized that many of the patients suffered recurrent bouts of depression too brief to qualify as "major depression" or "dysthymia" in ***DSM*** terminology. In the *European Archives of Psychiatry* in 1985, Angst proposed the diagnosis "recurrent, brief depression" (RBD) as a subtype of affective disorder. (The series of articles in which they suggested the diagnosis began in 1984.)

See also **CATECHOLAMINE HYPOTHESIS OF DEPRESSION.**

DEREALIZATION. *See* **DEPERSONALIZATION.**

DIAGNOSTIC AND STATISTICAL MANUAL OF MENTAL DISORDERS. *See* ***DSM***.

DISSOCIATIVE DISORDERS. *See* **DEPERSONALIZATION; MULTIPLE PERSONALITY DISORDER.**

DOPAMINE. Dopamine is a **neurotransmitter** belonging chemically to the class of catecholamines. The efficacy of many antipsychotic drugs is thought to reside in their success in blocking the receptors for dopamine in the brain, especially the D2 receptor. In 1957, Swedish neuroscientist Arvid Carlsson (1923–) discovered the role of dopamine as a neurotransmitter, and his article appeared in *Science* in 1958. (For the basic scientific narrative in these neurotransmitter discoveries, *see* **IPRONIAZID AND THE MONOAMINE OXIDASE INHIBITORS; NEUROTRANSMITTER; RESERPINE.**) In 1961, Julius Axelrod (1912–) and co-workers at the **National Institute of Mental**

Health discovered a reuptake mechanism for norepinephrine (NE)—and for dopamine (as the precursor of NE, dopamine is also a neurotransmitter in its own right)—announcing the discovery in *Science*. (Axelrod won a Nobel Prize in 1970 for research that also included this work.)

In 1975, Solomon Snyder and co-workers discovered the existence of a receptor for dopamine, making the announcement in *Life Sciences*. And the following year, 1976, the Snyder group announced in *Science* that the potency of antipsychotic drugs was a function of their ability to block this dopamine receptor. (Two months later, Philip Seeman [1934–], a pharmacologist at the University of Toronto, came forward in *Nature* with the very same discovery.) In 1976 as well, Snyder and colleagues ventured the "dopamine hypothesis" of schizophrenia in the *American Journal of Psychiatry*, using among other evidence the information that amphetamines, which are "dopaminergic" (i.e., potentiate the action of dopamine), made schizophrenia worse. Similar to the fate of the "**catecholamine hypothesis**" of depression, the dopamine hypothesis of schizophrenia is no longer strictly believed. Yet, it stimulated much important research on dopamine and its role in psychiatric illness.

DSM: DIAGNOSTIC AND STATISTICAL MANUAL OF MENTAL DISORDERS, American Psychiatric Association (from 1952). (*See also* **"ST. LOUIS SCHOOL OF PSYCHIATRY"; SPITZER.**) This series of diagnostic handbooks, coming from a country that was not yet a world power upon the psychiatry stage, began with a low international profile. By the time the most recent version appeared in 1994, the *DSM* (also referred to as "the *Manual*" in this text) had become the global standard of diagnosis, placing the competing *ICD* series (*International Classification of Diseases*) of the World Health Organization in the shade.

***DSM* "One"** (1952). Called "*DSM-I*" of course only in retrospect, this initial guide to classification was heavily under the influence of **Adolf Meyer** of Johns Hopkins University. It referred to most conditions as "reactions" and gave only thumbnail sketches of each. Internationally, it went unheralded. George N. Raines (ca. 1908–1959), director of psychiatry at Georgetown University Medical Center, was head of the Committee on Nomenclature and Statistics. *DSM-I* contained 106 diagnoses.

DSM-II (1968). This second edition reflected more the influence of psychoanalysis, then at the height of its influence upon American psychiatry. The conditions were mostly listed as "neuroses" rather than "reactions." The descriptions of each entity continued to be brief and without much indication of the clinical criteria required to fulfil the diagnosis. Ernest M. Gruenberg (1915–1991), an epidemiologist and professor of psychiatry then at Columbia University, was head of the nomenclature committee. **Robert Spitzer** advised the committee as a "consultant." *DSM-II* contained 182 diagnoses.

The "St. Louis criteria" of psychiatric illness (1972). As part of the diagnostic rethinking leading up to ***DSM-III***, John Feighner and the other members of the **St. Louis school** published in 1972 in the *Archives of General Psychiatry* an article on "Diagnostic Criteria for Use in Psychiatric Research." The authors, who included **Eli Robins, Samuel Guze**, Robert Woodruff (1934–), **George Winokur**, and Rodrigo Muñoz (1939–), proposed "formal diagnostic criteria," in place of "best clinical judgment," that clinicians would have to apply in making a diagnosis. The illnesses were limited to 14, and the operational criteria were laid out in point form in what was to become classic *DSM-III* style. For example: "At least three of the following manifestations must be present for a diagnosis of 'definite' schizophrenia," the authors said, and listed five criteria. (*See also* "**FEIGHNER DIAGNOSTIC CRITERIA.**")

The Research Diagnostic Criteria (1978) as a preview of *DSM-III* (1980). **Robert Spitzer**, Columbia University psychologist Jean Endicott (1936–), and **Eli Robins**, building on the work of the **St. Louis school**, proposed in 1978 in the *Archives of General Psychiatry* a revised list of diagnoses to be used in research. Called the Research Diagnostic Criteria, the RDC system included "panic disorder," described as similar to anxiety neurosis; they identified "generalized anxiety disorder with significant depression" (the mirror image of their concept "minor depressive disorder with significant anxiety") and maintained previous concepts of phobia. Because of Spitzer's centrality in the production of ***DSM-III***, which appeared 2 years later, the RDC criteria set the stage, to some extent, for *DSM-III* (yet not entirely; *see* **DEPRESSION: RECENT CONCEPTS: *DSM-III*** [1980]).

DSM-III (1980). This third edition of the *Manual* recognized the growing importance of diagnosis in American psychiatry and was drastically revised, instituting detailed operational criteria that had to be met to qualify for a diagnosis. The conditions were changed from "neuroses" to "disorders," although at the bidding of the psychoanalytic community the word "neurosis" was included in parentheses after many "disorders." The *Manual* laid out five "axes" on which diagnoses might be made: axis I for most mental disorders except those in axis II, which were personality and developmental disorders; axis III for physical disorders; axis IV for "severity of psychosocial stressors"; and axis V, "highest level of adaptive functioning past year." In practice, axis I was used far more often than any of the others, and with time the convention became adopted that axis I meant drug-treatable, and axis II meant lifelong character pathology and basically untreatable. **Robert Spitzer** was chair of the task force on nomenclature. Within a short time, *DSM-III* became the worldwide gold standard of psychiatric diagnosis. By May 1982, a little more than 2 years after its launch in February 1980, it had gone through eight printings, each averaging about 30,000 copies. *DSM-III* contained 265 diagnoses.

DSM-III-R (1987). This revised version ("R") of the third edition changed very little, although it was, at 567 pages, considerably longer than the previous version (*DSM-III* was 494 pages; *DSM-I* was 132 pages). **Robert Spitzer** remained the head of the nomenclature "work group." *DSM-III-R* contained 292 diagnoses.

DSM-IV (1994). This version was substantially unchanged from the previous, except for being longer still (886 pages), with ever more diagnoses and descriptions of criteria that had to be met. Allen Frances (1942–) of Columbia University was head of the "task force" that devised it. *DSM-IV* contained 307 diagnoses.

DUTCH PIONEER COMMUNITY CARE IN PSYCHIATRY (from 1945). Although the Dutch Mental Hygiene Movement (Nederlandsche Vereeniging ter Bevordering der Geestelijke Volksgezondheid) had been founded in 1924, it remained an anemic organization with little influence. In August 1945, however, just at the end of hostilities, the Minister of Social Affairs asked the mental hygienists to suggest a national program in mental hygiene for knitting back a country that had been badly rattled by wartime events. The organization responded with proposals focusing on group treatment, early treatment, and community care. At the International Congress on Mental Health in London in 1948, the large Dutch contingent led by Henricus Cornelis Rümke (1893–1967), professor of psychiatry at the University of Utrecht between 1936 and 1963 and who had been prominent in the "Utrecht School" of phenomenology and anthropology, returned home filled with determination to promote not merely mental hygiene but mental health. This reformist vigor penetrated the various Roman Catholic, Protestant, and "non-confessional" "pillars" of health care into which Dutch society was then split (the famous "pillarization" system of Dutch social organization). One scholar writes, "Beginning in the sixties, most [pillarized] psychiatric hospitals witnessed an astounding proliferation of all kinds of therapeutic communities, rehabilitation units, short and long term treatment programs, substance abuse clinics, and services for people with behavioral problems and personality disorders" (Schnabel, in Porter, ed., *Culture of Psychiatry*, p. 32). These were not, however, linked to deinstitutionalization, a process that began later in The Netherlands.

Then in 1982, the ties with the various pillars were cut, and under the influence of Kees Trimbos (1920–1988), professor of social psychiatry in Rotterdam, and like Rümke a Catholic, outpatient psychiatric services became organized into community health-care centers focusing on psychotherapy and called "RIAGGSs," the Dutch equivalent of Regional Institute of Ambulatory Mental Health Care. More attuned to patients with lesser psychiatric problems, the RIAGGS kept their distance from patients with serious disorders. Yet, the almost 60 RIAGGS that developed became what was probably the world's first well-integrated system of ambulant mental-health care. Finally, in the 1990s, they did move closer to the hospitals in the context of deinstitutionalization.

DYSMORPHOPHOBIA, or body dysmorphic disorder (from 1891). Uneasiness about one's looks is probably as old as the human condition. The French poet Baudelaire described in the late 1850s in "Scattered thoughts" (*"Pensées éparses"*): "The man who believes himself ugly, or who sees in himself an imaginary deformity . . . Obsession."

In 1891, Italian psychiatrist **Enrico Morselli** (1852–1929) attached a medical term to the phenomenon, coining dysmorphophobia in an article in the *Bulletin of the Royal Medical Society of Genoa* (*Bolletino della Reale Accademia Medica di Genova*); by it he meant unrealistic fear of personal ugliness, an omnibus concept to which some authorities today now reckon anorexia nervosa. (*See* **BODY IMAGE: DISTURBANCES OF.**) He wrote in 1891, "The dysmorphophobic patient is, in fact, truly tortured: in the midst of his daily routines, of speeches, while reading, during lunch, thus anywhere and at any time of day, he is struck by the suspicion of a deformity that might have appeared on his body and without his knowledge: he fears that he has or might have his forehead pressed in and flattened [depressa e schiacciata], his nose ridiculous, his legs crooked" (p. 111).

Morselli's diagnosis started to receive international currency when **Emil Kraepelin** tucked it into the eighth edition of his textbook, the volume published in 1915. Making it part of obsessive-compulsive neuroses, Kraepelin said, "Some patients cannot rid themselves of the thought of having something conspicuous or ridiculous on their bodies, arousing the attention or ridicule of passers-by with the strangely shaped nose, crooked legs or a repellent odor" (*Psychiatrie*, 8th ed., IV, p. 1861). Kraepelin used Morselli's term but did not mention Morselli himself.

Dysmorphophobia came into ***DSM-III-R*** in 1987 as "body dysmorphic disorder (dysmorphophobia)" in the "somatoform disorders" section, "a preoccupation with some imagined defect in appearance in a normal-appearing person." The drafters did not like the "-phobia" part because the suffix suggested "phobic avoidance," which was not the case here (the patients are glued to the mirror rather than avoiding it). If the misbelief was of psychotic intensity, "delusional disorder" would be a better diagnosis, it was noted in the *Manual*.

E

EATING DISORDERS. *See* **BODY IMAGE: DISTURBANCES OF: anorexia nervosa; BULIMIA.**

ELECTROCONVULSIVE THERAPY (ECT) (from 1938). Although medicine had known applications of electricity for mental symptoms since the late eighteenth century, only in the mid-1930s did the accelerating interest in somatic therapies sparked by the success of **insulin coma therapy** and **convulsive therapy** with Metrazol cause Ugo Cerletti (1877–1963), professor of psychiatry in Rome, to start thinking about the therapeutic induction of convulsions with electricity. After he and three of the assistant physicians in his clinic—Ferdinando Accornero (1910–?), Lucio Bini (1908–1964), and Lamberto Longhi (1909–?)—had established the safety of the procedure through animal research, on April 20, 1938, they treated the first psychiatric patient with ECT, a forty-ish man with schizophrenia of recent onset who responded well to a series of shocks over the next few days. Cerletti wrote up the findings in an article entitled "Electroshock" ("L'Elettroshock") in the *General Archives of Neurology* (*Archivio generale di neurologia*) in 1938. It was not the effectiveness of convulsions as such that these Italian investigators established, for countless applications of Metrazol (Cardiazol) had already clinched the point that convulsive therapy was effective, but rather, as American ECT researcher Richard Abrams (1937–) puts it, "that such convulsions could be induced safely, reliably, and inexpensively by electrical means" (*Electroconvulsive Therapy*, 4th ed., 2002, p. 6).

In diffusing news of the effectiveness of ECT, a refugee German physician named Lothar Kalinowsky (1899–1992)—his mother was Jewish—who had been an assistant in Cerletti's clinic, played a key role, helping to establish its use in England in 1939 at Warlingham Park Hospital in London. Though Kalinowsky did not introduce it to the United States, he became a central figure in demonstrations of it at the the New York State Psychiatric Institute. (Who introduced ECT to the United States remains controversial. According to psychiatry historian Walter Barton it was Cincinnati psychiatrist Douglas Goldman [1906–1986] in 1939. Goldman was clinical director at Longview State Hospital. Many authorities give credit to David J. Impastato [1903–1986] and Renato J. Almansi [1909–2000] at Columbus Hospital in New York City in February 1940.) Later, the main individual behind the diffusion of ECT in the United States was **Max Fink**, who learned the technique in the Army during the war and in 1952 began using it as a resident at Hillside Hospital in Glen Oaks, New York.

To moderate the risk of fracturing vertebrae during a convulsion, in 1940 Omaha psychiatrist Abram Bennett (1898–1985) suggested in the *Journal of the American Medical Association* the drug curare as a way of blocking the nerve–muscle junction. This gain in safety permitted the expansion of ECT to larger numbers of depressed patients. Almost from the beginning, clinicians started administering **barbiturate** anesthetics to reduce patients' anxiety, particularly in partial seizures, and to diminish the force of the grand mal seizures, in which the patients were at risk of spinal fractures. In 1942,

Impastato and Almansi described in the *Journal of Nervous and Mental Disease* the use of phenobarbital and Sodium Amytal in order to "overcome the most dreaded complication of the method—fractures of the spine or limbs" (p. 400). In 1952 two Swedish researchers, Carl *Gunnar* Holmberg (1919–) and *Stephen* Wilhelm Thesleff (1924–) at the Karolinska Institute in Stockholm, proposed in the *American Journal of Psychiatry* using the less risky drug succinylcholine as a means of preventing spinal fractures.

In 1978, the American Psychiatric Association (APA) issued its first timid acceptance of ECT in a report on *Electroconvulsive Therapy*. Following a consensus conference on ECT in 1985 at the National Institute of Mental Health, in the late 1980s the APA convoked a new Task Force on ECT, endorsing it more enthusiastically in *The Practice of Electroconvulsive Therapy: Recommendations for Treatment* (1990). In 1999, the APA reconvened its Committee on ECT (formerly the Task Force), and in 2001 issued a second edition of its 1990 report. The committee noted that, "The clinical literature establishing the efficacy of ECT in specific disorders is among the most substantial for any medical treatment." They concluded, "Severe major depression with psychotic features, mania . . . and catatonia are conditions for which there is a clear consensus favoring early reliance on ECT" (pp. 5–6).

When ECT is properly administered, about 85% of patients with serious depression respond to it. In 2003, assessing the effectiveness of ECT in a series of depressed Israeli patients, Bernard ("Benny") Lerer (1948–), director of the Biological Laboratory of Hadassah University Hospital in Ein Karem, Israel, said to a journalist from the newspaper *Haaretz*, "Have you ever asked yourself how it is that a treatment with such a terrible stigma, a treatment that the public is afraid of and is said to be primitive and unhelpful—has, despite all this, survived into the 21st century, and not in obscure little places but in the world's most advanced medical centers? The answer is simple. Because it works."

ELECTROENCEPHALOGRAPHY. *See* **BERGER, HANS.**

ELKES, JOEL (1913–). A pioneer psychopharmacologist, Elkes was born in Königsberg, Germany, the son of a prestigious physician in Kovno in neighboring Lithuania. His father, head of the Jewish community in the Kovno ghetto, died in Dachau in 1943; his mother, the daughter of a well-to-do grain merchant, survived the Holocaust and died in Israel. In 1930, Elkes left Kovno to study medicine at St. Mary's Hospital in London, graduating, after a period of financial difficulty caused by interruption of communications in the war, in 1941. He joined Alistair Frazer (1909–1969) as research assistant in the department of pharmacology at the University of Birmingham, shortly getting charge of the research unit on mental disease; there, in the late 1940s, he established a "Drugs and the Mind" program. After spending a year in the United States as a Smith Kline & French Fellow and Fulbright Fellow, Elkes returned to Birmingham in 1951 as head of the first department of experimental psychiatry in the world, with a mission of bridging basic research and clinical psychiatry. The department was supported by the Rockefeller Foundation and the Medical Research Council of England. It comprised experimental animal laboratories plus a clinical arm, the "Uffculme Clinic," with 40 beds. Situated in the former Cadbury mansion in Birmingham, the clinic was modeled on the "Peckham Experiment" in London and was designed to provide comprehensive care, including an outpatient unit, a day hospital, and a home visiting service. The department was among the first research facilities in the world in psychopharmacology. In research begun in 1951 (and reported in *Clinical Neurophysiology* in 1953), Elkes and Philip Bradley (1919–) implanted electrodes in animals to study neuropharmacology. It was at Winson Green Hospital in Birmingham that Charmian Elkes and Joel Elkes conducted the first blind controlled trial of **chlorpromazine** in chronic psychotic patients, which was published in the *British Medical Journal* in 1954. (*See* **WOMEN IN PSYCHIATRY: Charmian Elkes.**)

In 1957, Elkes moved to the United States at the invitation of Seymour Kety (1915–2000) and Robert A. Cohen (1909–?) of the **National Institute of Mental Health** to set up a clinical neuropharmacological research center (CNRC) at **St. Elizabeths Hospital** in Washington, D.C. He was simultaneously professor of psychiatry at George Washington University. At the CNRC, some important early work in the metabolism of **dopamine** was carried out, and such clinical investigators as German emigré psychiatrist Fritz Freyhan (1912–1982), previously at a mental hospital in Delaware, and British psychiatrist Anthony Hordern (1925–), who had just finished training in London, undertook clinical trials. In 1963, Elkes became the Henry Phipps professor of psychiatry at Johns Hopkins University, succeeding Seymour Kety. In line with Elkes' views about extending research in psychiatry from the experimental to the clinical, he renamed the department from "psychiatry" to "psychiatry and behavioral sciences." He retired from that post in 1975. As biographer Thomas Ban remarked, "The impact of Elkes' professional activities on the development of neuropsychopharmacology through training of professionals is unparalleled. The list of the people who passed through his laboratories reads like a Who's Who of American Psychopharmacology" (in *Elkes Selected Writings*, p. 20). In 1958, Elkes also opened up the whole area of receptorology—at a time when few were interested in the subject—with his insight that the neurotransmitters ("neurohumoral transmitter substances") might have a specific effect on different kinds of receptors in the brain. (The paper was published in a Ciba Foundation *Symposium on the Neurological Basis of Behavior.*)

ENGEL, GEORGE L. (1913–1999). Coiner of the phrase "biopsychosocial model," Engel was born in New York City and graduated with an M.D. from Johns Hopkins University in 1938. He trained in internal medicine at Peter Bent Brigham Hospital in Boston, then in 1946 was appointed to the departments of medicine and psychiatry of the University of Rochester, where he remained. As his interest in psychoanalysis strengthened, in the years 1949 to 1955 he underwent training at the New York Psychoanalytic Institute and the Chicago Institute for Psychoanalysis. Engel set out to apply psychoanalytic doctrine, where appropriate, to medical illnesses and became noted for his thoughtful integration of psychosocial issues in the care customarily provided in internal medicine. (*See* **DELIRIUM.**) It was, however, for his coinage of the term "biopsychosocial model"—as opposed to the "medical model"—in an article in *Science* in 1977 that he became most celebrated. The title was: "The need for a new medical model: a challenge for biomedicine," and the concept was not merely that social aspects of care must be considered but that the system of care itself should be revamped. Engel argued in particular that psychiatry had come to a crossroads: "Psychiatry's crisis revolves around the question of whether the categories of human distress with which it is concerned are properly considered 'disease' as currently conceptualized and whether exercise of the traditional authority of the physician is appropriate for their helping functions." Engel concluded, "The dominant model of disease today is biomedical, and it leaves no room within its framework for the social, psychological, and behavioral dimensions of illness" (pp. 129, 135). These words became a banner for many medical reformers in their efforts to make medicine more patient-centered, and psychiatrists often came to pride themselves on using the "BPS" model, although it was in stark contradiction to the teaching of the **St. Louis School** and the views of **Samuel Guze** that "psychiatry is a part of medicine." Indeed, Anthony W. Clare (1942–), at the Institute of Psychiatry in London, later slaked such BPS thinking as "a voice hostile to medicine. This voice preaches 'holism' and beckons psychiatry out into the soft, doughy area of gestalt psychology and encounter therapy to minister to the needs of people less ill than dissatisfied and more appropriately classified as demoralised than disordered." He said this, without mentioning the BPS model as such, in a 1982 volume that **Michael Shepherd** edited called *Psychiatrists on Psychiatry*, p. 21.

EPILEPSY. Called "the falling sickness," epilepsy was once seen primarily as a psychiatric illness, one of **William Cullen's** "neuroses." Seizure patients who also had psychiatric symptoms often landed in asylums and were included in psychiatric textbooks. Epilepsy as a so-called neuropsychiatric condition thus has a place in the history of psychiatry, even though in a strict sense epilepsy is defined as seizures associated with sudden electrical discharges of the brain (thus implicitly placing it in the province of neurology because neurology has inherited all behavioral disorders—such as Parkinson's disease—associated with specific brain lesions). Interestingly, virtually all antiepileptic medications turn out to have significant uses in psychiatry.

Although many of the symptoms of epilepsy had been well characterized since the Ancients, only in the nineteenth century did the current classification evolve that distinguishes between primary generalized (often idiopathic) seizures and partial seizures (often associated with a specific lesion).

In his 1815 article "On Epilepsy" ("De l'épilepsie"), **Étienne Esquirol** said that in the hospitals they were now differentiating between "le grand et le petit mal," in other words, in today's parlance, between tonic-clonic convulsions (grand mal seizures) and absence seizures (petit mal seizures) (Esquirol, I, p. 281). Then, in 1824, Esquirol's student Louis-Florentin Calmeil (1798–1895), in his doctoral dissertation *On Epilepsy (De l'épilepsie)*, supplied "absence" seizures as a synonym for petit mal. Calmeil also introduced into medicine the term "état de mal," translated into English as "status epilepticus," a series of uninterrupted seizures having a poor outcome. During the years, grand and petit mal have both been considered "true" epilepsy because the cause was unknown and at autopsy the brain seemed to be normal.

A major concept to emerge in the nineteenth century was "focal" seizures: symptoms beginning on one side of the body caused by a specific brain lesion. Codifying focal into a larger theory of epilepsy was the work of English neurologist John Hughlings Jackson (1835–1911), who from 1862 to 1906 studied convulsive phenomena at the National Hospital for the Relief and Cure of the Paralysed and the Epileptic in Queen Square in London (later called the National Hospital for Nervous Diseases). In the 1860s, Jackson worked out the notion of unilateral epilepsy: partial, or focal, fits originating from a lesion in the basal ganglia or cerebral cortex and then tracking to other muscle groups. This later became known as "Jacksonian" epilepsy. In Jackson's concept of the hierarchy of layers in the central nervous system, fits associated with the brainstem ("pontobulbar") originated at the lowest level; "epileptiform" fits, later called Jacksonian, originated from the middle level; and "epilepsy" as such came from the highest level, or cerebral cortex. In an article in 1875, reprinted in his *Selected Writings*, Jackson revived previous medical thinking about sensory "dreamy" state seizures, later called temporal lobe epilepsy, or psychomotor epilepsy. Jackson's work was spread through a myriad of dispersed articles, and an excellent guide to it is the magisterial study of medical historian Owsei Temkin, *The Falling Sickness* (1945; second enlarged edition, 1971). (*See also* **POSITIVE VS. NEGATIVE SYMPTOMS.**)

The investigation of epilepsy was placed on a modern footing with the development of electroencephalography by **Hans Berger** in the 1920s.

As for the treatment of epilepsy, London physician Charles Locock (1799–1875) proposed the use of bromide salts at a meeting in 1857 of the Royal Medical and Chirurgical Society. Of note as well, the bromide salts also had some efficacy as sedatives in the treatment of what was then called "hysteria." The landmark drug for the treatment of convulsions was the barbiturate phenobarbital (Luminal), which was patented by the Bayer company in 1911 and launched the following year. (*See* **BARBITURATES.**) Phenobarbital was also the classic long-acting sedative drug of the pre-**benzodiazepine** period. In 1938, at the instigation of Boston neurologist and neurosurgeon Tracy Jackson Putnam (1894–1975), the Parke-Davis company launched the nonsedating anticonvulsant phenytoin (Dilantin), which later showed efficacy in the treatment of mania.

In the 1990s and after, a number of anticonvulsant drugs started to be indicated as "mood stabilizers" in mania, notably valproic acid, first synthesized in 1882. Valproic acid's antiepileptic properties were discovered serendipitously in 1963, and shortly thereafter the sodium salt of the drug, called sodium valproate (Depakine) was marketed as an anticonvulsant and antimanic; another formulation, semi-sodium valproate, called sodium divalproex (Depakote), was introduced to the United States in 1983 as effective in epilepsy; it was later indicated for mania, and in 1997 was approved by the U.S. Food and Drug Administration for migraine headache. Epilepsy thus remains integrated with psychiatry at the level of pharmacotherapy. It has never been convincingly demonstrated that epilepsy itself is a source of psychiatric symptoms or represents a distinctive kind of personality, contrary to the conventional wisdom of the nineteenth century.

ERIKSON, ERIK (1902–1994). A psychoanalyst who said that human development continues throughout life, Erikson was born out of wedlock in Frankfurt, Germany. He never knew his birth father, but when his mother, who was Danish, married pediatrician Theodor Homburger when Erik was 3 years old, he took the name Erik Homburger.

His adoptive father was Jewish, his mother Lutheran; Erik Homburger was raised as a Jew. Taunted as a schoolboy for his "Jewishness," despite his starkly Nordic features, Erik Homburger became interested from early on in "identity crises." His high school graduation in Karlsruhe represented his highest academic degree. In 1927, at the suggestion of his friend Peter Blos, Erik Homburger went to Vienna to help Blos and the American psychoanalyst Dorothy Tiffany-Burlingham (1891–1979) found a progressive school for children. There he demonstrated that he had a "knack," in his term, for dealing with children; **Anna Freud** became involved in the school and also analyzed Erikson (he was subsequently trained at the teaching institute of the Vienna Psychoanalytic Society). Sensing a Nazi cataclysm in the offing, in 1933 he emigrated to the United States and set himself up as a child analyst in Cambridge, Massachusetts; he also joined the Harvard medical faculty. After a sojourn at Yale University as professor at the medical school and the Institute of Human Relations, in 1938 he left for the West Coast, where he began to theorize about child development as a response to societal prompts, rather than just inwardly driven by sexuality. (In 1939, he began calling himself Erikson rather than Homburger.)

In 1950, Erikson wrote *Childhood and Society,* for which he became widely celebrated, arguing that development continued throughout life in a series of eight stages—involving a "crisis" of identity in each—rather than just terminating at age 5 in some hard and fast mold. The book also helped build bridges from psychoanalysis to cultural anthropology and to social psychology. Erikson additionally became celebrated for two "psychobiographies" (a term he did not coin): *Young Man Luther* (1958) and *Gandhi's Truth* (1969). In 1950, he left the University of California rather than sign a loyalty oath and went as senior staff member to the Austen Riggs Center in Stockbridge, Massachusetts. In 1960, he returned to Harvard as a professor of human development, retiring in 1970. Erikson was said to be the first child analyst in the United States.

EROTOMANIA. Erotomania is the delusional belief that one's love for someone else is reciprocated. In the non-French world today, it is considered to be part of paranoia or schizophrenia, but in France, "Clérambault's syndrome" retains the status of an independent psychiatric diagnosis. The term "erotomania" in the sense of excessive sexual desire has a long history, going back at least to the seventeenth century. In the early nineteenth century, **Étienne Esquirol** gave it a second meaning, the delusional belief that one is loved by someone else: In his 1838 essay on "monomania," he wrote that, "Erotomania belongs to the medical disorders. It is a chronic cerebral disorder , characterized by excessive love, either for a known object or for an imaginary object. In this disorder, only the imagination is troubled; there is no lesion of thought" (*Des maladies mentales,* II, 32). In his *Clinical Lectures on Mental Diseases* (1883), Thomas S. Clouston (1840–1915), superintendent of the Edinburgh asylum, called it "old maids' insanity" and deemed it of ovarian origin. **Emil Kraepelin**, in his 1896 textbook, considered erotomania a form of "paranoia." The international literature of the time regarded excessive sex desire and delusional sexual ideas both to be forms of erotomania.

With the work of Parisian psychiatrists Paul Sérieux (1864–1947) and Joseph Capgras (1873–1950) on "Les folies raisonnantes" (intelligent insanity) in 1909 (*see* **FRENCH CHRONIC DELUSIONAL STATES**), French writing on the subject of erotomania diverged from the international literature: "erotic delusions" (le délire érotique) became a distinctive form of delusional thinking ("délire d'interprétation") without hallucinations and without progressing to madness. The French version became sharply chiseled by the beginning of the First World War: patients with incurable, well-tailored delusional systems about romancing a victim and who are neither demented, nor "paranoid" schizophrenics, nor any other kind of schizophrenic.

In 1920, Gaétan Gatian de Clérambault (1872–1934), head of the psychiatric emergency service of the Paris Prefecture of Police, assigned erotomania to the "passional psychoses," meaning any paranoid conviction held with intense feeling; thereafter, erotomania also became known as "Clérambault's syndrome" (written sometimes as "De Clérambault's syndrome). (*See* **FRENCH CHRONIC DELUSIONAL STATES: mental automatism** [1920].) (Note that Gatian de Clérambault is the correct form of Clérambault's family name, but it is seldom used.) He described the case of a woman who believed that the King of England was in love with her. Clérambault proposed a mechanism for the disorder—a toxic insult to the brain that he called "mental automatism." In making erotomania part of an autonomous category of psychiatric illness—the "passional psychoses" (les délires passionnels)—he asserted that they possessed their own distinctive laws of evolution separate from those of delusional thinking. In doing so, he aligned himself with the tradition of Paris neurologist **Jean-Martin Charcot,** who sought to identify the iron laws governing such presumably natural disorders as hysteria. (Clérambault gave his first account of an erotomania case in the December 1920 issue of the *Bulletin of the* [*Paris*] *Society of Clinical Mental Medicine* [*Bulletin de la Société Clinique de Médecine Mentale*], but only in the February 1921 issue did he spell out his ideas about the inevitable evolution of the disorder.)

Since Clérambault, erotomania has been seen as a form of schizophrenia or paranoia in Anglo-Saxon circles. It surfaced in ***DSM-III-R*** (1987) as "delusional disorder: erotomanic type," yet remains a distinctive illness entity in France. The disorder itself tends to be much in the media as stalkers of various public personalities—including such figures as Brad Pitt, Madonna, Gwyneth Paltrow, and Steven Spielberg—make the lives of their prey miserable until they become objects of a court order or confinement.

ESQUIROL, JEAN-ÉTIENNE-DOMINIQUE (1772–1840). Founder of the French tradition of psychiatric nosology, Esquirol was born in Toulouse into a noble family—his father was president of the chamber of commerce—and began his medical studies there in 1792. In 1799, he went up to Paris and started auditing **Philippe Pinel**'s courses at the **Salpêtrière hospice.** "It was that day that decided his fate," wrote psychiatrist René Semelaigne (1855–1934) many years later in his dictionary of French psychiatrists. "These two elite beings felt their mutual attraction to each other. Esquirol became Pinel's favorite student. Each day, Esquirol went to the Salpêtrière, accompanying his chief on rounds, helping him in his work. It was Esquirol who wrote [Pinel's] treatise of *Clinical Medicine* (*La Médecine clinique*), the first edition of which came out in 1802 (I, p. 126). As a result of all these interruptions, only in 1805 at age 33 did Esquirol manage to defend his doctoral dissertation on *The Passions . . . as a Cause of Mental Illness* (*Les Passions considérées comme causes . . . de l'aliénation mentale*) and graduate with an M.D. He argued, as Pinel had done, for the gentle treatment of those with mental illness and said they were not unlike patients with other kinds of medical illnesses.

In 1811, Esquirol joined Pinel on the medical staff of the Salpêtrière, where he remained until 1825 when the post of chief-physician at the national asylum in the Paris suburb of Charenton became vacant. Meanwhile, in 1802 Esquirol began taking a few wealthy patients into his private house across from the Salpêtrière. In 1827, he moved this establishment to vast new grounds at Ivry, and in his later years divided his time between Charenton and his private sanatorium, where he regularly entertained his students with memorable meals. (Semelaigne remembered Jacques-Joseph Moreau, called Moreau de Tours [1804–1884], at age 80, speaking almost with tears in his eyes of those Sunday dinners.) Although Esquirol was much involved with medical education (he initiated France's first course of psychiatry lectures in 1817) and with the reform of France's asylums, in retrospect he has mainly been remembered for his attempts to refine psychiatric diagnosis with such terms as "monomania" and "lypemania" (*see* **PSYCHOSIS: EMERGENCE: Esquirol's monomania, [1816, 1838]; DEPRESSION: EMERGENCE: lypemania** [1820]). In a three-volume work, *On Mental Illness* (*Des maladies mentales*), published in 1838, he reprinted a number of his earlier essays, bringing some of them up to date. Esquirol really represents the beginning of all classification in psychiatry, given that **William Cullen** had so little experience and classified on the basis of abstract principles.

EUGENICS. *See* **PSYCHIATRIC GENETICS.**

EXPOSURE THERAPY. *See* **COGNITIVE-BEHAVIORAL THERAPY.**

EXTRAPYRAMIDAL SIDE EFFECTS (EPS). "Extrapyramidal" means the tracts of the spinal cord involved in the involuntary movement of muscles: the pyramidal tract is for voluntary movement; "iatrogenic" means medically caused. Iatrogenic symptoms such as shuffling gait; tremor of the hands, tongue and facial muscles; and "oculogyric crises" (involuntary rolling upward of the eyes) caused by the effect of antipsychotic medication on these extrapyramidal tracts are referred to as extrapyramidal side effects, or EPS; they are also sometimes called extrapyramidal "signs," "symptoms," or "syndrome."

The term "extrapyramidal motor reactions" goes back to British neurologist Samuel Alexander Kinnier Wilson's (1874–1937) article on "the old motor system and the new" in the *Archives of Neurology and Psychiatry* in 1924. Yet, the first clinical observations of EPS in connection with antipsychotic drugs date from the mid-1950s. In 1954, Hans Steck (1891–1980), professor of psychiatry at the university clinic at Céry-Lausanne in Switzerland, called attention in the *Annales médico-psychologiques* to an "extrapyramidal syndrome" in patients on **chlorpromazine** and **reserpine**. As well, in 1954 Hans-Joachim Haase (1922–), then a staff psychiatrist at the mental hospital in Oberwil-Zug, also in Switzerland, reported in the *Nervenarzt* that chlorpromazine patients were developing a "Parkinsonian" syndrome. (*See* **PARKINSONISM: NEUROLEPTIC INDUCED; TARDIVE DYSKINESIA.**)

EY, HENRI (pronounced EYE) (1900–1977). Originator of the "organo-dynamic" school of thought in French psychiatry after the Second World War, Ey was born in a village in southwest France, finished his medical studies in Paris, and interned in the psychiatric hospitals of the Seine Department (Paris). In 1925, he became professor **Henri Claude's** (1869–1945) chef de clinique (comparable to an assistant professor who also has a junior hospital appointment) at **Ste.-Anne mental hospital**, then moved to Bonneval asylum (Eure-et-Loir department) in 1931 as chief psychiatrist. He would remain at Bonneval for the next 30 years. Ey promulgated an "organo-dynamic" view of psychiatry in which brain biology (on the model of John Hughlings Jackson's "hierarchy of distintegration") rubbed shoulders with psychoanalysis. Despite his rustic post, Ey remained an influential figure in Paris because of the Wednesday seminars that he held at Ste.-Anne, which had great influence upon the whole generation of French psychiatrists who came of age in the 1950s and 1960s. (The library where he gave these is now called the Henri Ey Library.)

Ey was said to have scorned the introduction of the new psychopharmaceuticals in the 1950s and after (even though they revolutionized his practice at Bonneval). His ideas about psychopathology, involving Jacksonian **positive and negative symptoms** across the whole range of psychosis and neurosis, appeared in his three volumes of *Psychiatric Studies* (*Études psychiatriques*) between 1948 and 1954. In 1960, Ey coauthored with Paul Bernard (qualified 1938) at the Ste.-Anne mental hospital and Charles Brisset (qualified 1944) at the Hôpital Rothschild an important *Textbook of Psychiatry* (*Manuel de psychiatrie*), and he was editor of the journal *L'évolution psychiatrique* from 1947 to 1971. Said Swiss psychiatrist Christian Müller (1921–) of Ey's influence, "If I had to make a choice . . . and say who around the year 1960 most authoritatively influenced European psychiatry, I would certainly name for Germany **Kurt Schneider**, for England **Aubrey Lewis**, and for France Henri Ey."

EYSENCK, HANS JÜRGEN (1916–1997). Born in Berlin, the child of an actor father (who was Protestant) and a film-star Protestant mother (who was Jewish by ethnicity), Eysenck was denied admission to the University of Berlin and in 1934 emigrated to England, where from 1936 to 1940 he studied psychology under the tutelage of Sir Cyril Burt (1883–1971) in London; he received a Ph.D. in psychology in 1940, briefly served as an air-raid warden, then from 1942 to 1946 did research in psychology at Mill Hill Emergency Hospital (an extension of the **Maudsley Hospital**) in London. In 1946, he joined the Maudsley proper and in 1947 became director of the hospital's psychology division. When in 1948 the postgraduate medical federation of the University of London enlarged the academic unit at the Maudsley, so that it became the Institute of Psychiatry, Eysenck became head of its psychology department; from 1955 he was professor of psychology until being emerited in 1983.

Rejecting Freudian doctrines in favor of biology and behaviorism, Eysenck is associated with shifting the discipline of psychology in England from psychological testing to clinical psychology, genetic research, and statistical methods. He is said to have been the founder of clinical psychology in the United Kingdom and to be the most-cited mental-health writer after Freud. His theory of behavioral therapy was based on personality types involving extraversion and introversion among others. (*See* **PERSONALITY DISORDERS: Eysenck's dimensions of personality** [1948].)

Together with American psychologist Burrhus Frederick Skinner (1904–1990), Eysenck presided over a massive expansion of clinical psychology, so that behaviorism passed from the hands of such Russian researchers as the physiologist Ivan Petrovich Pavlov (1849–1936), who in 1904 received the Nobel Prize for his discovery of the conditioned reflex, to a corps of office-practice psychologist–therapists. His many books and articles made him popular with the public, but such academic landmarks as *The Biological Basis of Personality* (1967) made him a towering scientific figure as well, despite his controversial approaches to such matters as hereditarianism in crime and the link between IQ and race, as well as to feminism and left-wing politics. His views about the "general intelligence factor," which in 1939 he called "g," and about what in 1952 he termed "psychoticism" ("P"), gave grist for research to a generation of psychologists. In 1964, he introduced the Eysenck Personality Questionnaire, based on his Maudsley Personality Inventory of 1959; the "EPQ" became a standard instrument in psychological testing. In propagating behavior therapy, Eysenck adopted the position that neurosis stems from learning experiences originally acquired to avoid anxiety, and what is learned can be unlearned. In 1965, he and Canadian psychologist Stanley Rachman published *The Causes and Cures of Neurosis: An Introduction to Modern Behaviour Therapy Based on Learning Theory and the Principles of Conditioning.* (*See* **COGNITIVE-BEHAVIORAL THERAPY** [from 1963].)

F

FALRET, JEAN-PIERRE (1794–1870). Born in the south of France, Falret studied medicine first at Montpellier University, then starting in 1811 in Paris; here he drifted into the orbit of **Philippe Pinel** and **Étienne Esquirol** and began working in Esquirol's private nervous clinic in the rue Buffon. Falret graduated with an M.D. in 1819. (In 1822, Falret and Félix-Auguste Voisin [1794–1872] founded their own private clinic in the suburb of Vanves.) In 1831, Falret landed at the **Salpêtrière hospice**, where he remained. Falret is known best for originating along with Baillarger the diagnosis manic-depressive illness. (*See* **MANIC-DEPRESSIVE ILLNESS: circular insanity** [1850].) He was a keen advocate of institutionalization, believing that the "isolation" of mental patients from their normal milieux in treatment-oriented mental hospitals would aid their recovery.

"FEIGHNER DIAGNOSTIC CRITERIA" (also called "the St. Louis criteria") (1972). Motivated by a desire to identify real psychiatric illnesses rather than the vague impressions then fashionable in American psychiatry, in 1972 a team of researchers in the department of psychiatry of Washington University School of Medicine in St. Louis suggested that, in terms of stability over time, family history, and well-defined clinical features, there were a small number of natural disease entities (in fact, 15). In the mood area, the researchers accepted depression and mania as "primary" disorders, plus reactive depression as a "secondary" disorder. They listed specific operational criteria the patient would have to meet to qualify for the diagnosis, such as sad mood, in addition to five of a list of eight other symptoms; for example, sleep difficulty, recurrent thoughts of death, or suicide. Chief author of the landmark article in the *Archives of General Psychiatry* was John Feighner (1937–), who had been a resident in that department. Among the co-authors were the leaders of the **St. Louis school** responsible for the revival of biological thinking in American psychiatry, such as **Eli Robins** (1921–1995), **Samuel B. Guze** (1923–2000), Robert A. Woodruff, Jr., (1934–), George Winokur (1925–1996), and Rodrigo Muñoz (1939–).

FENICHEL, OTTO (pronounced FEN-ee-kel) (1897–1946). Born in Vienna into a lawyer's family, Fenichel was a systematizer of psychoanalytic theory, especially the theory of neurosis. He graduated in medicine from Vienna in 1921, then became involved in the youth movement, especially those aspects stressing sexual liberation. Having audited Freud's lectures at the university during the First World War, in 1919 he organized in the medical faculty a psychoanalytically inspired Seminar for Sexology. Fenichel did psychoanalytic training analyses with Paul Federn (1871–1950) in Vienna and **Sándor Radó** in Berlin, and in 1924 in Berlin he organized a "child seminar" outside the framework of the local psychoanalytic institute. In Berlin, Fenichel sympathized with fellow psychoanalyst Wilhelm Reich's (1897–1957) communist associations: "Marxism and psychoanalysis counted alike for him as scientific disciplines," as one observer put it (quoted in Mühlleitner, *Biographien*, p. 94). In 1933,

Fenichel went into exile, first to Norway (where in 1934 he became secretary of the Danish-Norwegian Psychoanalytic Society), then to Prague, then after 1938 to the United States, where, like so many psychoanalysts, he settled in Los Angeles. His 1931 book, *Hysterien und Zwangsneurosen: Psychoanalytische Spezielle Neurosenlehre,* actually about hysteria and obsessive-compulsive disorder, was translated into English in 1934 as *Outline of Clinical Psychoanalysis.* In 1945, Fenichel's principal work was published, *The Psychoanalytic Theory of Neurosis,* with which he established himself as the "Encyclopaedist of Psychoanalysis." (*See also* **FREUDIAN INTERPRETATION OF OBSESSION: Otto Fenichel** [1945].)

FINK, MAXIMILIAN (MAX) (1923–). The leader of the movement to bring electroconvulsive therapy (ECT) back into American psychiatry, Fink was born in Vienna, the son of a physician. His parents moved shortly after his birth to the United States, and in 1945 Fink graduated with an M.D. from New York University. Between 1948 and 1953, he trained in psychoanalysis at the William Alanson White Institute, while simultaneously doing a psychiatry residency at Montefiore, Bellevue, and Hillside hospitals; he certified in neurology in 1952 and in psychiatry in 1954. In 1954, Fink was appointed director of research (and after 1956 director of the department of experimental psychiatry) at Hillside Hospital in Glen Oaks, New York. Between 1962 and 1966, he was director of the Missouri Institute of Psychiatry in St. Louis, then returned to New York where he was professor of psychiatry at New York College of Medicine. From 1972 until his retirement in 1997, he taught at the State University of New York campus at Stony Brook.

When Fink came to the largely psychoanalytically oriented Hillside Hospital as a resident in 1952, he was assigned to **electroconvulsive therapy**, and upon qualifying in psychiatry 2 years later, he became chief of the ECT and the **insulin coma** treatment service. In 1954, he received from the **National Institute of Mental Health** a grant for the study of electroencephalography (EEG) in electroconvulsive therapy, thus beginning his research career. In 1959, he and **Donald Klein** began at Hillside a random-assignment study of **imipramine**, **chlorpromazine**, and placebo, determining in several articles beginning in 1961 the antidepressant action of chlorpromazine and the effects of both drugs in various diagnoses. Fink studied the EEG effects of chlorpromazine (1955) and imipramine (1957) in patients and in normal volunteers. This marked the beginning of research in pharmaco-EEG. At a scientific congress in Rome in 1958, Fink met Turan Itil (1924–), a psychiatrist at the University of Nuremberg. (At that meeting, the two of them, together with Dieter Bente [1921–1983], also at Nuremberg, formed the International Pharmaco-EEG Group [IPEG].) At Fink's invitation, in 1963 Itil came to the Missouri Institute of Psychiatry, and the two of them began collaborating on a computer system for analyzing EEGs.

Fink's efforts to re-legitimize ECT, then under a cloud as a result of the **antipsychiatry movement**, began in 1967 as he and collaborators Richard Abrams (1937–) and Jan Volavka (1934–) of Prague began a systematic study of ECT supported by the National Institute of Mental Health. In 1972, together with Seymour Kety (1915–2000), then at Massachusetts General Hospital, and James McGaugh (1931–) of the University of California's Irvine campus, Fink organized the NIMH Conference on the Psychobiology of Convulsive Therapy (proceedings published in 1974). Fink's involvement with the American Psychiatric Association's task force on convulsive therapy, which met for the first time in 1975, represented a step forward in his efforts to rehabilitate ECT. (The task force's report on ECT appeared in 1978.) From 1980 to 1982, Fink served on the collaborative ECT project of the National Institute of Mental Health, and in 1985 he became founding editor of the journal *Convulsive Therapy*. Fink was the author of the then standard guide to ECT: *Convulsive Therapy: Theory and Practice* (1979) as well as of several later books on the subject.

FOLIE À DEUX. Referring to the contagion of psychological symptoms, the term was coined in 1877 by **Ernest-Charles Lasègue** and Jules-Philippe-Joseph Falret (1824–1902) in an article in the *Annales médico-psychologiques*. "It has been said that mental illness is contagious and that the company of mental patients should not be considered exempt of danger for those who live in contact with them" (p. 322). There were, the authors allowed, certain circumstances in which this statement is not entirely false. When delusional patients succeeded in imposing their views on a second person, this latter person had several characteristics: "That he be of weak intelligence, more disposed to passive docility than to emancipation; second, that he lives in constant contact with the patient; thirdly, that he be enlisted [in the delusion] by the lure of some kind of personal gain. . . . One gives into the pressure of madness only if it causes one to glimpse the realising of a cherished dream" (p. 326).

The German equivalent, "induced insanity"* (induziertes Irresein), was described by Georg Lehmann (1855–1918), then an assistant psychiatrist in the provincial asylum at Saargemünd in the former French province of Lorraine, in 1883 in the *Archiv für Psychiatrie und Nervenkrankheiten*. He concluded that the second person was usually constitutionally predisposed to mental illness. In 1894, Evariste Marandon de Montyel (1851–1908) at the Ville-Evrard asylum near Paris, in an article on "morbid mental contagion" in the *Annales médico-psychologiques*, identified three forms of the disorder: la folie communiquée (a concept that he took from Jules Baillarger [1809–1890] meaning approximately one person causing the symptoms of another, or induced insanity); la folie simultanée (two people exposed to the same cause who simultaneously become ill); and la folie imposée (a psychotic conveys his delusional ideas to someone who stands in a dependent relationship to him). ***DSM-III*** (1980) described folie à deux, with a nod to the French phrase, as "shared paranoid disorder": "The essential feature is a persecutory delusional system that develops as a result of a close relationship with another person who already has a disorder with persecutory delusions" (p. 197). In ***DSM-III-R*** (1987), this became "induced psychotic disorder"—with no mention of "folie à deux"—and in ***DSM-IV*** (1994) "shared psychotic disorder (folie à deux)."

FOREL, AUGUSTE (1848–1931). Known for his histological interests and his writings on hypnotism and sexuality, Forel was born on his parents' farm in Waadt Canton in Switzerland, acquired scientific interests (especially in ants) early in life, and, after

---

* In his *Psychopathology (Die Psychopathologie)* in 1913, **Karl Jaspers** considered epidemic hysteria to be a form of "induced insanity (the psychic epidemics)" (p. 340).

hearing Gustav Huguenin's and Bernhard von Gudden's lectures at the **Burghölzli** in Zurich, resolved to study psychiatry. After training in neurohistology with **Theodor Meynert** (1833–1892) in **Vienna** from 1871 to 1873, he got a post as assistant physician with Gudden (who had in the meantime come to Munich as professor of psychiatry) at the Provincial Asylum of Upper Bavaria, doing his Habilitation in Munich in 1877 on neuroanatomy. In 1879, he returned to Zurich and became soon thereafter professor of psychiatry and director of the university psychiatric clinic. In 1887, almost simultaneously with the Leipzig anatomy professor Wilhelm His (1831–1904)—who also was of Swiss origin—Forel developed the "neuron theory" of communication in the central nervous system. He did so via a procedure called "experimental degeneration," cutting a brain tract then observing the results.

In 1898, Forel resigned his professorship and retired to rural Switzerland where, having abandoned his neuroanatomical work, he devoted himself to research on sexual problems; his 1905 book, *The Sexual Question* (*Die Sexuelle Frage*) sold more than 100,000 copies in German and was translated into 11 languages. In addition to his research on sexuality and neuroanatomy (he was so familiar with brain architecture that he described the location of his own stroke), Forel was known for his hostility to alcohol and for an interest in hypnotism; he was also an international authority on ants.

FREE ASSOCIATION. *See* **FREUDIAN PSYCHOTHERAPY: TECHNIQUE.**

FRENCH CHRONIC DELUSIONAL STATES (from 1909). In France, there had been a long tradition of regarding delusions as the essence of psychosis, as witnessed in the work of **Valentin Magnan**. Yet around the time of the First World War, Magnan's distinction between degenerative and nondegenerative illnesses started to be played down. This compelled a whole reworking of the delusional diagnoses. As well, French psychiatrists were at pains to distance themselves from such German concepts as schizophrenia, which emphasized flattening of affect and other kinds of affective pathology. Delusional states became therefore catalogued on the basis of presumed mechanism (whether hallucinations or delusions were paramount). **Pierre Pichot** provides a useful explanation of these French diagnostic divergences in an article in *Psychological Medicine* (1982).

Chronic nonhallucinatory delusional states: delusional thinking (Le délire d'interprétation) (1909). Paris psychiatrists Sérieux and Capgras in their book *Intelligent Insanity: Delusional Thinking* (*Les folies raisonnantes: le délire d'interprétation*), hived these off from the larger block of delusions on the grounds that the absence of hallucinations and the failure to progress to dementia were important diagnostic features. (For details, *see* **PARANOIA**.)

Chronic imaginative psychosis (1910). This second member in the triad of French nondeteriorating delusional disorders, a classification that has survived to the present, was published by Ferdinand-Pierre-Louis-Ernest Dupré (1862–1921), then a staff psychiatrist at the Hôtel-Dieu hospital in Paris, and his student Benjamin Logre, in *L'Encéphale* under the title "Les délires d'imagination," meaning roughly elaborate confabulations. At a congress in 1910, they suggested "imagination," in the sense of fabrication, as a mechanism alongside hallucinations and interpretative delusions: "The imaginative patient is just as indifferent [as the delusional patient] to sensory impressions and logical demonstrations. . . . Creating fully formed his associations of ideas, the patient transposes upon the exterior world his subjective creations, giving them the character of objectivity. . . . The point of departure of his error is not the notion of an external fact, true or false . . . but a fiction of endogenous origin, a subjective creation. The delusional patient proceeds like a scholar, the imaginative patient like a poet" (*L'Encéphale*, 1911, p. 211). Many years later, and in apparent ignorance of Dupré's work, the American Psychiatric Association considered making "pathological lying" an official diagnosis.

Chronic hallucinatory psychosis (la psychose hallucinatoire chronique) (1911). Psychiatrist Gilbert-Louis-Siméon Ballet (1853–1916), who ran the service for "difficult psychopaths" at the Hôtel-Dieu hospital in Paris, proposed in 1911 in the journal *L'Encéphale* chronic hallucinatory psychosis combined with delusions as a distinct disease entity caused by heredity. The term was already familiar but, Ballet said, when properly circumscribed (as a singular noun) it represented a nosologically distinct disease. As with the Sérieux and Capgras formulation, Ballet's disease did not run downhill either, and other mental functions remained intact. The diagnosis was much debated in France, little adopted abroad, yet remains today a familiar construct.

Mental automatism and the passional psychoses (les psychoses passionnelles) of Gatian de Clérambault (1920). In 1920, Gaétan-Henri Gatian de Clérambault (1872–1934), often referred to as Clérambault rather than by his full last name, long-standing psychiatrist of the psychiatric emergency ward for the city of Paris (L'Infirmerie spéciale of the Prefecture of Police), published two important articles on delusional psychosis: the first, appearing in April in the *Bulletin of the Psychiatric Society* (*Bulletin de la Socíeté Clinique de Médecine Mentale*), proposed a possible mechanism for all of the delusional psychoses. Clérambault called it mental automatism and believed it similar to the underlying mechanism driving neurosyphilis, a profoundly organic cause of psychosis that literally took over the brain, producing "automatically" delusions and hallucinations.

A second article by Clérambault in December 1920 in the same journal introduced a new class of delusional disorders alongside the above-mentioned triad. Clérambault called them "the passional psychoses," meaning those with deep emotional conviction at their core; the psychosis springs fully formed into life, he said. Clérambault included among them erotomania, often called thereafter "Clérambault's syndrome," often confused with mental automatism as another "Clérambault's syndrome." (*See* **EROTOMANIA.**) Clérambault believed the whole range of these chronic systematized, or well-defined, psychoses to be driven by mental automatism.

Both concepts—mental automatism and the passional psychoses—had a large impact on French psychiatry, although Clérambault's doctrine of mental automatism has not survived, and the passional psychoses are no longer seen as independent entities.

FREUD, ANNA (1895–1982). One of the founders of the psychoanalysis of the child, she was born in Vienna the third daughter—and youngest of six children—of **Sigmund Freud**. She qualified in Vienna as a teacher, was analyzed between 1918 and 1921 by her father, and followed in his wake as a theorist of psychoanalysis, joining the Vienna Psychoanalytic Society in 1923. She opened a private psychoanalytic practice next to her father's in the family's spacious apartment at Berggasse 19 and wrote and lectured widely about the techniques of child analysis, publishing her first article on the subject—it was her introductory lecture to the Psychoanalytic Society in Vienna—in 1923. Her collected lectures appeared in 1927 as *Introduction to the Technique of Child Analysis* (*Einführung in die Technik der Kinderanalyse*). According to psychoanalysis historian Elke Mühlleitner, "For her father, sick with cancer from 1923 on, she took over a variety of duties, traveling in his stead to congresses, conducting negotiations, and accepting on his behalf a variety of prizes, including the Goethe Prize in 1930" (*Biographisches Lexikon*, p. 101). After Helene Deutsch emigrated in 1935 (*see* **WOMEN IN PSYCHIATRY**), Anna Freud became head of the psychoanalytic training institute of the society. Her main work appeared in 1936, *Das Ich und die Abwehrmechanismen* (*The Ego and the Mechanisms of Defense*), which became one of the foundation stones of "ego psychology." After the Nazi Anschluss with Austria in 1938, Anna fled with her father to London, where, in collaboration with James Strachey, she supervised the preparation and translation of her father's collected works.

In England, she became a major figure in the psychoanalysis of the child, first at the kindergarten Hampstead War Nurseries, open between 1941 and 1945; she then founded in 1947 the Hampstead Child Therapy Course and in 1952 a clinic attached to it, the Hampstead Clinic, which she directed until her death. From 1945 on she helped edit the journal *The Psychoanalytic Study of the Child*, and published in 1965 *Normality and Pathology in Childhood*. She was also known for conflicts with Vienna-born child psychoanalyst **Melanie Klein** who had settled in London in 1926 and viewed Anna's arrival with displeasure.

FREUD, SIGMUND (1856–1939). The originator of psychoanalysis, Sigismund Schlomo Freud was born in Freiberg, Moravia, the son of a merchant. Four years later, the family settled in Vienna, and Freud began medical studies in Vienna in 1873, finishing in 1881. He took so long to graduate because he had become intrigued by research in the basic sciences, especially with the work of physiologist Ernst Wilhelm von Brücke (1819–1892). Between 1882 and 1885, Freud did postgraduate training in various departments of the Vienna General Hospital, becoming a lecturer (Privatdozent) in 1885. The winter of 1885–1886 Freud spent as a fellow at the **Salpêtrière hospice** in Paris under **Jean-Martin Charcot**.

Yet, rather than continue with an academic career, in 1886 Freud started private practice in Vienna as a psychiatrist–neurologist, or Nervenarzt (he had never trained specifically in psychiatry). His academic interests, however, continued: In 1887, his friendship with the Berlin family doctor Wihelm Fliess (1858–1928) began, in the course of which Freud worked out the basic doctrines of psychoanalysis. In 1895, Freud published, together with his collaborator the Viennese family doctor Josef Breuer (1842–1925; pronounced BROY-er), *Studies in Hysteria* (*Studien über Hysterie*), to which Breuer contributed the case history of "Anna O" (Bertha Pappenheim, 1859–1936), and Freud several case histories of his own. This book marks the beginning of Freud's seeking the origins of patients' current problems in remote past events. In 1896, in a paper on "Heredity and the Etiology of the Neuroses," published in French, Freud used the term "psychoanalysis" for the first time, and in the following year abandoned the view that patients' seduction memories were owing to actual past occurrences.

Psychoanalysis as a doctrine was really launched with Freud's book *The Interpretation of Dreams* (*Die Traumdeutung*) in 1900. In 1902, Freud received the coveted appointment of associate professor (ausserordentlicher Professor) and thus the right to be addressed as "Herr Professor," on which he insisted thereafter. In 1902 as well, Freud founded the Psychological Wednesday Society, the beginning of psychoanalysis as a movement. In the coming years, such supporters as **Carl Jung** and Karl Abraham (1877–1925) were enlisted as acolytes, though Jung remained only briefly. In 1908, the Wednesday group was transformed into the more formal Vienna Psychoanalytic Society; simultaneously, the first international congress of psychoanalysis took place in Salzburg, followed by a second congress in 1910 in Nuremberg, and a third in 1911 in Weimar. In the first of many schisms, in 1911 Alfred Adler (1870–1937) left the Vienna Psychoanalytic Society; Jung's alienation from Freud would become manifest the following year. In 1913, there was a fourth international congress of psychoanalysis in Munich.

After the First World War, psychoanalysis grew inexorably as an international movement. Psychoanalytic outpatient clinics were opened in Berlin in 1920 and in Vienna in 1922. With the Nazi march into Austria of March 1938, psychoanalysis in Austria came to a brutal end, its practitioners forced into exile. Soon thereafter, the Freud family fled to London, where the Freuds took a house in the suburb of Hampstead. Freud died the following year of a maxillary cancer that had plagued him since 1923 at least (the year of his first operation); his personal physician Max Schur (1897–1969) ended his suffering with several injections of morphine. (For Freud's doctrines, *see* **FREUDIAN . . .** ; as well as specific psychoanalytic terms in their alphabetical order; *see also* **NARCISSISM; PARANOIA: Freud's view;** and **PERSONALITY DISORDERS: Freud and the "anal character"** [1908].)

FREUDIAN DOCTRINE OF HYSTERIA (1892 and after). The word "hysteria" accompanied Freud throughout his career. For him, it always meant physical symptoms having a psychological causation, yet his conception of the mechanism changed greatly during the years. In one of his earliest articles, "A Case of Hypnotic Healing" ("Ein Fall von hypnotischer Heilung") in the *Journal of Hypnotism and Suggestive Therapy* (*Zeitschrift für Hypnotismus, Suggestionstherapie*) (vol. 1, 1892–1893), he spoke of hysteria as involving "dissociation of consciousness."

Freud considered "conversion disorders" a particular form of hysteria. In his 1894 essay on the "Defensive Neuropsychoses" Freud explained that, in contrast to phobias and obsessions, in hysteria the intolerable memories of past events are detoxified in the mind by transmuting the sum total of their excitability into physical symptoms, "for which process I should like to propose the term 'conversion'" (*see* **"CONVERSION"**) ("Die Abwehr-Neuropsychosen," published in the *Neurologisches Zentralblatt*) (*Gesammelte Werke*, I, p. 63.)

Then in 1895, in *Studies in Hysteria* (*Studien über Hysterie*), which he co-authored with Viennese family doctor Josef Breuer (1842–1925), Freud argued that "traumatic hysteria" was caused by remote traumatic events and was treatable with cathartic therapy. It was here that Freud dilated upon the term "conversion symptom": "The hysterical nature of the defense [against intruding past memories] . . . consists in the conversion of the agitation into a somatic innervation, the benefit of which is that an unbearable idea is repressed from consciousness" (*Gesammelte Werke*, I, p. 181).

In 1905, in his "Fragment of an Analysis of Hysteria" ("Bruchstück einer Hysterie-Analyse") in the *Monatsschrift für Psychiatrie und Neurologie,* Freud showed in a case study that hysteria was intimately linked to the patient's underlying sexual life. "The psychopathology is, to put it bluntly, the patient's sexual life" (*Gesammelte Werke,* V, p. 278). Freud also said that sexuality in and of itself possessed biological components.

Finally in 1926, toward the end of his most productive theoretical years, in *The Problem of Anxiety* (*Hemmung, Symptom und Angst*) that appeared as a book, Freud called hysteria "the necessary defense against the libidinous demands of the Oedipus complex" (*Gesammelte Werke,* XIV, p. 146). Thus hysteria had become an intrapsychic mechanism for coping with anxiety, and subsequent psychoanalytic writing would *see* conversion symptoms as a way of binding anxiety.

FREUDIAN INTERPRETATIONS OF OBSESSION AND COMPULSION (from 1896). Aside from hysteria, obsession and compulsion constituted the core psychoneuroses (symptoms having an unconscious mechanism) that psychoanalysis sought to explain.

Freud first articulated his concept of obsessional neurosis (Zwangsneurose) in a paper "Further Observations on the Defense-Neuropsychoses" ("Weitere Bemerkungen über die Abwehr-Neuropsychosen") in the *Neurologisches Zentralblatt* in 1896. He explained that (all following translations are those of James Strachey), "the nature of the obsessional neurosis [is that] obsessional ideas are invariably transformed self-reproaches which have re-emerged from repression and which always relate to some sexual act that was performed with pleasure in childhood" (Freud, *Standard Edition,* III, p. 169).

In 1909, Freud enlarged this definition somewhat in "Notes upon a Case of Obsessional Neurosis" (Bemerkungen über einen Fall von Zwangsneurose), published in the *Yearbook of the Psychoanalytic Movement* and often referred to as "The Rat Man Case." Freud now wrote, "The compulsion . . . is an attempt at a compensation for the doubt and at a correction of the intolerable conditions of inhibition to which the doubt bears witness" (*Standard Edition,* X, p. 243; *Gesammelte Werke,* VII, p. 459). In this case, Freud viewed the process of regression as a special feature of the obsessional neurosis.

In 1926, in *The Problem of Anxiety* (*Hemmung, Symptom und Angst*), Freud spelled out the various defense mechanisms of the psyche against the intrusion of unwanted feelings, especially anxiety: "It is perhaps in obsessional cases more than in normal or hysterical ones that we can most clearly recognize that the motive force of defense is the castration complex and that what is being fended off are the trends of the Oedipus complex" (*Standard Edition,* XX, p. 114; *Gesammelte Werke,* XIV, p. 144). Freud said that the function of repression in patients with obsessional neurosis was to isolate the toxic affects from consciousness rather than to repress them by total amnesia, as in hysteria.

Otto Fenichel (1945) supplied the ultimate psychoanalytic formulation of obsessive neurosis in his textbook, *Psychoanalytic Theory of Neurosis* (1945). He began his chapter on "Obsession and Compulsion" with: "In all psychoneuroses the control of the ego has become relatively insufficient. . . . In compulsions and obsessions, the fact that the ego governs motility is not changed [unlike conversion disorders], but the ego does not feel free in using this government power. It has to use it according to a strange command of a more powerful agency, contradicting its judgment. It is compelled to do or to think, or to omit certain things; otherwise it feels menaced by terrible threats" (p. 268).

FREUDIAN INTERPRETATIONS OF PSYCHOSIS AND SCHIZOPHRENIA (1907 and after). Freud's fellow psychoanalyst Karl Abraham (1877–1925), who was just finishing a term as assistant physician at Bleuler's service in Zurich's **Burghölzli psychiatric clinic** and about to establish himself as a privately practicing psychiatrist in Berlin, attempted in 1907 a psychoanalytic explanation of adolescent sex dreams in dementia praecox, published in the *Zentralblatt für Nervenheilkunde und Psychiatrie* (he wrote a second article in 1908 on the difference between hysteria and dementia praecox).

Freud's own views of psychosis (1911). In 1911, Freud set himself for the first time to the task of explaining psychotic illness in terms of libido theory. (*See* **PARANOIA.**) In analyzing the autobiography of the jurist and politician Daniel Paul Schreber (who in 1903 had written a book about his nervous illness), Freud determined that paranoia and dementia praecox (schizophrenia) had different unconscious mechanisms. (Freud believed, however, that Schreber had paranoia, not schizophrenia.) Freud accepted **Emil Kraepelin's** construction of dementia praecox, as well as **Eugen Bleuler's** emendation of it. Yet, Freud disliked the terms the two men had devised, and explained dementia praecox in terms of a retreat of the libido from the outside world. He preferred the term "paraphrenia" (*Gesammelte Werke,* VIII, p. 313). Freud's paper "Psychoanalytic Remarks About an Autobiographically-Described Case of Paranoia (Dementia paranoides)" ("Psychoanalytische Bemerkungen über einen autobiographisch beschriebenen Fall von Paranoia [Dementia paranoides]"), appeared in the *Yearbook of Psychoanalytic Research* (*Jahrbuch der psychoanalytischen Forschung*) in 1911.

Psychoanalytic interpretations of psychosis resumed with the writings of Vienna psychoanalyst Paul Federn (1871–1950), especially his "Analysis of Psychosis" in the *International Journal of Psychoanalysis* ("Psychosenanalyse," *Internationale Zeitschrift der Psychoanalyse*) in 1933; then in the New World, these analytic efforts to confront psychosis were continued by, among others, the neo-Freudian **Harry Stack Sullivan.**

Psychoanalytic concept of "border-line" psychosis (1924). When he joined the Vienna Psychoanalytic Society in 1924, Robert Wälder (1900–1967), a Viennese lay-analyst, gave a paper entitled "Über den Mechanismen und Beeinflussungsmöglichkeiten der Psychosen." The paper was published in English in the *Journal of Psycho-Analysis* (1924) as "The Psychoses: Their Mechanisms and Accessibility to Influence." Wälder said he wanted to understand "the conditioning factors by which a psychosis comes about or is avoided in those 'border-line' characters in whom the phenomena of transition to a psychosis are so readily observed"* (p. 260).

---

* Wälder's "border-line" patients were not at all the same as the "border line" patients that New York psychoanalyst Adolph Stern (1879–1958) later described in a 1937 paper, published in 1938 in the *Psychoanalytic Quarterly*. (*See* **PERSONALITY DISORDERS: borderline** [1938].) By the term, Stern meant patients who were neither psychotic nor psychoneurotic but whose common characteristic was that they failed psychoanalysis. Stern suggested that these patients had 11 traits in common, including "narcissism" and "a state of deep organic insecurity or anxiety." (*See also* **BORDERLINE STATES.**)

FREUDIAN PSYCHOTHERAPY: TECHNIQUE (1893–1930s).

The "cathartic method" of Breuer and Freud (1893, 1895). In an article for the *Neurological Central Journal* (*Neurologisches Centralblatt*), Freud and Josef Breuer (1842–1925) reported the case of a young female patient with hysterical symptoms whom Breuer in the early 1880s had on successive occasions hypnotized, persuading her to shed her symptoms each time by coaxing her to recall her psychic condition at the origin of the symptom, thus achieving a "catharsis." As the two authors wrote in their 1893 "Preliminary Communication" (in James Strachey's translation), "The injured person's reaction to the trauma only exercises a completely 'cathartic' effect if it is an adequate reaction—as, for instance, revenge. But language serves as a substitute for action; by its help, an affect can be 'abreacted' almost as effectively" (p. 59 of Penguin edition). In 1895, Breuer and Freud published *Studies in Hysteria* (*Studien über Hysterie*); in his part of the book, Breuer reported this case more extensively, identifying the patient with the pseudonym "Anna O." (As English psychiatrist and psychoanalyst **Ernest Jones** revealed years later in his biography of Freud, her real name was Bertha Pappenheim [1859–1936].)

In his own practice, Freud began using the cathartic method, with or without hypnosis, then gradually going over to free association as a way of eliciting buried memories. In the conclusion of *Studies in Hysteria*, Freud said, "I have often in my own mind compared cathartic psychotherapy with surgical intervention. I have described my treatments as psychotherapeutic operations; and I have brought out their analogy with the opening up of a cavity filled with pus, the scraping out of a carious region, etc." (p. 392). Yet, it turns out that not all the details that Breuer reported of the Anna O. case were historically correct, and interested readers may wish to review her real tale, which the German medical historian Albrecht Hirschmüller has rescued from the records of the Swiss sanatorium "Schloss Bellevue" in Kreuzlingen, where she was subsequently admitted after Breuer's treatment (*see* his biography of Josef Breuer, published in 1978).

Freud's psychoanalytic method (1904 and after). (*See also* **ID.**) Although Freud's techniques evolved steadily from the time of the cathartic therapy (early 1890s) onward—and may be gleaned from his various case studies, only around 1904 does he start to explain the technique of psychoanalysis. In a paper he published in a volume that Munich psychiatrist Leopold Löwenfeld (1847–1924) edited, on *Psychic Compulsive States* (*Psychische Zwangserscheinungen*), Freud laid out what he called "Freud's Psychoanalytic Method" ("die Freudsche Psychoanalytische Methode"), explaining that he places his patients in a comfortable recumbent position on a sofa, with Freud seated on a chair behind them. Speaking of himself in the third person, Freud continued, "He reminds them, before they get into a detailed recounting of their case history, to say out loud everything that runs through their head in this connection, even if they believe it to be unimportant or irrelevant, or that it is nonsense. With special emphasis, however, they are called upon not to exclude any thought or recollection from the account on the grounds that this information could be shameful or embarrassing." The analyst then sees what has been left out of the account, or repressed, in an act of resistance. The significance of the resistance must then be interpreted (Deutung), the details of which Freud said he was not yet ready to make public (*Gesammelte Werke*, V, pp. 5–7).

According to psychoanalysis historian Reuben Fine, Freud's psychoanalytic technique evolved through four stages: (1) making the unconscious conscious (1886–1905), (2) working through transference and resistance (1905–1914), (3) plumbing the architecture of the psyche, in terms of ego and id (1915–1923), and (4) the function of analysis as creating a proper setting for ego functioning (1923–1939) (*see* Fine, *History of Psychoanalysis*, p. 499).

Stekel's "brief" psychoanalytic technique (1919).* One innovative idea of **Vienna** psychoanalyst and heretic Wilhelm Stekel (1868–1940), over which the official psychoanalytic movement has passed largely in silence, is Stekel's notion of ending psychoanalytic treatments successfully within 3 to 4 months. He adumbrated this view in an article in *Today's Therapeutics* (*Therapie der Gegenwart*) in 1919, saying "Anxiety neuroses have a good prognosis and are curable in four to six weeks" (p. 339). Then in his 1938 book about technique (*Technik der analytischen Psychotherapie*), Stekel returned to the theme more fully: "Many years ago I called attention to the fact that one can achieve splendid results in a short time (in 2–3 months). Patients who came to me from abroad and were unable to remain in Vienna more than 6 to 8 weeks were freed of their complaints and were made well again in a personal and social context. As counterexamples I knew of many interesting foreigners who had been in daily analysis over a year and even five years (!) without improving an iota." Referring to his brief, interventionist technique as the "active method," he said the analyst must follow his intuition in quizzing the patient (otherwise forbidden in classical psychoanalysis), because: "The patient is an actor, who plays a part both to himself and to us and believes that he is getting the better of us. Of course Freud believes in the unconscious. I no longer believe in the unconscious. Thirty years of experience have proven to me the contrary" (pp. 7–9; exclamation in original).

Ferenczi's "active" psychoanalytic technique (from 1920). In a speech at the Sixth International Congress of Psycho-Analysis at The Hague in 1920, Hungarian analyst Sandor Ferenczi (1873–1933), a family doctor in Budapest who brought psychoanalysis to Hungary and was one of Freud's closest co-workers, described "active therapy," a technique he said he was "further" characterizing, thus intimating that it was Freud who had first come up with it. But in contrast to Freud's "passive" technique, Ferenczi's "active" methods involved giving patients all kinds of interactions: "I soon had the opportunity to apportion to a patient tasks that consisted in her renunciation of certain hitherto pleasurable activities (onanistic stimulation of the genitals . . .). The result was that new memories became accessible and the progress of the analysis was visibly accelerated" (Ferenczi, *Further Contributions*, English translation, 1927, p. 201). In fact, Ferenczi was full of prompts for his patients, giving them orders—later "suggestions"—and prohibitions, encouraging them to vent their negative feelings

---

* The beginning of brief psychotherapy is usually associated with psychoanalysts Otto Rank (1884–1939) and Sandor Ferenczi (*see* below), who in their 1924 book, *The Development of Psychoanalysis* (*Entwicklungsziele der Psychoanalyse*), argued that analyses could be shortened if the analyst renounced the goal of illuminating every last aspect of the patient's personality structure: "It was a fateful error to believe that no one can be completely analyzed who has not been theoretically enlightened about all the details of one's own abnormalities" (p. 50). Yet, Stekel clearly preceded them.

toward their therapists, even kissing some of them. The idea was, in the words of Ferenczi's young colleague Sandor Lorand (1893–1987), "to request the patient—in addition to using free association—to act or behave in a certain way, in the hope of increasing tension, thereby mobilizing unconscious material." Ferenczi had the view that some very intractable patients required "love," in order for them to restore contact with their psychic condition before the trauma occurred (Lorand, in Alexander, ed., *Psychoanalytic Pioneers*, pp. 20, 23).

Kohut's "self psychology" (1971). Heinz Kohut's self-psychology was one of the three streams into which classic Freudian psychoanalysis broke (the other two being ego psychology, which is a continuation of the classic tradition, and object relations theory, which is associated with the United Kingdom and rival subcamps having as their quarrelsome historic leaders **Melanie Klein**, **Anna Freud**, and Donald Woods "D. W." Winnicott (1897–1971). Self-psychology made a large impact in the United States in the 1970s and 1980s after the publication of Kohut's book, *The Analysis of the Self* (1971).

Heinz Kohut (1913–1981), a Vienna-born physician who had fled Austria to come to the United States in 1941 (where he resumed his medical career as a resident in neurology in Chicago), believed that classic psychoanalysis did not work for the kinds of help that patients were increasingly seeking. Rather than requesting relief for classical psychoneurotic symptoms, U.S. patients were having problems with relationships or experiencing a sense of meaningless. Kohut labeled this new pattern of complaints with Freud's term "narcissism" (*see* **NARCISSISM; PERSONALITY DISORDERS: *DSM-III*** [1980]) and recommended an empathic kind of psychotherapy to fill the patient's "self." Kohut wrote in *The Analysis of the Self* of these narcissistic personalities: "The spontaneous establishment of one of the stable narcissistic transferences [**transference** permits depth psychotherapy to take place] is the best and most reliable diagnostic sign which differentiates these patients from psychotic or borderline cases, on the one hand, and from ordinary transference neuroses, on the other" (p. 4). As for symptoms, Kohut said, "The patient will describe subtly experienced, yet pervasive feelings of emptiness and depression. . . . The patient will attempt to let the analyst know that . . . he is not fully real, or at least that his emotions are dulled; and he may add that he is doing his work without zest, that he seeks routines to carry him along since he appears to be lacking in initiative" (p. 16). Addressing these kinds of complaints in urban post-1970s America procured for Kohut a large following.

Sifneos's "short-term psychotherapy" (1972). In his role as director of the Psychiatry Clinic of the Massachusetts General Hospital from 1954 to 1968, Peter E. Sifneos (1920–) developed a short-term psychotherapy technique based on the principle of provoking anxiety through challenging questions rather than assuaging it. In his book *Short-Term Psychotherapy and Emotional Crisis* (1972), Sifneos called his technique "similar in theory" to long-term psychoanalytic psychotherapy but focused on solving the patient's main emotional problem. The crisis-intervention phase lasted up to 2 months and the "short-term anxiety provoking" part 2 to 12 months. Sifneos added, "Psychoanalysis, of course is anxiety-provoking psychotherapy of long-term duration" (p. 71).

FRONTAL LOBES. Among the lobes of the brain, the frontal lobes have the main responsibility for executive functions; neuropsychiatric lesions of the frontal lobes are likely to result in disinhibition, apathy, and executive deficits such as lack of persistence and perseveration (too much persistence). This kind of knowledge was built up in years of experience with head trauma: noting the deficits that a particular injury produced. (*See* **BODY IMAGE: DISTURBANCES OF: Head** [1918].) Yet, in functional psychiatric illness (depression, schizophrenia, and other major disorders without a known structural cause), the frontal lobes have a particular role as well. In 1913, in the eighth edition of his textbook, **Emil Kraepelin** noted that the histological findings of a number of researchers pointed to some kind of lesion in the frontal lobes (*Psychiatrie,* 8th ed., III [2], p. 903). Yet, the light microscopes used by that generation of investigators were unable to spot differences in the size of various brain structures in health and illness: They could only note disorder in the various cell layers of the cerebral cortex.

With the advent of sophisticated techniques of **neuroimaging** in the 1970s and after, however, it became possible to detect differences in the size and function of various brain structures in schizophrenics compared to controls. At this point, investigators revived the "hypofrontality" hypothesis of schizophrenia. In 1974 in the *Acta Psychiatrica Scandinavica,* David H. Ingvar (1924–2000) and Göran Franzén (1929–), of the departments of clinical neurophysiology and psychiatry at Lund University, using radionuclides, noted abnormalities in blood flow in the frontal lobes of schizophrenic patients. In 1985, in a volume on localizing schizophrenia that was edited by **Nancy Andreasen**, Daniel Weinberger (1947–), then chief of the section on neuropsychiatry at the **National Institute of Mental Health**, asked "Is schizophrenia a frontal lobe disease?" and mobilized the evidence that pointed to yes. Nancy Andreasen's own magnetic resonance imaging study, completed in 1986 and published in the *Archives of General Psychiatry*, added further evidence to the rapidly growing incrimination of the frontal lobes. This work on "hypofrontality" represents an interesting, if unwitting, confirmation of the ideas about the frontal lobes of the classic psychiatric tradition.

G

GATIAN DE CLÉRAMBAULT, GAETAN-HENRI. *See* **EROTOMANIA; FRENCH CHRONIC DELUSIONAL STATES: mental automatism** (1920).

GENETICS. *See* **PSYCHIATRIC GENETICS.**

GERMAN "ROMANTIC" PSYCHIATRY. Several prominent German psychiatrists who flourished in the last years of the Romantic movement (the early nineteenth century) were called by their opponents "Romantic" psychiatrists because of the prominence they gave to moral values. These psychiatrists held "romantic" views because of the almost mystical links that they glimpsed between psychiatry and philosophy and because of a belief in the psychogenesis of illness (as opposed to the somatogenic beliefs of the biological psychiatrists). The Romantic psychiatrists were entirely eclipsed by the continued surge of biological thinking in the 1860s and after, and they are important historically only because they represent an initial eruption of psychological thinking into psychiatry. Among prominent Romantic psychiatrists were the following individuals.

Johann Christian Reil (pronounced RILE) (1759–1813). Born into a pastor's family in East Friesia, Reil is remembered for introducing psychological approaches to German psychiatry. He graduated with an M.D. from Halle in 1782, received his Habilitation in Berlin, then after 1788 was professor of medicine in Halle and head of the clinical institute. Called in 1810 to be professor of medicine in Berlin, he died 3 years later in a typhus epidemic after the battle of Leipzig. In addition to his practical efforts to have city asylums founded in Berlin and Halle, Reil is known for his book *Rhapsodies on the Application of the Psychic Method of Cure in Mental Disorders* (*Rhapsodien über die Anwendung der psychischen Curmethode auf Geisteszerrüttungen*) that he published in 1803. He argued for "psychic" approaches to mental illness in addition to the standard physical therapies of the day: Physicians used "psychic," or psychological, methods "when they act upon states of mind [Seelenkräfte], ideas, feelings and desires in such a manner as to produce changes in the patient's organization of mind, through which their illnesses are healed" (p. 25). Given that medicine already had two main treatment orientations—surgical and medical—"it is now time to add a third, the psychic" (p. 27). Reil suggested using the whole atmosphere of the asylum, rather than some particular psychotherapeutic scheme, as the best way of influencing the patients' thoughts.

Filled with notions of the "animal magnetism" of his day, Reil understood psychology as the study of the "anomalies of the self-consciousness of subjectivity," as for example doubting the realness of one's own personality "or confusing our ego [unser Ich] with that of another person" (pp. 71–72). He described somnambulism and multiple personalities as psychological disorders. Medicine, he said, concerned itself with the natural sciences. But "a medical psychology would be something else entirely, the quintessence of empirical and psychological understanding, conceived with constant attention to the reciprocal relationship of both of these sides of the human condition and staying in the closest possible relationship to the task of healing" (pp. 38–39).

Romantic in all this was Reil's insistence on the primacy of free will over passion. Reil saw insanity as limiting the freedom of the patient's will: "The relationship of the parts of the mind [das Seelenorgan] to one another is based on a certain distribution of psychic energy in the brain and the entire nervous system. If this relationship is disturbed, dissonance arises: leaps of thought, abnormal ideas . . . fixed rows of ideas, and the corresponding drives and actions. The capacities of the mind [Seelenvermögen] cease to be responsive to the freedom of the will" (p. 46). The best way to make the mind obedient again to the will was to subject the patients to iron discipline in mental institutions, he said.

Reil is, ironically, probably best known to medical students for having described a particular brain structure, the "island of Reil," or insula, which forms part of the boundary of the auditory sensory area.

Johann Christian August Heinroth (1773–1843). Born of a medical family in Leipzig, Heinroth exemplified the moralizing side of Romantic psychiatry, with its doctrine of self-control over the passions. He began medical studies in Leipzig in 1791, finally graduating after numerous interruptions in 1805. He earned his Habilitation the following year with a work on "medical anthropology," then in 1811 received a lectureship in psychiatry at Leipzig University, and in 1827 was appointed professor of psychiatry. Although his big *Textbook of Disturbances of Mental Life* (*Lehrbuch der Störungen des Seelenlebens*), published in 1818 and translated into English in 1975 by George Mora, was permeated by a kind of pietistic mysticism, it did attempt a new classification of psychiatric illnesses that tried to delineate many specific subtypes. His moralizing approach to illness received perhaps its fullest expression in his *Textbook of Mental Hygiene* (*Lehrbuch der Seelengesundheitskunde*), published in 1825 and filled with such observations as, "The passions are like glowing coals hurled into the house of life, or serpents that spew poison into the veins, or vultures that devour the innards. From that moment on, when people let themselves be transported by passion, order comes to an end in the economy of their lives" (p. 591).

Carl Wilhelm Ideler (pronounced EE-del-er) (1795–1860). Born into a pastor's family, Ideler studied medicine in Berlin, qualifying in 1821. In 1828, he was summoned from private general practice to supervise the psychiatry beds of the Charité Hospital in Berlin; the invitation came from an official of the Prussian government who had read Ideler's book *Anthropology for Physicians* (*Anthropologie für Ärzte*), which was published in 1826. In 1830, psychiatry at the Charité became a separate division, with Ideler at its head. He received the Habilitation as a university lecturer the following year. In 1839, he was appointed professor of psychiatry and remained in office until his death in 1860, "like a ruined castle from the past looming into the present," as someone said. Although Ideler was not an innovator in asylum management—relying upon forcible techniques of confinement in order to encourage the patients to fight off the evil influence of passion—he did emphasize the psychological aspect of psychiatric illness. For example, in an article in the *General Journal of Psychiatry* (*Allgemeine Zeitschrift für Psychiatrie*) in 1846, he pleaded for a revival of psychological thinking and for less emphasis on pathological anatomy. Ideler was often thought of as a disciple of Heinroth's, with the same moralizing bent and desire to use the power of confinement in order to drive the devil out of his patients.

Because of their metaphysical orientation, some of the German Romantic psychiatrists were often referred to as the "psychic school" (Psychiker), in contrast to the somatically oriented school (Somatiker), who saw psychiatric illness as medical illness. Among prominent Somatiker of the pre-1860 period were Karl Wigand Maximilian Jacobi (1775–1858), director of the Siegburg asylum, and Johann Baptist Friedreich (1796–1862), professor of psychiatry in Würzburg. The rather philosophical debate between these two schools subsided with the ascendancy of the medical-empirical approach to psychiatry as represented by Berlin professor **Wilhelm Griesinger**, who took over Ideler's chair at the Charité in 1865.

GESTALT THERAPY. "Gestalt," meaning in this context wholeness of form, became a kind of therapy associated with the human potential movement of the 1960s and 1970s. Although the concept of wholeness of form—and the persistence of the whole despite changes in it—goes back to the Ancients, the term "Gestalt" was revived in 1890 by the German philosopher Christian von Ehrenfels (1859–1932). In the years between the World Wars, a school of German psychologists adopted the concept as a way of thinking about visual and auditory perception, and it retained considerable currency even after the Second World War when in 1952, in the journal *Studium Generale,* Klaus Conrad (1905–1961), professor of psychiatry at Homburg University in the German province of Saarbrücken, suggested the psychologists' recent work on "Gestalten" might offer psychiatry a useful third way of proceeding, beside Jaspers's "infrapsychic" biological approach and the "ultrapsychic" invocation of archetypes: "I propose that the analysis of psychopathological events from the viewpoint of Gestalt-theory be called "Gestalt analysis [Gestaltanalyse]" (p. 49).

Yet, the concept of "Gestalt therapy" came to the United States via psychoanalyst Fritz Perls (1893–1970), who had studied medicine in Berlin, undergone there several training analyses, and then in 1926 gravitated to Frankfurt am Main to continue his analysis and to work as an assistant in neurologist Kurt Goldstein's (1878–1965) Institute for Neurology. It was Goldstein who introduced Perls to Gestalt psychology. In 1933, Perls migrated from Germany to South Africa and there in 1941–1942 wrote a manuscript, published only in 1945 in London as *Ego, Hunger and Aggression*, that outlined the principles of Gestalt therapy, directed toward the reestablishing of wholeness in the battered psyche. In 1946, Perls migrated to the United States, landing after many peregrinations in 1966 as resident psychiatrist at the Esalen Institute in Big Sur, California. He also founded institutes for Gestalt therapy in New York and in British Columbia. His book *Gestalt Therapy: Excitement and Growth in the Human Personality* (1951) made him a forerunner of the human potential movement, whereby he accentuated "unlimited spontaneity." (*See* **PSYCHOTHERAPY: Carl Rogers**.) The basic premise of Gestalt therapy is that the neurotic's conceptual field is cluttered with Gestalten, or intuitive forms, and that he is unable to make sharp differentiations about what he or she really wants. The therapy restores him to a position where need satisfaction is possible.

GRIESINGER, WILHELM (pronounced GREE-sing-er) (1817–1868). Considered the virtual founder of the first wave of biological psychiatry because of his views on the organicity of mental illness, Griesinger was born in Stuttgart. He graduated in 1838 in medicine at Tübingen with a particular interest in infectious diseases and served between 1840 and 1842 as an assistant of Ernst Albert Zeller (1804–1877) at the Winnenthal asylum. On the basis of this experience, he wrote an article in 1843 on "psychic reflex actions" (in the *Archiv für physiologische Heilkunde*), which might be considered important as setting the stage for looking at the brain physiologically rather than spatially (neurology gets the spatial perspectives). Then in 1845 at the age of 28, he published a psychiatry textbook, *Mental Pathology and Therapeutics* (*Die Pathologie und Therapie der psychischen Krankheiten*), a manual that expressed Griesinger's organicist view: "All mental illness [alles Irresein] is based on brain disease," he said (p. 7).

Yet, the manual enjoyed no particular reknown. Returning to Tübingen, he completed his Habilitation at the medical clinic in 1847, with the right to lecture in general pathology. At this point, Griesinger began a long series of wanderings: 1849 to Kiel as Ordinary professor and director of the outpatient clinic, then 1850 to Cairo as director of the Egyptian medical services, then 2 years later back to Germany again where in 1854 he became director of the medical clinic in Tübingen. In 1860, he was called to Zurich, where he became director of the cantonal hospital and, in addition, took over the headship of the city asylum, beginning in 1863 a series of lectures in psychiatry. In 1861, he published a second and greatly revised edition of his earlier textbook; this much more influential edition had a role in shifting psychiatry onto a more biological basis. Griesinger's migrations came to an end in 1865 as he moved to Berlin as Ordinary professor, director of the university's medical clinic in the Charité hospital (which he gave up in 1867), and simultaneously director of the psychiatric clinic, where his heart now lay. Together with Ludwig Meyer (1827–1900), professor of psychiatry in Göttingen, and *Carl* Friedrich Otto Westphal (1833–1890), at the time an assistant in the psychiatric clinic of the Charité, in 1867 he founded an important new psychiatric journal, the *Archive of Psychiatry and Nervous Diseases* (*Archiv für Psychiatrie und Nervenkrankheiten*), the first issue of which appeared in October of that year (although "1868–70" is printed on the title page of the first volume). In October 1868, Griesinger died of appendicitis at age 51.

The intellectual achievements for which Griesinger is remembered were mainly crowded into the brief period at the end of his life: First, he wanted to break with the tradition of **German "Romantic" psychiatry**, exemplified by his predecessor at Berlin, Carl Wilhelm Ideler, and to make a scientific, clinically oriented psychiatry the intellectual equal of the other medical specialties, indeed to revive the teaching of psychiatry to medical students in a downtown urban clinic rather than in outlying rural asylums. Another achievement was the second edition of his textbook, *The Pathology and Treatment of Mental Illnesses*, in 1861, expanding as it did the concept that the brain was the seat of mental illness. Finally, Griesinger's new journal, the *Archive*, in the hands of Meyer and Westphal quickly became the leading research journal in psychiatry internationally; it was explicitly dedicated to work on the underlying neurological nature of psychiatric illness. In retrospect, Griesinger figures as the founder of the first "biological psychiatry" (the second surfacing in our own time).

GROUP THERAPY. *See* **PSYCHOTHERAPY: group psychotherapy** (1939); **"therapeutic community"** (from 1939).

GUZE, SAMUEL BARRY (pronounced Goo-ZAY) (1923–2000). Born in New York City, in 1945 Guze earned his M.D. at Washington University in St. Louis. He trained in internal medicine at Barnes Hospital (one of the teaching hospitals of Washington University) and at a Veterans Administration hospital in Connecticut. It was at Barnes that he became interested in psychiatry while working in the consultation-liaison service; there he encountered staff psychiatrist George Saslow (1906–), who was very hostile to psychoanalysis.

In 1951, Guze joined the psychiatry department at Washington University as an instructor, ultimately succeeding **Eli Robins** in 1975 as head of psychiatry; he retired from the post in 1989. As one of the founders of the **St. Louis school**, Guze like Robins was convinced that psychiatry must again become part of medicine; he rejected the "biopsychosocial" model of psychiatry propagated by University of Rochester internist and psychiatrist **George L. Engel** and argued for the medical model in his 1992 book, *Why Psychiatry is a Branch of Medicine*.

Guze is particularly known for his 1962 work on chronic **hysteria**, later called somatization disorder, in which he linked a family history of hysteria on the female side of a family tree to sociopathic behavior on the male side; it was published in the *New England Journal of Medicine*, with Guze's resident Michael Perley (1936–) generously listed as the main author. (Perley went on to have a career as endocrinologist and nephrologist.) In 1970, Guze baptized chronic hysteria "Briquet's syndrome," after the French psychiatrist Pierre Briquet (1796–1881), whose 1859 book, *Traité clinique et thérapeutique de l'hystérie*, was one of the first quantitative studies of the disorder. (Yet, it was in 1881 that Briquet enunciated his concept of hysteria as a chronic familial illness.) (*See* **HYSTERIA: "Briquet's Syndrome"** [1881].) Guze was a coauthor, with resident John Feighner, of a 1972 paper on psychiatric diagnosis published in the *Archives of General Psychiatry* that introduced operational criteria for making diagnoses. In 1974, Guze and Donald Goodwin (1931–1999), another member of the St. Louis school, wrote a book on *Psychiatric Diagnosis* that has been described as "the manifesto" of the St. Louis school. In that year, Guze was offered the chair of psychiatry at Johns Hopkins University but decided to stay at Washington University and "look after Eli." Robins and Guze stressed the concept of "validation" of psychiatric diagnoses. Guze in particular insisted on "external" validation. This led to a falling out between the St. Louis school and **Robert Spitzer** and the ***DSM-III*** drafters, who sought "reliability," meaning agreement among users.

H

HALLUCINATION. *See* **FRENCH CHRONIC DELUSIONAL STATES; PSYCHOSIS: EMERGENCE; SCHIZOPHRENIA: EMERGENCE; SCHIZOPHRENIA: RECENT CONCEPTS.**

HALLUCINOGEN. Drugs to induce hallucinations experimentally—even therapeutically—were introduced in psychiatry in the 1940s under the label "psychotomimetics" or "psychodysleptics." The prehistory: In 1845, Paris psychiatrist Jacques-Joseph Moreau (1804–1884) (called "Moreau de Tours," after the city where he began his medical studies) initiated the study of experimental psychosis through his work on *Hashish and Mental Illness* (*Du hachisch et de l'aliénation mentale: études psychologiques*). The subject rested then for many years, to be resumed again by the great Berlin pharmacology professor Louis Lewin (1850–1929) in his 1924 study *Phantastica: the Sedative and Excitatory Drugs of Pleasure* (*Phantastica: die betäubenden und erregenden Genussmittel*), where he did experimental work on opium, cocaine, and cannabis indica, among other drugs. (Lewin, who refused to convert to Christianity, never received a proper professorship and had been only "titular professor" at Berlin's Technical University [Technische Hochschule], "honorary professor" at the time he wrote this book.)

Kurt Beringer (1893–1949) at Heidelberg was known for writing in 1927 the classic work, his Habilitation, on mescaline intoxication (*Der Meskalinrausch*)—the first work on experimental psychosis as a way of studying psychopathology. In 1934 in the *American Journal of Psychiatry*, Erich Lindemann (1900–1974), then a resident at the University of Iowa, explained how they had used mescaline, hashish, cocaine, and Sodium Amytal on schizophrenic and psychoneurotic patients at the university psychiatric hospital.

Yet, the modern era of using drugs to investigate brain function was arguably introduced in 1943 by lysergic acid diethylamide, referred to as "LSD-25," which Albert Hofmann (1906–), a chemist at Sandoz Limited in Basel, Switzerland, together with a colleague, synthesized in 1938 in an effort to find drugs that act on the uterus in the same manner as ergot. In 1943, Hofmann returned to the compound and serendipitously noted that it made him dizzy; then, curious about its brain effects, he carried out a systematic self-experiment, discovering it to be a powerful hallucinogen. Up to that point, no compound had been known in psychiatry with such an ability to transform perception. In 1947, psychiatrist Werner Stoll, the son of the Sandoz pharmacology director Arthur Stoll (1887–1971), did a controlled clinical study of LSD (6 schizophrenic patients and 16 normal controls) at the **Burghölzli** mental hospital (published in the *Swiss Archives of Neurology and Psychiatry*), and Sandoz made it available as the investigational drug Delysid, said to improve patients' ability to recall distant memories in psychotherapy. In 1949, Gion Condrau (1919–) at the Burghölzli tried it on a wider range of diagnoses and reported in the *Acta Psychiatrica Neurologia* that most patients were actually quite unresponsive, unlike the dramatic effects on controls.

Thereafter, therapeutic use of the hallucinogens went in two directions: as a low-dose "psycholytic" on neurotic patients; *see* the first therapeutic study of LSD in the United States in 1950 by Anthony K. Busch (1905–) of the St. Louis State Hospital and Warren C. Johnson (1923–) of Washington University, who concluded in *Diseases of the Nervous System* that "L.S.D. 25 may offer a means for more readily gaining access to the chronically withdrawn patients. It may also serve as a new tool for shortening psychotherapy" (p. 243).

The other direction was as a high-dose "psychedelic"; the term was suggested in 1957 by Humphrey Fortescue Osmond (1917–2004), the superintendent of Saskatchewan Hospital in Weyburn, Saskatchewan, in the *Annals of the New York Academy of Sciences*: "I have tried to find an appropriate name for the agents under discussion," said Osmond, "a name that will include the concepts of enriching the mind and enlarging the vision. . . . My choice, because it is clear, euphonious, and uncontaminated by other associations, is psychedelic, mind-manifesting" (p. 429). Osmond initiated the use of psychedelics on chronic alcoholics, among other patients; see the 1965 review of medical uses of LSD in *Clinical Pharmacology and Therapeutics* by Abram Hoffer (1917–), a psychiatric researcher then at University Hospital in Saskatoon, Saskatchewan, who had worked with Osmond at Weyburn.

In 1953, Osmond famously introduced mescaline to novelist Aldous Huxley (1894–1963), who remained curious about mind-transforming drugs, having featured them so prominently in his novel *Brave New World* (1932), a totalitarian society in which people are controlled by drugs. As the *New York Times* reported in Osmond's obituary, Huxley had proposed his own term for such drugs to Osmond:

> To make this trivial world sublime,
> take half a gram of phanerothyme.

Rejecting that, Osmond responded,

> To fathom Hell or soar angelic,
> Just take a pinch of psychedelic.

In 1954, Herman C. B. Denber (1917–2000) of Manhattan State Hospital on Ward's Island in New York, and Sidney Merlis (1925–) of the Central Islip State Hospital on Long Island, initiated efforts to use mescaline therapeutically. They published in *Psychiatric Quarterly* a clinical trial of 10 patients with various diagnoses who had taken the drug together with chlorpromazine, and then were studied electroencephalographically. "In general, anxiety and tension disappeared following the mescaline-chlorpromazine injections," they reported. "Agitation gave way to complacency. The depression, where present, lifted and the mood lightened" (p. 639). They obtained supplies from the drug house Smith, Kline & French Laboratories, which apparently had mescaline in development.

In 1965, Sandoz stopped distributing LSD-25 because of a rising epidemic of street use (yet it remains available for medical use in Switzerland at the time of the present writing). Knowledge of the ability of a chemical compound to transform brain and mind function, especially what researchers believed at the time was its ability to produce "model psychoses," catalyzed research in psychopharmacology, making LSD-25, along with **chlorpromazine**, one of the germinative drugs of the discipline.

In 1964, just before the eclipse of LSD, one medical reader poetized tongue-in-cheek in the *Journal of the American Medical Association*:

> Give me a chalice of lysergic
> To quaff when day is done,
> That I may get a perceptual kick
> From my diencephalon.
>
> . . .
>
> So hey! It's off for the visions bizarre,
> Past the ego boundary,
> For a snort at the psychedelic bar
> Of the new psychiatry.

HAMILTON, MAX (1912–1988). Creator of widely used rating scales for depression and anxiety and a pioneer of British psychopharmacology, Hamilton was born in Offenburg (Hesse, Germany) and came with his parents to England at the beginning of the First World War. He graduated in medicine in 1934 at University College London and became interested in mental illness during the Second World War when assigned to an engineering unit, many of whose members had been placed there because of emotional problems. He started to read about psychology, then trained in psychiatry after the war, coming under the tutelage of psychologist Sir Cyril Burt (1883–1971) at University College Hospital, who began to teach him about statistics. "Within a couple of years," said Hamilton later, "I was probably the only psychiatrist in the country who knew psychometrics, rating scales and theories of measurement."

In 1953, Hamilton went to the medical school at Leeds as senior lecturer, where he began intensive work on scales, of which few existed in psychiatry at that point. When **chlorpromazine** was introduced in England in 1953, the firm May & Baker asked him to conduct a clinical trial. Then in the mid-1950s, he organized another trial of the antianxiety drug meprobamate, which had just been introduced. He devised a scale to measure decreases in the levels of patients' anxiety. When the trial was over, "We still had the patients," he said later. "We still had to see and treat them. Then something profoundly interesting happened: Two or three of these patients, carefully selected and diagnosed as anxiety states, became severely depressed and had to be given ECT, and responded very well. That set me thinking." So Hamilton devised a depression scale (later known as "HAM-D"). The anxiety scale was published in 1959 in the *British Journal of Medical Psychology*, the depression scale in 1960 in the *Journal of Neurology, Neurosurgery and Psychiatry*.

In fact, the timing of these publications led to some confusion: In another article on clinical syndromes in depression, cowritten with Jack Morrison White (M.B. 1941) at Stanley Boyd Hospital in Wakefield, and published in 1959 in the *Journal of Mental Science*, Hamilton said he had devised a depression scale and cited its forthcoming appearance as "1959." Yet, as mentioned above, it was not published until 1960.

Both scales are "household words," in a manner of speaking, in today's psychiatry. Hamilton became chair of psychiatry at Leeds in 1963 and retired from that department in 1977. Because he was a member of the Communist Party, the psychiatric establishment in London never really warmed to him, and he remained in Leeds. (Others attribute it to Hamilton's abrasive style.) His colleague, British psychopharmacologist

Merton Sandler (1926–) later said, "Max should have been the successor of **Aubrey Lewis** at the **Maudsley**" (Healy, *Psychopharmacologists*, II, p. 389).

HEIDELBERG. The Heidelberg university's department of psychiatry was the epicenter of the phenomenology movement in Germany and a source of much innovative thought, including key editions of **Emil Kraepelin**'s textbook.

The university psychiatric and neurological clinic (Psychiatrische und Neurologische Klinik der Ruprecht-Karl-Universität) was opened in 1878, the first professor of psychiatry Carl Fürstner (1848–1906) having been appointed in 1877.

After Fürstner stepped down in 1891 to go to Strasbourg, there followed the clinic's glory years: Emil Kraepelin was professor between 1891 and 1903, recruiting **Franz Nissl** and **Alois Alzheimer** as staff physicians. Gustav Aschaffenburg (1866–1944), considered the founder of forensic psychiatry in Germany, served as a resident, then staff psychiatrist, from 1890 to 1900. Ernst Rüdin (1874–1952), the geneticist (whose work in Munich during the Nazi period brought him under a cloud), was a staff psychiatrist around 1901–1902. Robert Gaupp (1870–1953), later professor of psychiatry in Tübingen, was a staff psychiatrist at Heidelberg from 1900 until he followed Kraepelin to Munich in 1904. Willy Hellpach (1877–1955), social psychologist and later German politician, operated his psychological laboratory from 1901 to 1903.

Kraepelin's immediate successor in 1904 was Karl Bonhoeffer (1868–1948), who left to become professor in Berlin almost as soon as he came. It was Bonhoeffer who had implemented Möbius's distinction between exogenous and endogenous illness. (*See* **DEPRESSION: EMERGENCE: exogenous vs. endogenous** [1909].)

In the years 1904–1918, **Franz Nissl** (1860–1919), the great neurohistologist, served as professor and head of the clinic. Under Nissl's aegis, the Heidelberg "phenomenology school" blossomed. As **Aubrey Lewis** later wrote of this period: "[Nissl] was a conscientious clinician but he had little sympathy or understanding for the psychopathological approach to the problems of psychiatry. Nevertheless, he collected a group of able young people around him, who recognized the relative sterility of [the neuropathological] approach . . . and he gave them his puzzled approval to follow their lights" (*Psychological Medicine*, 1977, p. 11).

The main concern of these young investigators was to overcome the limitations of the Kraepelinian system of "diseases." Foremost among them was **Karl Jaspers**, then in his mid-twenties, who had been a medical student at Heidelberg; in 1908 he entered the psychiatry clinic as an unpaid assistant (he did research) and remained there until 1915. Karl Wilmanns (1873–1945), a specialist in schizophrenia and in the problem of vagrancy, returned from Munich in 1904. Schizophrenia researcher Hans Gruhle (1880–1958) came to Heidelberg in 1905 and remained until 1934. Gruhle's notion was that one should study an illness such as psychosis on the basis of psychopathology (form of experience) and not on the basis of artificial physical speculations.

In his posthumous autobiography (1977), Jaspers has left a portrait of the intense collegiality and enthusiasm of this group: "It was a remarkable world of mutual spontaneity, with an awareness we all shared of participating in a tremendous expansion of knowledge, with all the arrogance of those who know too much, but also with a kind of radical criticism that subverted every position" (p. 19). After Nissl went to Munich in 1918 to Kraepelin's recently founded German Psychiatric Research Institute (Deutsche Forschungsanstalt für Psychiatrie), the Heidelberg dean asked Jaspers if he would like the professorship of psychiatry. Jaspers refused for reasons of health, and the chair went to Wilmanns.

In the years of the "phenomenology era," 1918–1933, Karl Wilmanns (1873–1945) was the professor. Under Wilmanns served some well-known members of the phenomenology group, such as **Wilhelm Mayer-Gross**. Mayer-Gross was not enthusiastic about Jaspers's distinction between erklären (explaining-rational) and verstehen (understanding-empathic), because he said everything could come under the latter, and preferred instead Jaspers's distinction—an Aristotelian one—between form and content. The former was psychiatry's assignment. Hans Prinzhorn (1886–1933) collected the patients' art in his tenure there between 1919 and 1924.

In 1928, Mayer-Gross and Kurt Beringer (1893–1949) founded the journal *Nerve Doctor* (*Nervenarzt*), which contained much of the productivity of the Heidelberg colleagues and encouraged contributions in psychopathology. Beringer was known for writing in 1927 the classic work, his Habilitation, on mescaline intoxication (*Der Meskalinrausch*): the first twentieth-century work on experimental psychosis as a way of studying psychopathology. (*See* **HALLUCINOGEN.**)

The volume on schizophrenia that Wilmanns edited in 1932 (*Die Schizophrenie*) in Oswald Bumke's series *Handbook of Psychiatric Illnesses* (*Handbuch der Geisteskrankheiten*) is seen as emblematic of the Heidelberg school's approach to the disease.

There followed the professorship between 1933 and 1945 of Carl Schneider (1891–1946). At the end of the Nazi period, Schneider committed suicide. Finally, in the years 1945–1955, **Kurt Schneider** became chair. After the Second World War, he became the chief representative of phenomenological thinking, but the school as it existed before 1933 in Heidelberg had long been dissolved.

HITZIG, JULIUS EDUARD (1838–1907). The codiscoverer, along with Gustav Theodor Fritsch (1838–1927), of the principle of the electrical excitability of the brain, Hitzig was born in Berlin, into the family of a well-known architect. After gaining his M.D. from Berlin in 1862, he received his Habilitation in internal medicine there in 1872; 3 years later he was called to Zurich as professsor of psychiatry and director of the university psychiatric clinic. In 1879, he went to the University of Halle as professor of psychiatry and director of the Nietleben asylum (Halle received an independent university psychiatric clinic only in 1885, of which Hitzig became head.) He was emerited in 1903 and died in a diabetic coma 4 years later. His best known publication was his epochal discovery of the electrical excitability of the motor cortex of the brain. At the April 5, 1870, meeting of the Berlin Medical Society, he told colleagues that, assisted by Fritsch, he had mapped a good portion of the motor cortex. The historic article was published in the *Berlin Clinical Weekly* (*Berliner Klinische Wochenschrift*) in 1870.

HOCHE, ALFRED ERICH (pronounced HO-ka) (1865–1943). One of **Emil Kraepelin**'s fiercest opponents, Hoche was born in Wildenhain in Saxony, studied medicine in Berlin and Heidelberg, and passed the qualifying exams in 1888; he became an assistant doctor at the outpatient clinic in **Heidelberg**, later in 1890 switching to the psychiatric clinic under Carl Fürstner (1848–1906). In 1902, he became the head of the department of psychiatry (Ordinary professor) in Freiburg in southwest Germany, remaining there until he resigned in 1934 at the time of the Nazi takeover. Hoche has been much reproached for having written in 1920 with jurist Karl Binding (1841–1920) a tract on the desirability of euthanizing children born with severe mental retardation (*On Permitting the Euthanasia of Life That Is Unworthy of Life* [*Die Freigabe der Vernichtung lebensunwerten Lebens*]). Whatever may be said about his judgment in having coined that phrase (that did give intellectual justification to later Nazi euthanasia), Hoche himself did not systematically encourage euthanasia. He detested the Nazis and committed suicide in Baden-Baden in 1943. His signal accomplishment was his "doctrine of symptom complexes," or syndromes (Syndromlehre), in contrast to Kraepelin's construction of large diseases such as dementia praecox. (*See* **MANIC-DEPRESSIVE ILLNESS: manic-depressive illness** [1899]; **SCHIZOPHRENIA: EMERGENCE: schizophrenia** [1893].) He believed that certain patterns of symptoms might recur in syndromes but that they did not represent fixed diseases and certainly did not correspond to any underlying patterns of brain biology.

HOMOSEXUALITY, GENDER IDENTITY DISORDER, AND PSYCHIATRY. In some areas, psychiatry has striven to be as scientific as possible, in studying the genetics of schizophrenia or the neurotransmitters involved in depression. In other areas, however, the discipline has proven very much a handmaiden of its cultural and political masters. Sexual behavior is one such area, and psychiatry's tendency to drift with the prevailing winds is seen no more clearly than in the area of homosexuality. (But, *see also* **MASOCHISM; SADISM.**) Although there has never been a moment since the Ancients when society smiled upon homosexuality, in the nineteenth century it became the object of medical censure in particular.

Carl Friedrich Westphal and "contrary sexual feeling" (1870). Westphal (1833–1890), born in Berlin as the son of a high government official, graduated in medicine there in 1855. In the late 1850s, he worked as an assistant physician under Carl Wilhelm Ideler (*see* **GERMAN "ROMANTIC" PSYCHIATRY**) in the psychiatric division of the Charité; later, he served under **Wilhelm Griesinger**. In 1869, after Griesinger's death, Westphal became head of the psychiatric and neurological services at the Charité, and in 1873 professor of psychiatry. In 1887, he fell ill with what seems to have been neurosyphilis and died 3 years later in the Binswanger family's private nervous clinic in Kreuzlingen in Switzerland. (*See* **ANXIETY: Westphal's agoraphobia-panic** [1872]; also **OBSESSIVE-COMPULSIVE DISORDER: "obsessive ideas" [Zwangsvorstellungen]** [1877].)

In 1870, Westphal published an article in the *Archives of Psychiatry and Nervous Diseases* (*Archiv für Psychiatrie und Nervenkrankheiten*) on "Contrary Sexual Feeling: The Symptom of a Neuropathic (Psychopathic) Condition" ("Die conträre Sexualempfindung: Symptom eines neuropathischen [psychopathischen] Zustandes"). He began the article, "In the cases of illness that I communicate in following, the main finding emerged as a symptom which, as such, has been hitherto little or not at all described: an inborn perversion of sexual feeling with the patient aware of its pathological nature." The symptom was derangements of proper sexual identity: in one patient, the desire of a young lesbian admitted to the Charité for sexual intercourse with other women; in another, a cross-dressing male patient who felt himself to be a woman, denying the desire for sex with other men. Westphal found it significant that there was a history of depression in the woman's family and that the man was subject to epilepsy, both being signs, he said, of a hereditary predisposition to pathology.

With the term "contrary sexual feeling," Westphal said he did not intend necessarily to identify just the sex drive "but also the simple feeling [Empfindung] of being alienated from one's own sex on the basis of one's entire internal being" (p. 107). Westphal declared explicitly that he was not proposing homosexuality to be a disease.

The male case, at least, constitutes an early description of what would later be called "gender identity disorder."

Krafft-Ebing sees homosexuality as evidence of degeneration (from 1877). While he was still professor of psychiatry at Graz University, **Richard von Krafft-Ebing** occupied himself with "contrary sexual desire"; in an article in 1877 in the *Archive of Psychiatry and Nervous Diseases* (*Archiv für Psychiatrie und Nervenkrankheiten*), he argued that same-sex attraction between men resulted from a constitutionally based disorder of sexual identity, a mixture of female and male traits, and that it constituted evidence of degeneration in the central nervous system.

In 1886, shortly after his arrival in Vienna as professor of psychiatry, he brought out the first edition of what was to become his massive encyclopedia of sexual perversion, *Psychopathia sexualis*. Here he discussed, "lack of sexual feeling towards the opposite sex with substituted sexual desire [Geschlechtsgefühl] and sexual drive [Geschlechtstrieb] to one's own sex." The characteristic of this psychopathic disorder was a "lack of sexual feeling toward the opposite sex to the point of horror. . . . Also, the man-loving man assigns to the member of his sex the sexual role of the woman," ditto for the woman who loves other women (pp. 56–57). The disorder could be inborn or acquired, yet even the acquired cases possessed some kind of a predisposition.

Among the evidence for homosexuality being a form of degeneration was (to take the first three points on Krafft-Ebing's list of six) (1) that the behavior begins early in life, and with unusual intensity; (2) that the sex organs themselves are not deformed: the disorder stems from the "character and entire emotional feeling" of the individual; (3) that the affected individuals also manifest other suspicious anomalies (pp. 59–60).

As Krafft-Ebing's book evolved through subsequent editions, "contrary sexual feeling" acquired an ever more prominent place, appearing even in the title. The twelfth edition, published in 1902 just after his death, had more than 100 pages on the subject (up from 16 pages in the first edition).

Yet, at the end of his life, Krafft-Ebing underwent something of a conversion: In 1901, a year before his death, he declared that homosexuality was "not an illness but rather an anomaly." He commented in an article, published in a gay-identified journal (*The Yearbook for Sexual Transition States* [*Jahrbuch für sexuelle Zwischenstufen*]) that science had finally approached the viewpoint of homosexuals themselves, that their "singular sexual orientation," though minoritarian, nonetheless represents for them "an adequate, natural and thus legitimate" mode of sexuality. Krafft-Ebing did not, however, revise his previous opinions in the twelfth edition of *Psychopathia sexualis*, the preface of which he signed in December 1902, weeks or days before his death (perhaps he was too weak to change the text). The subsequent editions of *Psychopathia sexualis* were unchanged, and the fourteenth, published in 1912, was reprinted in the 1990s. Krafft-Ebing's interpretation of homosexuality, as articulated in *Psychopathia sexualis*, remained dominant in psychiatry for decades to come.

Gay psychiatrists and medical writers who opposed the degeneration view of homosexuality (from ca. 1900):

Marc-André Raffalovich (1864–1934). Although Raffalovich was not actually a physician, he had studied medicine and spent much of his life as a medical journalist. Of Russian origin but circulating between Paris and London, he was openly gay and in numerous publications vehemently denied that homosexuality was a sign of degeneration. He is best known for *Uranism and Unisexuality: A Study of Different Manifestations of the Sexual Instinct* (*Uranisme et unisexualité: Étude sur différentes manifestations de l'instinct sexuel*), published in 1896, a book that presented homosexuality on the spectrum of normal sexual behavior. Raffalovich wrote, "The normal sexual invert is not necessarily sick or criminal; he is no more at the mercy of his sexual instinct than any other civilized man who has principles, duties and conventions to observe. There are criminal sexual inverts. . . . But one may not refuse to recognize the existence of the sexual invert who is not mentally unbalanced, not degenerate" (p. 25). According to sexuality historian Vernon A. Rosario, it was Raffalovich who introduced the modern concept of homosexuality as same-sex desire to France. (Uranism was a contemporary coinage for homosexuality.) (Note: There was a lively discussion over homosexuality within the French medical community in these years, with such prominent figures as forensic-medicine specialist Ambroise-Auguste Tardieu [1818–1879] dead set against it.)

Paul Näcke (1851–1913). Näcke was a German psychiatrist who came as close to acknowledging his own bisexuality as one could without actually coming out of the closet. Näcke, born of a German father and French mother, graduated in medicine from Würzburg University in 1873, then from 1880 occupied various staff positions in a series of asylums, ending as medical director of Colditz asylum (well-known because of its conversion to an Allied prisoner-of-war camp during the Second World War from which several high-profile escapes occurred). He had lived in France for a number of years and was fluently bilingual. From 1901, Näcke began writing a series of articles in such venues as the main French and German journals for criminal anthropology that betrayed an astonishingly close familiarity with the gay scene focused about public urinals in Paris, Berlin, and other cities. (Although Näcke was well disposed to Raffalovich's book, he found it improbable that the Russian author could know much about the actual life in Paris.) Näcke denied that homosexuality represented a degenerative phenomenon. He argued that men and women were basically born bisexual, and that their subsequent development was really almost a matter of chance. Said to be "happily married," he nonetheless declaimed upon such themes as gay tongue-kissing and shoe fetishism. As he wrote in 1910 in the journal *Sexual Problems* (*Sexual Probleme*), "At the present time, one finds Urnings at most abnormal, but certainly not sick or degenerate, and it is evident that the mere existence of contrary desire does not conceivably represent a stigma of degeneration" (p. 591). Moreover, Näcke insisted that it was mainly the educated classes who found homosexuality repellent and that "among the common people the subject is usually received with great indifference" (*Archiv für Kriminal-Anthropologie*, 1910, p. 79). In an article published posthumously, in the *Archive of Psychiatry and Nervous Diseases* (*Archiv für Psychiatrie und Nervenkrankheiten*) in 1914, Näcke allowed that he had had "a pretty considerable personal experience" with homosexuality (p. 323).

Havelock Ellis (1859–1939). Ellis, the English physician–sexologist whose monumental anthropological investigation of sex appeared in his seven-volume series, *Studies in the Psychology of Sex*, between 1897 and 1928. It began in German, in 1896 with a volume on "The Contrary Sexual Sense," which appeared in English in 1897. Ellis summed up his work in a final volume, called *Psychology of Sex*, in 1933. He referred to homosexuality in quite accepting tones: "Inversion [is] a congenital anomaly . . . which if it is pathological, is only so in [the] sense that pathology is the science not of diseases but of anomalies, so that an inverted person may be as healthy as a color-blind person. Congenital sexual inversion is thus akin to a biological variation" (pp. 228–229).

Note: There were numerous gay psychiatrists who remained mute on the subject of homosexuality, such as Edward Mapother (1881–1940), superintendent of the **Maudsley Hospital** from 1923 until 1939.

Psychoanalysis sets itself against homosexuality. Sigmund Freud himself was quite tolerant of homosexuality and did not advocate the use of psychoanalysis to convert gays into straights. Freud believed that people were basically born bisexual, and that events in development determined which orientation they would seek out. As for a psychoanalytic explanation of the nature of homosexual desire itself, as Freud wrote in the fourth edition, published in 1920, of his 1905 book, *Three Contributions to the Theory of Sex*, "To be sure, psychoanalysis has not to the present produced any complete explanation of the origins of inversion, yet nonetheless we have discovered the psychic mechanism of its genesis. . . . We have discovered in all cases examined to the present, that those who later become inverts experience in the first years of childhood a phase of very intensive, but very brief, fixation upon a woman (usually the mother), and that after overcoming it they identify with the woman and make themselves into a sex object, meaning that, on the basis of narcissism, they hunt out youthful men as much like themselves as possible, whom they so love as their mothers had loved them" (*Drei Abhandlungen zur Sexualtheorie*, p. 44). (*See* **NARCISSISM**.)

Yet, later generations of psychoanalysts, particularly in the United States after the Second World War, did not share Freud's tolerance. In his discussion of " Sexual Deviations" in Silvano Arieti's big textbook, *American Handbook of Psychiatry* (1959), New York psychoanalyst Paul Friedman (1899–), an emigré from Switzerland and Paris, managed to make the whole subject of homosexuality—which he discussed together with coprophilia and pedophilia—sound as nasty as possible: "The anus here serves as a substitute for the maternal vagina. . . . There may be considerable latent hostility toward the father, with unconscious ideas of castrating him through homosexual intercourse" (p. 595). Friedman considered psychotherapy to convert these unfortunates into heterosexuals quite appropriate, to be sure psychotherapy of an unusually directive kind: The therapist must mandate the gay patient to be abstinent. But, quoting Freud, Friedman said there was some good news: "In a certain number of cases we succeed in developing the blighted germs of heterosexual tendencies which are present in every homosexual" (p. 607).

Psychoanalyst Edmund Bergler (1899–1962), who had emigrated from Vienna to New York in 1938, wrote an article in 1944 in the *Psychoanalytic Review* on "Eight Prerequisites for the Psychoanalytic Treatment of Homosexuality," announcing "The prognosis of analytical treatment of homosexuals is a favorable one" (p. 268). In

1956, Bergler brought out *Homosexuality: Disease or Way of Life?* a book that left little doubt which he thought it was. "The perversion has become more widespread through artificial creation of new recruits as a result of the dissemination of misleading statistics," he wrote, referring to the 1948 study *Sexual Behavior in the Human Male* by Alfred C. Kinsey (1894–1956) and co-workers. Bergler reemphasized the conclusion he had reached in 1944: "It has recently been discovered that homosexuality is a curable illness" (p. 7). Why would they need curing? "Without exception, deep inner guilt arising from the perversion is present in homosexuals. This is shifted guilt, and it belongs to the masochistic substructure" (p. 24). On other psychoanalysts who set themselves against homosexuality, the reader may consult Ronald Bayer's *Homosexuality and American Psychiatry* (1987).

Homosexuality counts as a "sexual deviation" in *DSM-I* (1952) and ***DSM-II*** (1968). Without further discussion, these early editions of the American Psychiatric Association *Manual* simply declared homosexuality to be deviant. Gender identity disorders were not even mentioned.

Homosexuality becomes a nondisease for psychiatry (1973). The reassessment of homosexuality within the American Psychiatric Association began after sustained attacks from within by such psychiatrists as Thomas Szasz (*see* **ANTIPSYCHIATRY: Szasz**) and Judd Marmor (1910–2004). (Both had been trained as psychoanalysts.) There were also increasing attacks from without: at the annual meeting in 1970 of the American Psychiatric Association (APA) in San Francisco, a group of gay activists interrupted the proceedings of a panel on "issues in sexuality," cursing at New York psychoanalyst Irving Bieber (1908–1991), who had argued for conversion therapy. Again, in May 1973, the APA at its annual meeting organized a symposium on "Should Homosexuality Be in the APA Nomenclature?" The presentations, which included that of gay activist Ronald Gold ("Stop It, You're Making Me Sick!") and psychiatrist Richard Green (who argued that "heterosexuality should be in the APA nomenclature"), were printed in the *American Journal of Psychiatry* in November 1973. At the instigation of **Robert Spitzer**, in December 1973 the board of trustees of the APA decided that homosexuality would no longer be considered a psychiatric illness; this decision was ratified in a vote by the membership the following year.

Ego-dystonic homosexuality appears in *DSM-III* (1980). The issue of homosexuality remained so controversial within APA, however, that the advisory committee on "psychosexual disorders" of the Task Force on Nomenclature that designed *DSM-III* was virtually torn apart by it. Finally, the committee agreed to stigmatize "ego dystonic homosexuality" as a psychiatric illness, stipulating that it be applied only to homosexuals unhappy with their condition yet unable properly to respond to heterosexual desire.

For the first time in the *DSM* series, *DSM-III* featured "gender identity disorders," such as "transsexualism," as psychiatric illnesses. A "gender identity disorder of childhood" was also created.

Homosexuality vanishes entirely from *DSM-III-R* (1987). This edition of the *Manual* made no mention of it. This edition also shifted gender identity disorder to the pediatric section of the manual ("disorders usually first evident in infancy, childhood, or adolescence").

"Sex and gender identity disorder" becomes an independent category in *DSM-IV* (1994). Clearly having great problems with the classification of sexual issues, the drafters of *DSM-IV* removed sexual identity disorders entirely from any kind of "perversion" section and instead made sexual **sadism** and **masochism** subordinate to "identity disorders." This state of affairs would clearly satisfy none of the players whose sexual preferences were still being labeled pathological. One may anticipate that future *DSM* editions will also de-pathologize such practices as sexual sadomasochism, now referred to in the community as "roleplaying," as well as transgendering, which is the subject of protective regulations on university campuses everywhere.

The American Psychiatric Association officially disapproves of "reparative," or "conversion" therapy, of homosexuals (1998). The board of trustees of the APA issued a position statement opposing any kind of "reparative" therapy based on the assumption that homosexuality per se is a mental disorder or that the patient should change his or her sexual orientation.

HYPERACTIVITY. *See* **ATTENTION DEFICIT HYPERACTIVITY DISORDER (ADHD).**

HYPOCHONDRIASIS. The notion of "hypochondriacal melancholy" goes back to the Ancients, signifying a particular form of melancholy in which the hypochondrium (area beneath the ribs) is mainly affected. Felix Platter (1536–1614), professor of medicine at Basel, described in his 1602 textbook "a melancholic filthy vapour troubling the spirits and affecting the head [that] breeds that species of melancholy which they call hypochondriacal," a vapor that—as psychiatry historian Stanley Jackson explains in his *Melancholia and Depression*—Platter believed to arise from "melancholy blood" in the hypochondrial region (p. 94).

Nosologist **William Cullen** of Edinburgh, in his *First Lines of the Practice of Physic* (1777), put the notion of "hypochondriasis or the hypochondriac affection" on a modern footing by kicking humors out of the picture: "In certain persons there is a state of mind distinguished by a concurrence of the following circumstances: A languour, listlessness, or want of resolution and activity with respect to all undertakings . . . . Such persons are particularly attentive to the state of their own health, to every the smallest change of feeling in their bodies; and from any unusual feeling, perhaps of the slightest kind, they apprehend great danger, and even death itself. In respect to all these feelings and apprehensions, there is commonly the most obstinate belief" (pp. 249–250, vol. III, of 1799 edition). (*See also* **DEPRESSION: EMERGENCE: hypochondria as a subform of depression** [1860]; **HYSTERIA-PSYCHOSOMATIC-SOMATIZATION.**)

HYPOMANIA AND MANIA IN THE MODERN SENSE (1881). In a monograph on mania (called *Mania* [*die Manie*]), Emanuel Ernst Mendel (1839–1907), who headed a well-known private nervous clinic in the Berlin suburb of Pankow and was said to be the last psychiatrist to master completely both psychiatry and neurology, proposed the existence of a disease entity that he called "hypomania": "indicating forms of mania with the typical clinical picture but in lesser degree."* The characteristics: "The

* The term "hypomania" had been used by previous writers to mean a lesser degree of insanity, not mania in the modern sense. See, for example, Henry Johnson (1805–1877), *On the Arrangement and Nomenclature of Mental Disorders* (1843), where he calls hypomania a useful synonym for **Esquirol's** concept of monomania, or "partial insanity."

patients begin, as they say, 'to really enjoy life.' Bars, theaters and dances they might previously have avoided are now sought out, trips planned and quickly taken." Mendel emphasized a kind of moral egotism (not part of what was later considered to be the typical "hypomanic triad" of elated mood, pressured speech, and increased motor activity): "With increased self confidence they brush aside the doubts about the possible difficulties facing their projects; they also cut off further discussion. In these cases their egotistical character is particularly striking; they treat the relatives with indifference. Everything is oriented . . . toward the satisfaction of their own wishes and desires." Then the characteristic excesses of mania emerge, Mendel said: "They pay little attention to money, throwing it out the window, and in short order they run through actually astonishing sums" (pp. 38–40).

Mendel also recast the definition of mania itself, not as a mood disorder but as a "pathological acceleration in the succession of ideas and the pathologically increased excitability of the brain's motor centers" (p. 175). Before Mendel, chronic mania meant basically agitated dementia, a disease that went progressively downhill; Mendel's mania and hypomania were recoverable. Mendel was also an authority on the pathology of neurosyphilis, but he is remembered for his work on mania in the modern sense and for his coinage of hypomania. (*See also* **MANIC-DEPRESSIVE ILLNESS.**)

HYSTERIA-PSYCHOSOMATIC-SOMATIZATION. In 1802, Paris psychiatrist Jean-Baptiste Louyer-Villermay (1775–1837), in an essay differentiating hypochondria from hysteria, described a young female patient, uncertain about romance, who, "at the sight of her loved one fainted, uttering plaintive cries and sobbing involuntarily as she drifted in and out of somnolence. As she slipped into total unconsciousness, uncoordinated contractions of her upper limbs began, a convulsive twitching of her chest, violent palpitations and spasmodic contractions at the throat, with a feeling of strangulation and 'globe hystérique [lump in the throat],' also a tetanic contraction of her lower jaw and occasional convulsions of its muscles" (pp. 40–41). Louyer-Villermay made the diagnosis of hysteria. Although the view is commonly heard that the term "hysteria" goes back to the Ancient Greeks, in fact it does not: the diagnosis filters into medicine only in the seventeenth century.

In the great gamut of "psychophysiological disorders," or breakdowns of the mind–body relationship, hysteria has always occupied a particular niche, defined as (a) a stigmatizing term that male physicians have always used for behavior in women that they do not understand; (b) a synonym for functional convulsive disorders, or "pseudoepilepsy"; (c) a synonym for psychosomatic illness, or "functional" illness, sometimes called "conversion symptoms," or "conversion disorder"; (d) latterly, as a kind of personality disorder, again, primarily in women. There follow some of the landmarks from the seventeenth century, when the term "hysteria" first started to be used, to 1980, when it officially was dropped from psychiatric terminology.

The vicissitudes of the term "hypochondriasis," meaning abnormal fear of illness or concern with bodily symptoms, have been so numerous that they will not be considered in this *Dictionary*. (*See,* however, **DEPRESSION: EMERGENCE: hypochondria as a subform of depression** [1860].)

Hysteria as a convulsive phenomenon, or fits (1667). In an *Essay of the Pathology of Brain and Nervous Stock,* the Oxford physician and lecturer Thomas Willis

(1621–1675), the founder of neurology, equated hysteria with convulsive phenomena (including doubtless a good deal of epilepsy): "The hysterical passion is of so ill fame, among the diseases belonging to women, that like one half damned, it bears the faults of many other diseases. . . . a choaking in the throat, a vertigo, an inversio, or rolling about of the eyes, oftentimes, laughing, or weeping . . . sometimes convulsive motions in the face and limbs, and sometimes in the whole body, are excited" (quoted in Hunter-Macalpine, *300 Years*, p. 189). Willis thus founded the doctrine of hysteria that would run through neurology for the next 300 years.

Hysteria as a synonym for medically unexplained symptoms (1682). For Thomas Sydenham (1624–1689), the great London physician who is considered the father of medicine based on observation, "hysteric disorders" were the counterfeiters of illness. As he wrote in 1681, "The frequency of hysteria is no less remarkable than the multiformity of the shapes which it puts on. Few of the maladies of miserable mortality are not imitated by it. Whatever part of the body it attacks, it will create the proper symptom of that part" (*Works*, II, p. 85). Further: "Almost all the hysterical women that I have ever seen complain of a dejection (a sinking as they call it) of the spirits; and, when they wish to show where this contraction (or sinking) exists, they point to the chest. . . . That hysterical women break out into immoderate fits, sometimes of laughing, sometimes of crying, and that without any manifest cause, is known all the world over" (p. 88). In his note on hysteria, Sydenham thus originated the concept that would inform much of psychiatry, and all of internal medicine, for the next 300 years.

In the interests of brevity, this *Dictionary* will skip over the numerous contributions to hysteria between the seventeenth century, when the above authors founded the doctrine, to the mid-nineteenth century, when the outlines of contemporary interpretations become discernible. It would also be unmanageable to mention the great medical literature of the nineteenth century on mind–body relations, details of which may be found in my book *From Paralysis to Fatigue: A History of Psychosomatic Illness in the Modern Era* (1992).

Charcot's doctrine of hysteria (from 1870). **Jean-Martin Charcot**'s involvement with hysteria at the **Salpêtrière hospice** began in 1870 when, as the senior physician at the infirmary of the hospice, he asked that a special ward be created for non-insane female patients from another service who had "hystero-epilepsy." As he began to study these patients systematically, he differentiated two forms of hysteria: one was "minor hysteria" (la pétite hystérie), represented by more or less permanent stigmata such as constricted visual fields, cutaneous anesthesia, or hypnotizability; the other was "major hysteria" (la grande hystérie), dramatic outbursts of passion and posturing as the patients supposedly evolved through the various stages of a major attack. For Charcot, hysteria was an inborn, constitutional illness of which men as well were at risk. His theory of hysteria, resting on the basis of artifactual phenomena, collapsed rapidly after his death in 1893. But his celebrity as a physician gave "hysteria," as a supposedly neurological, brain-based phenomenon, great international attention. His ideas were laid out systematically in his *Tuesday Lectures at the Salpêtrière, Outpatient Department, 1887–1888* (*Leçons du mardi à la Salpêtrière, Policliniques, 1887–1888*).

Briquet: hysteria as a constitutional illness (1881). In 1859, Pierre Briquet (1796–1881), an internist at the Charité Hospital in Paris, wrote a big book on hysteria,

Clinical and Therapeutic Treatise on Hysteria (*Traité clinique et thérapeutique de l'hystérie*), based on a quantitative analysis of more than 400 of his female patients. The book helped destroy some customary myths about the disorder, such as its imputed cause from sexual frustration ; the book also cast light on the role of emotions and stress in the genesis of physical symptoms. Yet, it was only in a paper that Briquet gave to the Academy of Medicine in 1881, the year of his death, that he highlighted the role of family "predisposition" in hysteria. Looking at symptoms such as migraine, chronic pain, poor digestion, cutaneous anesthesia and pseudoepilepsy, he determined that "predisposed" women, including those with more laden histories on the female side of the family tree, had an earlier onset and longer duration of hospitalization than did the non-predisposed, and that they tended to have more frequently such challenging symptoms as anesthesias and convulsions. Although most patients recovered from their current illness, many relapsed. He referred to hysteria as "the insanity of sensibility" (la folie de la sensibilité). (The paper "On the Predisposition to Hysteria" ["De la prédisposition à l'hystérie"] was published in the *Bulletin de l'Académie de médecine,* Paris, 1881.)

Silas Weir Mitchell identifies "hysterical motor ataxia" as a subform of hysteria (1881). **Mitchell**, who specialized in the functional affections of wealthy women, called attention in his *Lectures on Diseases of the Nervous System, Especially in Women* (1881) to "hysterical motor ataxia": "The real and singular want of power . . . seems to set this apart from cases of mere neurasthenia. . . . The disorder is one of those which adds many recruits to that large class which some one has called 'bed cases,' and which are above all things distinguished by their desire to remain at rest" (p. 48). This special form of hysteria remained common in this class of patient, called "sofa cases" as well, until around the time of the First World War.

Astasia-abasia (Blocq syndrome) (1888). Paul-Oscar Blocq (1860–1896), at the time a hospital intern in Paris, described in the *Archives de neurologie* in 1888 "a disorder characterized by astasia and abasia" (the inability to stand up or walk). He said that **Jean-Martin Charcot** and Paul-Marie-Louis-Pierre Richer (1849–1933) had already characterized it in 1883 under the term "loss of motor power in the lower limbs because of lack of coordination in standing and walking" (p. 24). Yet, it was Blocq's term that caught on, and not Charcot's. (*See also* **AKATHISIA**.)

Freud's concept of hysteria (1892 and after). *See* **FREUDIAN DOCTRINE OF HYSTERIA**.

Babinski's definition of "hysteria" (1901). For Joseph-François-Félix Babinski (1857–1932), a Parisian neurologist who had trained under Charcot but by 1901 was head of the neurology service at La Pitié Hospital, hysteria was any disorder that could be induced by suggestion and abolished by persuasion. By "suggestion" he meant mainly medical suggestion, such as encouraging the patients to think they had a certain form of hysteria; by persuasion he meant hypnotism or some other form of psychotherapy. As he wrote in 1901 in the *Neurological Review* (*Revue neurologique*), "Hysteria is a psychological state that renders patients capable of self-suggestion" (p. 1077). No subsequent formulation has improved upon this.

The term "somatization" is introduced to psychiatry (1924). It was Freud's excollaborator Wilhelm Stekel (1868–1940), a Viennese family doctor and psychoanalyst, who introduced "somatization" to psychiatry. As early as 1924 he wrote, "As a result of the somatization of this lack of feeling [Gefühllosigkeit] the patient develops a complete anesthesia in both arms." This note appeared in the first volume of his own journal, *New Research in Sexuality* (*Fortschritte der Sexualwissenschaft*). In 1932, he described "An Interesting Case of Somatization" ("Eine interessante Somatisation") in *Psychoanalytic Practice* (*Psychoanalytische Praxis*).

The "patient as a person" movement (from 1924). Within American internal medicine, in the 1920s the view arose that patients' somatic symptoms could be as much a result of stress and nervousness as of organic disease. Some internists advocated viewing the "patient as a person" in order to treat comprehensively the disorders both of body and mind. The firing gun in this movement was probably Francis Weld Peabody's (1881–1927) *The Care of the Patient* (1924). Peabody, professor of medicine at Harvard, said that the ultimate cause of these "symptoms for which an adequate organic cause could not be discovered . . . [was] to be found not in any gross structural change of the organs involved, but rather in nervous influences emanating from the emotional or intellectual life, which, directly or indirectly, affect . . . organs that are under either voluntary or involuntary control" (pp. 24–25). The apogee of the movement, just before the great marriage between biochemistry and internal medicine that occurred after the Second World War, was doubtless George Canby Robinson's (1878–1960) *The Patient as a Person: A Study of the Social Aspects of Illness*, which appeared in 1939. Robinson, lecturer in medicine at Johns Hopkins University and a specialist in gastroenterology, noted, "Man is a unity of mind and body, and medicine must consider this unity. Physiology, chemistry, and biology cannot alone or together explain all the intricacies of illness. The disturbances of mind and body cannot be dealt with separately; they form two phases of a single problem" (p. 10).

Alexander's doctrine of "psychosomatic specificity" (1934 and after). In 1932, the emigé Hungarian psychoanalyst Franz Alexander (1891–1964) founded the Chicago Institute for Psychoanalysis and also received a professorship for psychoanalysis at the University of Chicago. At the institute, he occupied himself intensely with problems of the mind–body relationship. In an article in the *Psychoanalytic Quarterly* in 1934, he identified functional gastric disturbances with "the wish to receive or take," colitis-type illnesses with "the wish to give or eliminate," and constipation with "the wish to retain" (p. 508). Alexander did not at this point use the term "psychosomatic" but talked rather of "predominant conflict-situations and their solutions in each group [gastric, diarrhoea, constipation types]" (p. 533). In his later book *Psychosomatic Medicine* (1950), Alexander developed a doctrine whereby certain kinds of intrapsychic conflicts expressed themselves on the sympathetic side of the autonomic nervous system (ANS), others on the parasympathetic side. He claimed that the sympathetic, or "fight" side of the ANS responded to conflicts with such "psychosomatic" illnesses as hypertension, diabetes, and rheumatoid arthritis; the parasympathetic, or "flight" side with ulcerative colitis and asthma. These doctrines were highly influential in American psychosomatic medicine for a number of years. For example, the Rochester internist **George Engel**, later responsible for the "biopsychosocial" model of medicine, had studied with Alexander.

Karl Menninger describes "polysurgical addiction" (1934). "We all know the facility with which the hysterical patient can produce symptoms which gratify his unconscious needs," **Menninger** wrote in the *Psychoanalytic Quarterly*. "And if that need can be further gratified through a surgical manipulation, the means will not fail him to bring about a condition which even the most conscientious surgeon will be inclined to regard as indicative, if not imperative, of surgical interference" (p. 176). Menninger found that this "compulsion to submit to surgical operations" represented an unconscious form of "self-destruction."

"Vegetative dystonia" (1934). Berthold Wichmann, a young assistant in the university psychiatric clinic in Münster, Germany, who had qualified in 1930, maintained in the *Deutsche Medizinische Wochenschrift* in 1934 that many functional internal disorders were owing to sympathetic and parasympathetic hyperarousal. He suggested the term "vegetative dystonia" (autonomic dystonia) for the varying headaches, feelings of dizziness, gastrointestinal upsets, hyperhidrosis (excessive sweating), heightened muscle excitability, changing pulse rhythm, and functional tremors that are common in primary care. Wichmann said the disorder was primarily constitutional, or organic, and not psychogenic, but that it could have secondary psychiatric effects as well. Although the diagnosis never caught on in the Anglo-Saxon world, it became popular on the Continent after the Second World War. For years, several Swiss drug companies marketed drugs specific for "vegetative dystonia," such as Sandoz's Bellergal (a mixture of ergotamine, belladonna alkaloids, and phenobarbital). In 1961, Geigy launched the tricyclic antidepressant opipramol (Insidon), a sigma-receptor ligand that they bought from the discoverer company Rhône-Poulenc; from the first they marketed it for vegetative dystonia ("a psycho-vegetative harmonizer"). In the Anglo-Saxon world, vegetative dystonia is understood as somatic manifestations of mixed anxiety–depression.

The term "psychosomatic" becomes accepted (1935). Helen *Flanders* Dunbar (1902–1959), who was cross-appointed in the departments of medicine and psychiatry at Columbia University, wrote a book in 1935 entitled *Emotions and Bodily Changes: A Survey of Literature on Psychosomatic Interrelationships, 1910–1933*. She had wanted to bring together the literature on what the *Index Medicus* was still calling "physical-mental relationships." The book encountered such an enthusiastic reception that in the preface of the second edition, published in 1938, she explained how she had coined the term (or she believed she had coined it, but its use goes back to the early nineteenth century): She said it was not that the body was split between a psyche and a soma. "The term 'psychosomatic' is descriptive rather of the observer in his endeavor to apprehend rather than of the organism observed. Psychic and somatic represent merely two angles of observation. Our understanding of disease rests on pictures taken from these two angles viewed simultaneously, united stereoscopically" (p. xix).

The term "psychosomatic illness" is popularized (1938). James Lorimer Halliday (1897–1983), regional medical officer of the department of health for Scotland and confronting the problem of rising rates of chronic invalidism among the insured, suggested in the *British Medical Journal* in 1938 the term "psychosomatic illness" to designate the way in which psychological changes, acting via the brain, the autonomic nervous system, and the endocrine system (the "bodily mechanism of emotion" as others had termed it) might bring about "changes in chemistry, rhythm, secretion, and even structure in one or more parts of the body." Psychosomatic illness was thus for Halliday not co-terminous with "functional" illness, meaning symptoms in which there were no organic changes. Halliday's book *Psychosocial Medicine: A Study* *of the Sick Society* (1948) made the concept of "psychosomatic affections" widely known.

"Hysteria" as a distinct syndrome, not just individual conversion disorders (1951). James J. Purtell (?–1949), a psychiatrist at Tufts College Medical School, **Eli Robins** at St. Louis (*see* **St. Louis school**), and Mandel Cohen (1907–2000) at Harvard concluded in a study of chronic functional illness published in the *New England Journal of Medicine* that hysteria was a distinct syndrome seen mainly in female patients with long histories of multiple body symptoms, an onset early in life, and a certain personality style. "No patient had fewer than 11 symptoms," they wrote.

"Psychophysiologic autonomic and visceral disorders" in *DSM "One"* (1952). This first edition of the *Diagnostic and Statistical Manual* of the American Psychiatric Association did not use the term "hysteria," avoided explicitly the term "psychosomatic disorders"—which expression they considered a "point of view" in medicine rather than certain specified illnesses—and chose the above rather complicated expression to identify "the visceral expression of affect" (p. 29). The *Manual* also admitted the classic psychoanalytic "conversion reaction," with the explanation that "the impulse causing the anxiety is 'converted' into functional symptoms in organs or parts of the body, usually those that are mainly under voluntary control" (pp. 32–33). Finally, it included the category of "dissociative reaction," grouped under "psychoneurotic disorders," for fugue states and the like.

Hysteria as a distinct "disease entity" (1962). Continuing the work at **St. Louis** that **Eli Robins** had begun with Purtell, in 1962 Michael Perley (1936–), a medical intern from the University of Minnesota who had a Public Health Service studentship at Washington University in St. Louis, and **Samuel B. Guze** published in the *New England Journal of Medicine* the results of a long-term follow-up study of 39 patients with hysteria according to the Purtell–Robins–Cohen criteria. They found that hysteria was a clinical syndrome, or "disease," involving "a dramatic, complicated medical history beginning before the age of thirty-five, with multiple symptoms involving many organ systems" (p. 423). The presentation was stable over time. Previous authorities, such as **Jean-Martin Charcot**, had also believed hysteria to be a definite disease. Yet, that thread was lost and the nosological view resumes with the **St. Louis school**.

Hysteria in *DSM-II* (1968). In this second and more psychoanalytically oriented edition of the American Psychiatric Association's *Manual*, hysteria returned under the "neuroses" as "hysterical neurosis": "an involuntary psychogenic loss or disorder of function." It was subdivided into "conversion type," and "dissociative type," thus encompassing the "dissociative reaction" of *DSM-I*. Unlike ***DSM-I***, this second edition also admitted hysteria as a **personality disorder**, called "hysterical personality (histrionic personality disorder)": it was characterized by "seductive" and "attention-seeking" self-dramatization (p. 43). *DSM-II* retained the "psychophysiologic disorders" of *DSM-I*.

"Somatization" is reintroduced to psychiatry in a nonpsychoanalytic sense (1968). After Stekel, somatization continued to be used within the psychoanalytic literature in a specialized way. Then in 1968, Zbigniew ("Bish") J. Lipowski (1924–1997), at the time a member of the psychiatric consultation service of the Royal Victoria Hospital and of the Allan Memorial Insitute of **McGill University** in Montreal, suggested in an article in *Psychosomatic Medicine* that somatization be redefined as "the tendency to experience . . . psychological states . . . as bodily sensations, functional changes, or somatic metaphors" (p. 413).

"Briquet's Syndrome" (1971). In 1881, Briquet (*see above*) identified a pattern of chronic psychosomatic illness in women, having a partially genetic nature and beginning early in life. A century later, writing in the *American Journal of Psychiatry* in 1971, **Samuel Guze** of the **St. Louis school**, together with collaborators Robert A. Woodruff, Jr. (1934–) and Paula Clayton (*see* **WOMEN IN PSYCHIATRY**) named the syndrome after Briquet. The authors noted that hysteria, or Briquet's syndrome, is a "polysymptomatic disorder that is seen nearly always in females, begins early in life . . . and is characterized by recurrent or chronic ill health, the complicated history of which is frequently described dramatically" (p. 134). Hysteria in women and antisocial behavior in men tend to crop up in the same families, the authors noted. Four years later, in the *American Journal of Psychiatry*, Guze observed that hysteria and sociopathy tended to occur in the first-degree relatives of these patients, hence, it evidently had a partially genetic basis.

Hysteria disappears from psychiatry in *DSM-III* (1980). Under the pressure of enlightened public opinion, which tended to see the word "hysteria" when applied to women as stigmatizing, the task force that designed ***DSM-III*** smashed hysteria into a number of fragments.

This edition banished psychosomatic symptoms—historically the core of hysteria—to a group of diagnoses called "somatoform disorders," or "physical symptoms suggesting physical disorder." Among the somatoform disorders were "somatization disorder" (what Guze had called "Briquet's syndrome") and "conversion disorder," a physical symptom that "is apparently an expression of a psychological conflict" (p. 244).

It was the psychoanalysts who had given "hysterical personality" its currency, and in *DSM-III* this became "histrionic personality disorder": "Individuals with this disorder are lively and dramatic and are always drawing attention to themselves. They are prone to exaggeration and often act out a role, such as the 'victim' or the 'princess,' without being aware of it" (p. 313). Dissocation remained essentially unchanged. Those forms of hysteria once thought partly under the voluntary control of the patient were classified as "factitious disorders." The psychiatric tradition of seeing some brief psychoses as "hysterical" was acknowledged in a diagnosis called "brief reactive psychosis." (The index of *DSM-III* listed it under the adjective "hysterical.") Thus, *DSM-III* abolished hysteria from psychiatry.

I

ID. The word "unconscious" (das Unbewusste) was familiar in nineteenth-century Central European psychiatry. Freud used it from his earliest writings (1888 in Albert Villaret's *Dictionary of Medicine* [*Handwörterbuch der gesamten Medizin*] being apparently his first mention of it). Yet, the psychoanalytic term for the unconscious layer of the psyche referred to as the id was introduced into analysis in 1917 by Georg Groddeck (1866–1934), owner of the private sanatorium Villa Marienhöhe in Baden-Baden and amateur of Freud's ideas. In a book on *The Psychic Predetermination and Psychoanalytic Treatment of Organic Illness* (*Psychische Bedingtheit und psychoanalytische Behandlung organischer Leiden*) that he published in Leipzig in 1917, Groddeck said, "In the discussion of individual dispositions, I want to call attention to one feature of the human unconscious, of the id (das Es), which one might term the 'cautiousness of the id'; indeed I am almost inclined to use the expression, 'the reason of the id,' so similar are its expressions to those of the conscious mind, only that they are far more powerful" (*Schriften,* 70). In his 1923 book, *Ego and Id* (*Das Ich und das Es*), Freud decided to follow Groddeck's usage: "An individual is now for us a psychic id, unknown and unconscious, and the ego sits superficially on the id . . . not entirely enveloping it, in that way that an [embryonic] germinal disk rests on an egg" (*Gesammelte Werke,* XIII, p. 251).

IDENTITY. *See* **ERIK ERIKSON.**

ILLUSIONS. *See* **PSYCHOSIS: EMERGENCE: differentiating . . .** (1832).

IMIPRAMINE AND THE TRICYCLIC ANTIDEPRESSANTS (from 1957). By the mid-1950s, a number of drugs had become available with some effectiveness in nonhospital depression, such as meprobamate (Carter-Wallace's Miltown, launched in 1955) or the amphetamines (*see* **ANTIDEPRESSANT: first-generation**) and the amphetamine–**barbiturate** combinations. Yet, hospital depression remained untreatable except with **electroconvulsive therapy**. With the "tricyclic" antidepressants—so named because of their chemical structure—for the first time in history, serious depression acquired a pharmacotherapy of its own.

The story begins: In 1899, chemist Johannes Thiele (1856–1918), at the time director of the organic division of the chemistry laboratory of the Bavarian Academy of Sciences in Munich, together with his associate Otto Holzinger, synthesized an iminodibenzyl nucleus: two benzene rings attached to each other by a nitrogen atom and an ethylene bridge; this was unlike the phenothiazine nucleus [*see* **CHLORPROMAZINE**], which had a sulfur bridge instead of ethylene. Their article appeared in 1899 in *Justus Liebigs Annalen der Chemie*. In the late 1940s, chemists from the Geigy pharmaceutical company in Basel synthesized a number of derivatives from this base in their search for new antihistamines.

Roland Kuhn (1912–), a staff psychiatrist at the Münsterlingen asylum in Switzerland, had a long-standing arrangement with Geigy to undertake drug trials for them.

In 1951, at a time of great interest in the potential of antihistamines as hypnotics, Kuhn had tested a Geigy compound (G 22150) that turned out to be a poor hypnotic but had some effect on schizophrenic psychoses. In 1954, he called this to the attention of the head of pharmacology at Geigy, Robert Domenjoz (1908–1998), asking Geigy in light of the recent success of chlorpromazine if the firm wished him to undertake a larger trial. He also asked what else they might have on the shelf. Later in 1954, Kuhn met Domenjoz in a hotel in Zurich, where Domenjoz spread out a chart with about 40 chemical formulas and asked Kuhn to choose one for testing. Kuhn chose G 22355.

In the late autumn of 1954, Kuhn undertook trials of G 22355 at Münsterlingen. The drug turned out to be unimpressive in schizophrenia, but as Kuhn continued the trial, he started giving it to patients with "vital," or endogenous, depression. On the morning of January 18, 1956, one such patient, Paula I., who had been on G 22355 for 6 days, woke up cured of her depression. Said Kuhn later, "She reported this to Anna Keller, the nurse on her unit, who recognized the complete remission of her depression from the patient's facial expression, her behavior and her total being" (Ban, *Psychopharmacology*, III, p. 303). Kuhn reported this to Geigy shortly thereafter: "It is possible that . . . G 22355 [has] better effects on depression than Largactil [**chlorpromazine**] and Serpasil [**reserpine**]. So far, this cannot be said for certain, however. Should this impression be confirmed, it would be of importance." Yet, the firm was largely uninterested and continued to press for trials in other clinics of G 22355 as a "neuroleptic" (antipsychotic) or possibly as a hypnotic.

By April 1956, Kuhn was continuing the trials of G 22355 in depression and now was waving large signal flags at Geigy: "Since depression is not only one of the most frequently occurring mental illnesses, but one of the most frequently occurring illnesses in general, I see an immense potential here," he wrote to them. By April 1957, Geigy was sending G 22355 out to a wide network of trialists, but for trials in schizophrenia. Meanwhile, the Second World Congress of Psychiatry in Zurich was looming for the coming September 1957. Kuhn was asked to prepare a paper for it, to be published simultaneously in the August 31 issue of the *Swiss Medical Weekly* (*Schweizer Medizinische Wochenschrift*), and did so on his experiences with G 22355 in vital depression. On September 6, Kuhn read his paper to a half-empty room. (Kuhn said later it was probably a mistake not to have explained "vital depression," a concept of **Kurt Schneider's** and not widely familiar outside of German-speaking Europe.) (*See* **DEPRESSION: EMERGENCE: vital . . .** [1920].) Later that year, Geigy launched G 22355 in Switzerland as imipramine; brand name Tofranil.

But nobody at Geigy really woke up to the fact that the company had a drug on its hands with the potential impact of penicillin until a year later, in September 1958 at the first International Congress of Neuropharmacology in Rome (the company had organized a symposium to which Kuhn was not invited), Kuhn ran into Robert Boehringer, one of the owners of Geigy. Said Kuhn later, "After I told him that on 16 February [1958] in Basel I had pointed out the significance of G 22355 for the treatment of depression, Robert Boehringer, who had a case of depression in his family, took some tablets of the drug to Geneva, where he resided. After he returned home a week later he found the patient recovered. He notified the direction of the firm, whereupon it was agreed to continue the cooperation with me."

Geigy brought imipramine out in the American market in 1959. (They had patented it in 1951.) **Heinz Lehmann** at Verdun Protestant Hospital in Montreal did the first North American trials together with staff psychiatrists Charles Cahn (1921–) and Roger Louis De Verteuil (1919–ca. 1971), publishing the results in the October 1958 issue of the *Canadian Psychiatric Association Journal.* In 1965, in *Pharmacological Reviews*, **Gerald L. Klerman** and Jonathan O. Cole (1925–), under the auspices of the Psychophamacology Service Center of the **National Institute of Mental Health,** conducted a large review of the safety and effectiveness of imipramine, considering various head-to-head studies of the tricyclic antidepressants vs. **electroconvulsive therapy** vs. the MAOIs (*see* **IPRONIAZID**) and vs. **chlorpromazine** and other phenothiazines.

The great success of imipramine prompted a host of other tricyclic antidepressants, some of which, together with their launch date in the American market, follow by year of patent:

- 1960: amitriptyline (Merck launched Elavil in 1961).
- 1962: desipramine (Geigy launched Pertofrane in 1965); this is one of the main active metabolites of imipramine.
- 1963: clomipramine (Ciba-Geigy* launched as Anafranil in the United States in 1990—earlier in other markets, with Switzerland and West Germany in 1968 being the first).
- 1965: doxepin (Pfizer launched as Sinequan in 1969).
- 1965: nortriptyline (Lilly launched as Aventyl in 1965); this is a major metabolite of amitriptyline.

Although the many tricyclic antidepressants had varying side-effects, none was ever demonstrated superior in efficacy to imipramine, which remains today, despite the proliferation of many different drug classes of "**antidepressants,**" the gold standard of antidepressant therapy.

In his pioneering work, Kuhn scorned rating scales such as those of **Max Hamilton** and believed that only close clinical observation of patients, informed by a knowledge of psychopathology, would identify homogeneous groups of drug responders.

INSULIN COMA THERAPY (ICT) (1927 and after). After the discovery of insulin in 1922, efforts to employ it in psychiatry at subcoma levels began almost immediately. Manfred Sakel (pronounced SOK-el) (1900–1957) won a place in the history of psychiatry because he used insulin to induce hypoglycemic comas (hence the term "insulin shock therapy") in the treatment of schizophrenia, some of which were accompanied by convulsions. This was the first treatment of even partial effectiveness for schizophrenia.

Sakel, who graduated with an M.D. from the University of Vienna in 1925, became assistant physician at an exclusive private nervous clinic in Berlin-Lichterfelde. In 1927, he began treating the symptoms of morphine withdrawal with insulin, accidently inducing a coma in one patient, and deliberately putting some of his patients

---

* Ciba and Geigy merged in 1970; in 1996 Ciba-Geigy, merged with Sandoz, becoming Novartis.

in comas thereafter. In 1930, he announced his insulin treatment of withdrawal symptoms in the *German Medical Weekly* (*Deutsche Medizinische Wochenschrift*), not mentioning that he was inducing comas in the patients. (In a more extensive account in the *Journal of Combined Neurology and Psychiatry* [*Zeitschrift für die gesamte Neurologie und Psychiatrie*] in 1933, he did say that many of the patients became comatose.)

In 1933, after the Nazi seizure of power, Sakel returned to **Vienna** and persuaded psychiatry chief Otto Pötzl (1877–1962) to let him try the insulin cure on schizophrenics. (Apparently, Sakel had treated schizophrenics successfully in Berlin as well—some say inducing comas by accident—without writing about it.) Beginning in November 1934, in a 13-part series in the *Vienna Medical Weekly* (*Wiener Medizinische Wochenschrift*), Sakel described what the local population of Vienna was already starting to celebrate as a "miracle cure" for schizophrenia. In 1935, Sakel brought his findings together in a book, *A New Method of Treating Schizophrenia* (*Neue Behandlungsmethode der Schizophrenie*). The following year, in 1936, Sakel traveled to the United States to treat a wealthy private patient with the new therapy and then soon thereafter emigrated to New York. It was not, however, Sakel who introduced the procedure to an American audience but Joseph Wortis (1906–1995), then a staff psychiatrist at Bellevue Hospital in New York, who began insulin coma therapy there in 1934 after watching Sakel conduct it in Vienna, reporting his first results at a meeting in November 1936, and thereafter in the *Journal of Nervous and Mental Disease* in 1937. Bernard Glueck (1883–) at Stony Lodge, a private psychiatric hospital in Ossining, New York, should also be mentioned, for he had journeyed to the cantonal hospital in Münsingen, Switzerland, and watched Max Müller (1894–1980) perform it, describing his very favorable impressions in the *Journal of the American Medical Association* in September 1936.

The true effectiveness of ICT was much debated at the time and remains controversial among historians today. It is fairly clear that the effective element in the therapy was the convulsions that the treatment occasionally induced and not the insulin itself. Sakel was parsimonious with numbers, and it was difficult to tell from his account to what extent ICT was superior to placebo. Kurt Kolle (1898–1975), head of psychiatry in Munich, said in an obituary of Sakel in the *German Medical Weekly* (*Deutsche Medizinische Wochenschrift*) that 45% of the schizophrenic patients at the Munich university clinic received "lasting full remissions" from ICT, compared to 10% who improved spontaneously. **Linford Rees** said in 1950 that in a trial with historic controls, ICT had beaten **electroconvulsive therapy** and **leukotomy** in the treatment of schizophrenia. But in 1953, Harold Bourne, a resident at the Fountain Hospital in London, had looked at the literature on insulin treatment vs. electroconvulsive therapy and, in an article in the *Lancet* entitled "The Insulin Myth," found it no more effective. (Bourne had little sympathy for somatic therapies of any kind and later found himself a central figure in the "therapeutic communities" movement.) The article was strongly challenged by **William Sargant, Rees,** and **Willi Mayer-Gross**, all of whom had had quite favorable experiences with insulin. In time, insulin coma clinics arose in psychiatric hospitals around the world. Yet, it was a randomly controlled trial of **chlorpromazine** and ICT at Hillside Hospital in Glen Oaks, New York, led by **Max Fink** and published in the *Journal of the American Medical Association* in 1958, that wrote the death sentence of ICT: the authors found that "chlorpromazine had the advantage of being safer, easier to administer, and better suited to long-term management" (p. 1846).

In 1941, **Sargant** and Nellie Craske (née Wilson, M.B. 1929) described in the *Lancet* "modified insulin therapy," or insulin subcoma therapy, for high-grade anxiety in war neuroses. Their basic procedure was to administer a small enough dose of insulin to produce "a state of drowsiness," then to break the session an hour or two later by giving the patients sugary tea. The effect was quite salutary on the "anxious, hysterical and depressive symptoms of a reactive type" in men "who had broken down in the Flanders retreat [Dunkirk] or as a result of other severe war stress" (p. 213).

Subsequently, giving schizophrenics small doses of insulin over longer periods of time came into vogue as well.

Historically, ICT is important because it represents the first of the somatic therapies for the "functional psychoses," namely schizophrenia and manic-depressive illness.

IPRONIAZID AND THE MONOAMINE OXIDASE INHIBITORS (MAOIs) (from 1957). This is an early class of drugs noted to have a significant effect on depression.

The prehistory: In 1937, Caecilia Pugh and Juda Hirsch Quastel (1899–1987) at the biochemical laboratory of Cardiff City Mental Hospital observed in the *Biochemical Journal* that the brain has a system for oxidizing (metabolizing) amines (chemicals that contain NH groups) and that this system deaminates, or removes amino groups from the higher amines. This is significant because the major **neurotransmitters** all contain amines and are referred to as the "monoamines." Then, in 1952 at Hoffmann-La Roche Laboratories in Nutley, New Jersey, in research reported in the *Journal of Organic Chemistry*, chemist H. Herbert Fox (1912–?), who was trying to create new compounds for the treatment of tuberculosis, synthesized from a form of isonicotinic acid a drug later called isoniazid (made from a hydrazine base, or two NH groups hooked together).* It turned out to be effective against tuberculosis (TB), and from isoniazid a variant was synthesized called iproniazid (the phosphate of iproniazid was given the trade name Marsilid). It was not capable of being patented.

As clinicians gave iproniazid to TB patients, they noticed psychiatric "side effects." In the first clinical trial of the drug in 1952 for TB, Irving Selikoff (1915–1992) at the Paterson Clinic in New Jersey, together with associates, noted in the *Journal of the American Medical Association* that some of their patients had experienced "mild euphoria"; the authors reported this as an example of "drug toxicity." (Selikoff won an Albert Lasker Award in 1955 for codiscovering the treatment for TB.) In 1956, George E. Crane (1912–), a psychiatrist in the pulmonary division of Montefiore Hospital in the Bronx,

---

* In 1953, two Cincinnati psychiatrists, Harry M. Salzer (1906–) and Max L. Lurie (1920–), suggested in an article in the *A.M.A. Archives of Neurology and Psychiatry* that isoniazid had a therapeutic effect on anxiety and depression. Yet, isoniazid is not an MAO inhibitor, and other researchers were unable to confirm that it improved the mood of tuberculosis patients. In retrospect, the antidepressant effect of isoniazid was probably more owing to the enthusiasm with which patients receive any new drug rather than to its pharmacological usefulness. (This is the reason for making controlled trials the gold standard of evidence in psychiatry, although impressive anecdotal evidence, such as Salzer and Lurie supplied, should at least raise the level of curiosity.)

noted in the *American Journal of Psychiatry* the psychiatric "side effects" of iproniazid in tuberculous patients with mental disorders. He viewed the patients' "elation" and other symptoms as problematical rather than advantageous: "Iproniazid causes profound changes on certain psychic functions in the direction of an increase of mental capacity and vitality. . . . This new vitality, however, disturbs the emotional balance of some individuals by breaking down defenses and reactivating suppressed conflicts" (p. 500).

Thus, when **Nathan Kline** of the Rockland State Hospital in Orangeburg, New York, took another look at iproniazid as a possible psychiatric drug, it constituted a fresh approach. At a meeting in April 1957 that was sponsored by the American Psychiatric Association at the Upstate campus at Syracuse of the State University of New York, Kline and co-workers reported that their depressed in- and outpatients had done very well on iproniazid; that it seemed to be a "psychic energizer." The paper was published in December 1957 in *Psychiatric Research Reports*.

Meanwhile, other researchers were trying to figure out how iproniazid worked. In 1938, Ernst Albert Zeller (1907–1987), then an assistant at the Physiology-Chemistry Institute of Basel University, separated monoamine oxidase from diamine oxidase, thus discovering the enzyme (*see* his article in *Helvetica Chimica Acta*). In 1952, Zeller, who had emigrated from Switzerland in 1948 and was now professor of biochemistry at Northwestern University in Evanston, Illinois, found that iproniazid inhibited monoamine oxidase. (Inhibiting the enzyme would make monoamines available longer to the brain.) (For Zeller et al., *see Experientia*, 1952, p. 349.)

The crucial discovery here—one that unlocked the whole study of the monoamines in depressive illness and their treatment with drugs such as iproniazid—was guided by Alfred Pletscher (1917–), a Roche scientist who in 1955 was a guest worker at Bernard B. Brodie's (1909–1989) Laboratory of Chemical Pathology of the National Heart Institute, part of the National Institutes of Health in Bethesda. Pletscher, Parkhurst A. Shore (1924–), and Brodie determined that giving rabbits reserpine drove down the levels of serotonin in their gut tissue. Because **reserpine** already had a history of psychiatric effectiveness, the authors wrote, in the August 26, 1955, issue of *Science,* that "some of the central [brain] effects of reserpine are mediated through the release of serotonin" (p. 375). But if reserpine drove serotonin down, what would maintain it?

Shortly thereafter the same team, but this time with Brodie as the senior author, confirmed that the *Rauwolfia* alkaloids (reserpine) reduced the level of serotonin in the brain, whereas iproniazid maintained it (*see* their article in the *Journal of Pharmacology and Experimental Therapeutics* in 1956). (Back in Basel at Roche later in 1956, Pletscher and his colleague H. Besendorf demonstrated that iproniazid's effect on brain serotonin was indeed a causal one; *see* their 1956 article in *Helvetica Physiologica Acta.*) This was really the beginning of pharmacological psychiatry: a drug that would maintain brain serotonin might be clinically useful.

The significance of monoamine oxidase in the brain started to become clearer after Sidney Udenfriend (1918–) and collaborators in the Laboratory of Chemical Pharmacology at the National Heart Institute of the National Institutes of Health (NIH) established in 1957 that monoamine oxidase converted serotonin to a breakdown product (5-hydroindole acetic acid). When they gave iproniazid to animals (thus inhibiting monoamine oxidase), the animals experienced a rise in serotonin (*see* Udenfriend et al., *Biochemical Studies on Serotonin*, 1957).

Ipronazid and the Monoamine Oxidase Inhibitors (MAOIs)

As Roche scientist William A. Davis (1908–) explained in the *Journal of Clinical and Experimental Psychopathology* in 1958, "The information that Marsilid [iproniazid], an energizer, was able to raise the level of serotonin in the brain and that reserpine, a tranquilizer, lowered serotonin in brain tissue stimulated much interest in the biochemistry of brain function" (p. 3). Indeed, these findings from the laboratories of NIH opened a kind of royal road in psychopharmacology that would lead to many subsequent discoveries.

It should be added that this progress at the National Heart Institute was achieved only because in these years Brodie, Udenfriend, and Robert L. Bowman (1916–), the chief of the laboratory of technical development at the Institute, had constructed a spectrophotofluorimeter, a device that let them analyze small amounts of monoamines in the brain. They were thus able to follow levels of serotonin after the administration of drugs like reserpine and iproniazid. The device was first described in an article in *Science* in 1955, of which Bowman was senior author.

In 1961, Marsilid was withdrawn as being too toxic for clinical use. Yet, other MAOIs came onto the market, including nialamide (Roerig-Pfizer's Niamid, patented 1959 to Pfizer; U.S. launch 1959); isocarboxazid (Roche's Marplan, patented 1959 to Roche; U.S. launch 1959); phenelzine (Parke-Davis's Nardil, patented 1959 to Lakeside; U.S. launch 1959); tranylcypromine (Smith Kline Beecham's Parnate, patented 1961 to Smith Kline & French; U.S. launch 1961); and pargyline (Abbott's Eutonyl, patented in 1962 to Abbott; U.S. launch 1963). Nialamide, isocarboxazid, and phenelzine are all hydrazine derivatives.

In 1968 Donald S. Robinson (1928–) and co-workers at the National Heart Institute determined in an article published in *Biochemical Pharmacology* that blood platelets are rich in monoamine oxidase, and they developed a simple test for measuring the blood level of MAOIs by monitoring the level of the enzyme in the platelets. This made it possible to titrate doses more effectively. Arising from this work, Robinson and Alexander Nies (1930–1989), an assistant professor of psychiatry at Vermont (where Robinson had in the meantime moved), conducted the first double-blind placebo-controlled trial of an MAOI—phenelzine—clearly establishing its effectiveness in depression-anxiety (*see* their article in *Archives of General Psychiatry*, 1973).

On the scientific pathway of the monoamine oxidases, an important step was separating the two chemical variants, called A and B. This matters because some drugs act only on one or the other. In making this differentiation, two scientists in different laboratories reported more or less simultaneously: Moussa Youdim (1940–) was one; he had trained in pharmacology at **McGill University** and in the United Kingdom. In various papers from 1969 onward with Merton Sandler (1926–), professor of chemical pathology at several London institutions, Youdim characterized the two forms of monoamine oxidase. Working with Pletscher and pharmacologist Willi Haefely (1930–1993) at Roche, Youdim developed the drug moclobemide (Aurorix in some markets) for affective disorders, the first "reversible" (short-acting) MAO-A inhibitor without a potentially fatal side effect that plagued some of the older MAOIs (known as the "cheese reaction"). The other scientist simultaneously at work on MAOI subtypes was Joseph Knoll (1925–), a Budapest pharmacologist who in 1972 developed the drug selegiline (Deprenyl, among other trade names) for depression and Parkinsonism; selegiline is an MAO-B inhibitor and does not cause the cheese reaction.

(See Knoll and K. Magyar's article in *Advances in Biochemical Psychopharmacology* [1972]; they were apparently unaware of Youdim's work.)

In sum, the iproniazid story represents the initial discovery that modifying brain neurotransmitters could influence the course of psychiatric illness. As Alfred Pletscher later commented, "Although iproniazid has not been a commercially successful antidepressant, it was a remarkable breakthrough for drug research. It started research on MAO-inhibitors, which is still going on. . . . Iproniazid was one of the first modern psychotropic drugs shown to cause an alteration of cerebral neurotransmitter dynamics in vivo [in humans and animals]. This finding supported the general hypothesis that such changes might be causally connected with the action of antidepressant drugs in man" (in Ban, editor, *Reflections on Twentieth-Century Psychopharmacology* [2004], pp. 177–178).

J

JANET, PIERRE-MARIE-FELIX (1859–1947). Known for the introduction in France of medical psychotherapy and for coining the term "psychasthenia," Janet was born in Paris but grew up in the provinces, the son of a legal editor and nephew of a well-known professor of philosophy at the Sorbonne. In 1879, he was admitted to the École Normale Supérieure, an elite teacher-training institution, and after passing the Agrégation in 1882, he taught high school for a number of years. In search of a subject for a doctoral dissertation, he discovered psychology and began interviewing patients, giving an initial paper in 1885 on hypnosis and somnambulism. (Writing a dissertation in 1889 on "psychological automatism," at the time he was interested in such phenomena as **multiple personality**; he had already published a major article on "the doubling of personality" in 1886.)

In November 1889, Janet began medical school and was taken under **Jean-Martin Charcot's** wing; Charcot created for Janet a laboratory for the study of experimental psychology at the **Salpêtrière hospice** and presided over the examination in 1893 of Janet's medical thesis on the psychology of hysteria. In 1897, Janet left the Salpêtrière and quit the high school posts where he simultaneously had been teaching to take the chair of experimental psychology at the Sorbonne; from there, he progressed in 1902 to the Collège de France. Janet continued to practice medicine on the side and until 1942 consulted at the **Ste.-Anne mental hospital.**

Janet initiated medical psychotherapy in France in his 1893 book on the *Mental State of Hysterics* (*L'état mental des hystériques*), where he considered the utility of "suggestion," meaning hypnotic and nonhypnotic psychotherapy; he is also remembered for his coinage of the term "psychasthenia," a variety of neurasthenia for which Janet postulated the mechanism of lowered brain energy leading to "abulia" (meaning loss of will-power). (Some authorities, however, consider neurasthenia to be emotional hyperesthesia, whereas they view psychasthenia as intellectual weakness of some kind.) For Janet, the concept of psychasthenia included almost all psychiatric symptoms except hysteria. His two-volume work on *Obsessions and Psychasthenia* was published in 1903.

JASPERS, KARL (1883–1969). Jaspers was born in Oldenburg in northern Germany, studied law, qualified in medicine in 1908 at **Heidelberg**, then from 1908 to 1915 served as a part-time assistant at the Heidelberg psychiatric clinic under **Franz Nissl**; he worked only part-time because he had bronchiectasis and avoided a demanding schedule. In the psychiatric clinic, he did research on psychological testing and blood pressure. However, Jaspers's commitment to psychiatry was brief. At the clinic, his interests inclined increasingly to psychology, doing his Habilitation in that subject in 1913, as well as to philosophy. In 1920, he received an appointment in philosophy at Heidelberg, becoming chair of the department (Ordinarius) in 1922. Under National Socialism, in 1937 he was forced to retire because his wife, whom he refused to divorce, was Jewish; in 1943, he was forbidden to publish further; and in 1945, he was reinstated in the Chair at Heidelberg. In 1948, he became Chair (Ordinarius) of the philosophy department in Basel, from which post he retired in 1961. Thus, Jaspers is thought of primarily as a philosopher, yet his early contributions to psychiatry were of great importance.

His 1910 paper on delusional jealousy (Eifersuchtswahn) in the *Zeitschrift für die gesamte Neurologie und Psychiatrie* (*see* **PARANOIA**) brought into psychiatry the distinction of German philosopher Wilhelm Dilthey (pronounced DIL-tai) (1833–1911) between rational ways of knowing things, in this case knowing patients' symptoms, and empathic (einfühlbar) ways. The rational grasping of causal relationships Jaspers called—in Dilthey's terms—"explaining" (begreifen—also sometimes called erklären). This was in contrast to the intuitive feeling of one's way into a patient's subjective world and called "understanding" (verstehen). "When we look at psychic life we have two pathways: We try to put ourselves in the other's shoes, we feel our way into the person (verstehen). Or we observe individual elements of the phenomenon in their relationship and causal order, . . . explaining without necessarily achieving empathy. We limit ourselves to 'explaining' (begreifen), as when we explain relationships in the physical world, in the sense that we think of an objective underlying process, a 'physical' one or an 'unconscious' one, where nature has inherently determined that we cannot empathize our way into it" (p. 602).

In the case of pathological jealousy, for example, verstehen would permit the physician to perceive psychologically that jealousy had always been part of the patient's personality development. Yet, if the jealousy had come out of the blue, as part of the onset of a sudden brain-disease process, the more rational act of begreifen would be appropriate. This distinction between the contemplation of causes and intuitiveness had a large impact on psychiatry: understanding implied to see meaning in motivated behavior, to understand (verstehen) "how affects arise out of certain moods," compared to the explaining (begreifen) of causal analysis, how memory loss or fatigue occur.

Jaspers later wrote in his autobiography (1977) of applying these distinctions in practice at Heidelberg: "We distinguished on the one hand the patient's biographical course as the development of his personality that evolved in an understandable way through the phases of life; and on the other the processes that might cause a person to become dramatically different in a wrenching break, for reasons that we considered to be organic without really knowing what they were" (p. 20). Later, followers of Jaspers talked about "life history" vs. "case history."

As a result of having already written several penetrating essays, in 1911 Jaspers was asked by his colleague Karl Wilmanns (*see* **HEIDELBERG**) (and by the Springer Publishers) to undertake a general textbook of psychopathology. Published in 1913, the year in which Jaspers received his Habilitation in psychology, *General Psychopathology* (*Allgemeine Psychopathologie*) would become the single most influential text in **psychopathology**, although Jaspers was not the originator of the term. The book went through a number of editions, Jaspers completing the ultimate version in 1942 with the help of Kurt Schneider but not allowed to publish it until 1946. The most recent reprint of this 1946 version came out in 1973 as the "ninth edition." The English translation of Jaspers's book was greatly delayed, and only in 1962 did Jan Hoenig and Marian Hamilton bring out the seventh edition as *General Psychopathology*. It remains the classic guide to the study of psychopathology.

JONES, ERNEST (1879–1958). Known as the Welshman who was closest to Freud's inner circle and as Freud's most prominent early biographer, Jones was born into the family of a mineowner in Wales. In 1901, he graduated with an M.B. from University College London and soon thereafter his brother-in-law, a surgeon, drew his attention to Freud's works. Given the depressed state of British psychiatry at the time, Jones is said to have been awed that there was "a man in Vienna who actually listened with attention to every word his patients said to him." In 1908, Jones attended the first international psychoanalytical congress in Salzburg, where he met Freud and decided to devote himself to Freud's doctrine. From 1908 to 1913, he lectured on psychiatry at the medical school in Toronto—one of the earliest psychoanalysts to teach in a faculty of medicine. From this Canadian outpost, he began to seed North America with psychoanalysts, and in 1911 helped found the American Psychoanalytic Association. Then in 1913, he set himself up in London as a practitioner of psychoanalysis and founded the London Psycho-Analytical Society, which in 1919 became the British Psycho-Analytical Society, as it was then called, of which Jones was president for many years. In 1953, the first volume of his source-based but hagiographical biography of Freud was published, *The Life and Work of Sigmund Freud*, the third and last appearing in 1957.

JUNG, CARL GUSTAV (1875–1961). The creator of a system of psychotherapy that once aspired to rival psychoanalysis, Jung was born in Kesswil, Switzerland, into a pastor's family. He finished his medical studies in Basel in 1900. (Jung's M.D. degree was from Zurich in 1902, with a dissertation on *The Psychology and Pathology of So-called Occult Phenomena* (*Zur Psychologie und Pathologie sog. Okkulter Phänomene*). After studying with **Pierre Janet** in Paris, in 1900 he entered training in psychiatry at the University Psychiatric Clinic (**Burghölzli**) in Zurich under **Eugen Bleuler**, and finished his Habilitation in 1905, which was published in 1907 as *The Psychology of Dementia praecox* (*Über die Psychologie der Dementia praecox*). In 1909, Jung gave up university teaching to enter private practice and to dedicate himself to his writing.

Jung had become inspired by Freud's ideas in 1903 after re-reading *The Interpretation of Dreams* (*Die Traumdeutung*, 1900), and in 1906 began corresponding with Freud. Freud and Jung met in Vienna in 1907. As early as 1906, Jung was doing empirical research on word association in an effort to confirm Freud's ideas (which his article that year in the volume *Diagnostische Assoziationsstudien* claimed to do). Yet in 1914, Jung resigned from the presidency of the International Psychoanalytic Association and broke with Freud.

Jung went on to develop his own "analytical psychology," in which infant sexuality played virtually no role but instead symbols of the "collective unconscious" occupied center stage. The symbols in the patient's psyche do not stem from the patient's personal experience, Jung said, but from the collective experiences of the human race. For these experiences, Jung chose the term "archetypes." In a Jungian analysis, the patient ultimately comes to realize that symbols previously perceived as personal and individual are in reality expressions of the collective unconscious. Jung began to articulate these notions in "Transformations and Symbols of the Libido: Contributions to the Developmental History of Thought," published in the *Psychoanalytic Yearbook* in 1911 ("Wandlungen und Symbole der Libido: Beiträge zur Entwicklungsgeschichte des Denkens," *Jahrbuch für Psychoanalyse und psychopathologische Forschung*). The first comprehensive statement of his ideas was *The Psychology of Unconscious Processes: An Overview of the Modern Theory and Method of Analytical Psychology* (*Die Psychologie der unbewussten Prozesse: ein Überblick über die moderne Theorie und Methode der analytischen Psychologie*, 1917).

Jung is also known for his typology of personality types. In his book *Psychological Types* (*Psychologische Typen*, 1921), he elaborated the difference between extraverted individuals, whose energy flows toward the outer world, and introverts, whose energy flows inward. For each type, there were four basic modes of functioning: thinking, feeling, sensation, and intuition, yielding an eight-box grid on which to classify personality variation.

Although Jung's analytical psychology was much overshadowed by psychoanalysis, it retained a certain international audience during the first half of the twentieth century, becoming more of a curiosity thereafter. Jung's reputation also suffered because of his sympathy with the National Socialist regime in Germany.

K

KAHLBAUM, KARL LUDWIG (1828–1899). One of the originators of the concept of schizophrenia—next to **Bénédict-Augustin Morel** and **Emil Kraepelin**—and pioneer of nosology, Kahlbaum was born in a small Prussian town into the family of a coachman. Although he had a bent toward the natural sciences, practical considerations steered him to medicine, and he received his M.D. from Berlin University in 1854. In 1856, he joined the staff of the Allenberg asylum in East Prussia and distinguished himself by his careful observation of patients. In 1863, he received his Habilitation in psychiatry at the University of Königsberg in East Prussia. Three years later, in 1866, after the Prussian ministry had denied him a clinical professorship in psychiatry, he took a post at a private nervous clinic in Görlitz, and in 1867 he became owner of the clinic. Here, he founded a service for pediatric psychiatry (Pädagogium für jugendliche Nerven- und Gemüthskranke), where he and his assistant Ewald Hecker (1843–1909), whom he had brought with him from Allenberg, had opportunity to examine a number of young people with acute schizophrenia. (Kahlbaum was married to a cousin of Hecker's.)

Kahlbaum was among the first researchers to separate out different disease entities in psychiatry on the basis of course. (*See* **SCHIZOPHRENIA: EMERGENCE** [from 1863].) The model of neurosyphilis was the inspiration of this entire generation of investigators: find other diseases that also had constantly changing symptom pictures at any given moment, yet all of which ineluctably end in death and dementia (or end in some other way, but which have a common course). In 1863, he published his Habilitation, *The Classification of Psychiatric Diseases* (*Die Gruppirung der psychischen Krankheiten*), which identified "typical insanity" (Vesania typica) as degenerating progressively into dementia. In 1874 his book, *Catatonia* (*die Katatonie: oder das Spannungsirresein*), placed motor symptoms in psychosis on the map. And an article of his in 1882 in *Der Irrenfreund* (*The Friend of the Insane*) described cyclothymia. (*See* **MANIC-DEPRESSIVE ILLNESS.**) In view of the enormous curriculum vitas that investigators compile today, it is worthy of note that Kahlbaum, whom Carl Wernicke (*see* **WERNICKE-KLEIST-LEONHARD PATHWAY**) considered next only to **Theodor Meynert**, had a lifetime record of publication of only 16 books and articles.

KLEIN, DONALD F. (1928–). One of the pioneers of psychopharmacology and nosology in the United States in the 1960s and after, Klein was born in New York City. He trained at Creedmoor State Hospital and served from 1953 to 1958 at the U.S. Public Health Service Narcotics Hospital in Lexington, Kentucky. From 1959 to 1976, he was a research psychiatrist at Hillside Hospital in Glen Oaks, New York, in the department of experimental psychiatry that **Max Fink** had founded in 1956, advancing to director of research and evaluation. In 1974, Hillside Hospital merged and became the Long Island Jewish-Hillside Medical Center. In 1976, he became professor of psychiatry at Columbia University medical school and director of research at New York State Psychiatric Institute. Although a candidate at the New York Psychoanalytic Institute between 1957 and 1961, Klein's interest, as he put it, "turned to other, more promising, directions."

In 1962, Klein and Fink at Hillside found in a placebo-controlled randomized trial that depressed patients benefited from **chlorpromazine**, a phenothiazine-class antipsychotic medication, just as well as patients treated with **imipramine**, the first tricyclic antidepressant. This finding, published in the *Archives of General Psychiatry*, further challenged* the distinction then forming between "antipsychotics" and "antidepressants." Two years later, in an article in *Psychopharmacologia* in 1964, Klein suggested on the basis of a double-blind placebo-controlled trial that "anxiety" was not a single affect. Spontaeous panic and anticipatory anxiety could be distinguished on the basis of response to medication. Hospitalized agoraphobic patients had their spontaneous panic attacks remit during imipramine treatment but maintained high levels of anticipatory anxiety and phobic avoidance. Furthermore, these patients did poorly on chlorpromazine, which was then considered a powerful agent in psychotic anxiety, as psychosis was then considered due to extreme anxiety.

The article marked the beginning of the emergence of **panic disorder** as an independent disease entity. Moreover, it opened a new chapter in psychopharmacology with "the use of patterns of drug response as dissecting tools" in delineating diseases. One of the earliest textbooks in the uses of psychotropic drugs, *Diagnosis and Drug Treatment of Psychiatric Disorders* (1969), was co-authored by Klein with John M. Davis (1933–), who was then a psychopharmacologist at the National Institute of Mental Health.

In 1974, Klein proposed in the *Archives of General Psychiatry* "endogenomorphic depression," a diagnosis that cut across the reactive vs. endogenous distinction, as a revision to the depression nosology. Although the diagnosis was not taken up in ***DSM-III***, the core criteria of loss of interest and pleasure were accepted. It also led to research in "atypical depression." (*See* **DEPRESSION: RECENT CONCEPTS: atypical depression (revived)** [1979].) At the New York State Psychiatric Institute, which is linked to the department of psychiatry of Columbia University, Klein was the senior figure in a group of researchers including Frederic Quitkin (1937–) and Michael Liebowitz (1945–). They devised innovative ways of looking at depressive and anxiety disorders, including "social anxiety disorder." They also called attention to the benefits of the then neglected monoamine oxidase inhibitor class of antidepressant drugs. (*See* **IPRONIAZID.**)

KLEIN, MELANIE REIZES (1880–1960). Leading theorist of the unconscious in early stages of infancy, Melanie Klein was born in Vienna, the daughter of a physician. She studied art and history at Vienna University, without graduating, then at the age of 21 married Arthur Klein, a chemist, and followed him to Budapest. Here, she became enthusiastic about the new discipline of psychoanalysis and underwent an analysis

* In 1959, John Mark Hinton, then a senior registrar at the **Maudsley Hospital** (and later successor to Denis Hill as professor of psychiatry at Middlesex Hospital), had already shown in the *Journal of Mental Science* that the antipsychotic perphenazine was effective in depression. There is also anecdotal evidence from Jean Sigwald's trial in 1953 that chlorpromazine had done well as an antidepressant.

with Freud's disciple Sandor Ferenczi (1873–1933), reading a paper on child development in 1919 to the Budapest Psycho-Analytical Society. In 1921, she separated from her husband, he moving to Sweden and she, at the invitation of psychoanalyst Karl Abraham (1877–1925), moving to Berlin, where she became involved in the psychoanalysis of children and started to develop the psychoanalytic play technique for which she became known. In 1925, at the invitation of English psychoanalyst **Ernest Jones**, she lectured on psychoanalysis in London, moving there the following year. It was in England that she developed her great reputation as a child analyst, later proceeding to the analysis of adults as well. Her theories polarized much of the membership of the budding British Psychoanalytic Society, the "Kleininans" endorsing her ideas about introjection and projection, as opposed to the rival theories of **Anna Freud**. In 1932, she published a major work, *The Psycho-Analysis of Children*. As her biographer, John Arnold Lindon explains, "Introjection and projection function from the beginning of postnatal life as some of the earliest activities of the ego. Introjection implies that the outer world . . . is experienced as taken into the self and thus becomes part of the infant's inner life." "Projection alters the infant's impression of his environment, and by introjection this changed picture of his environment influences what goes on in his mind. Thus an inner world is built up that is partly a reflection of the external one" (*Psychoanalytic Pioneers*, pp. 366–367). Other Kleinian concepts such as "splitting" and "projective identification" permitted Klein, a lay analyst, to build a bridge between the experiences of early childhood and the formation of psychiatric symptoms in the adult.

KLERMAN, GERALD L. (1928–1992). The epidemiology of depression and the description of a new form of psychotherapy represent the major achievements of "Jerry" Klerman, the consummate psychiatric insider. Born in New York City, Klerman graduated with an M.D. from New York University in 1954 and trained in psychiatry at the Massachusetts Mental Health Center in Boston in the glory days of psychoanalysis. From 1959 to 1961, Klerman worked as Jonathan Cole's (1925–) assistant in the Psychopharmacology Service Center of the **National Institute of Mental Health** (NIMH), then returned to Harvard as an instructor in psychiatry. In 1965, he joined the department of psychiatry of Yale University as an assistant professor, and in that year he and Cole showed in a paper in *Pharmacological Reviews* that **imipramine** did indeed have a therapeutic effect in depression. From 1970 to 1977, Klerman was professor of psychiatry at Harvard, then after a brief stretch as an administrator at the National Institutes of Health in Bethesda, he returned to Harvard from 1980 to 1985 as director of the Stanley Cobb Research Laboratories at the Massachusetts General Hospital. From 1985 until his death from diabetes, he was professor of psychiatry at Cornell University Medical College in New York (at the Payne Whitney Clinic). Also, from 1972 on, he headed the NIMH collaborative program on the psychobiology of depression, a large longitudinal study that concluded the incidence of depression was increasing. He also launched in 1977 the epidemiologic catchment area study, the results of which appeared in 1991 in a volume edited by Lee Robins (**St. Louis school**). Beginning in 1974, he and his wife, epidemiologist **Myrna Weissman**, together with several others, described the "interpersonal" system of the psychotherapy of depression: a "brief, focused, specific strategy," as per the subtitle of the book (1984) that emerged at the end of their project. (*See* **PSYCHOTHERAPY: interpersonal**

psychotherapy [from 1967].) In 1982, he became the leader of a major study of the drug alprazolam (Xanax), funded by the Upjohn company and described by his obituarist psychiatrist Martin Keller (1946–) of Brown University as "the largest multinational, multicenter controlled clinical trial in the history of psychiatry." (*See* **BENZODIAZEPINES.**)

KLINE, NATHAN SCHELLENBERG (1916–1983). Kline grew up in Atlantic City, New Jersey, in a family that owned a chain of department stores; his mother, Flora Schellenberg, was a physician. After studying psychology at Harvard graduate school in the late 1930s, Kline went into medicine and graduated with an M.D. from New York University in 1943. He began training in psychiatry at **St. Elizabeths Hospital** in Washington, D.C., served in the Second World War, and in 1946 worked as a research assistant at Columbia University's medical school. In 1950, he became research director at Worcester State Hospital in Massachusetts, one of the oldest state hospitals in the United States. He finally became a board-certified psychiatrist in 1953, shortly after leaving Worcester to become research director at Rockland State Hospital in Orangeburg, New York. At Rockland, he would stay for the rest of his days, until his death in New York City of an aortic aneurysm. In 1975, his unit became the Rockland Research Institute. Between 1957 and 1980, Kline also had an academic affiliation with Columbia.

One of the pioneers of psychopharmacology in the United States, Kline made two major discoveries. In 1954, he confirmed the effect of various extracts and alkaloids of the plant *Rauwolfia serpentina* Benthan, especially the alkaloid **reserpine** (already in use against hypertension), in chronically ill psychiatric patients. Using a placebo-controlled trial, Kline discovered that *R. serpentina* significantly reduced anxiety in psychotic patients, making them "able to talk more freely during psychotherapy." It also exerted a "tremendous[ly] relaxing and tranquilizing effect" on restless and tense patients, making **insulin coma therapy** unnecessary for some. As well, "dreams became vivid and easily remembered." Kline's report in the *Annals of the New York Academy of Sciences* launched reserpine on its brief career as an antipsychotic and antianxiety drug before it went out of fashion in psychiatry because of side effects (the accusation that it induced depression seems to have been a canard). In 1957, Kline won a Lasker Award for this work.

In 1957, Kline and two colleagues reported at a psychiatry meeting their clinical experience with the antituberculosis drug **iproniazid** on apathetic and depressed patients in hospital and in his private practice in Manhattan. Kline also recounted the drug's effect on himself. Contrary to what previous researchers had believed, iproniazid seemed effective in various psychoneuroses, and the researchers—who later ended up in ligitation over their various roles—called it a "psychic energizer." It was one of the early drugs that acted upon monoamine oxidase in the brain and hence were termed monoamine oxidase inhibitors, or MAOIs, useful especially in the treatment of depression. Kline published the work in June 1958 in the *Journal of Clinical and Experimental Psychopathology*, and for it he won a second Lasker Award in 1964.

In the often gray world of academic psychiatry, Kline cut an unusually colorful figure. He was frequently described as "hypomanic." "His private practice was like something out of a Hollywood movie," said **Michael Shepherd**. A grateful patient made it possible for Kline and fellow psychopharmacologists to meet every year in some luscious Caribbean setting, a convocation named in her honor as "the Denghausen Group." From this group emerged the idea of the first large international lithium trial. In 1955, Kline testified for the first time before the United States Congress on the need for federal support of psychopharmacology, and before long large sums were flowing into the coffers of the **National Institute of Mental Health**. There is no doubt that Kline's role as advocate hastened the adoption of psychopharmacology in the mainstream of American psychiatric practice at a time when psychoanalysis predominated.

KORSAKOFF'S PSYCHOSIS. *See* **DEMENTIA.**

KRAEPELIN, EMIL (pronounced Krep-LEEN) (1856–1926). The founder of modern psychiatric nosology, Kraepelin was born in the province of Mecklenburg in northern Germany into the family of a music teacher. Kraepelin finished his medical studies at Würzburg University in 1878. After 4 years at the Upper Bavarian Provincial Asylum in Munich under Bernhard von Gudden (1824–1886), Kraepelin became a staff psychiatrist in Leipzig under Professor Paul Flechsig (1847–1929), working at the same time in the laboratory of psychologist Wilhelm Wundt (1832–1920). In 1883, he wrote his Habilitation. After several years' work as an asylum psychiatrist in various places, in 1886 he was appointed Ordinarius professor of psychiatry at Dorpat (Tartu) University, then in the Russian Empire (later Estonia); in 1891, he returned to Germany to become the Ordinarius professor of psychiatry in **Heidelberg** and director of the university psychiatric clinic. At Heidelberg, where neurology was part of internal medicine (the chair held by neurologist Wilhelm Erb [1840–1921]), Kraepelin could follow his own tastes and devote himself entirely to psychiatry. What he wanted was a psychiatry with the neurology removed from it, a complete break with past traditions.

In 1903, Kraepelin moved to Munich as the Ordinarius professor of psychiatry and director of the university clinic there, new quarters for which opened the following year. He would remain in Munich thereafter, founding in 1917 in the Munich suburb of Schwabing the German Psychiatric Research Institute for Psychiatry (Deutsche Forschungsanstalt für Psychiatrie; DFA), which later came under the patronage of the nationwide sponsor of scientific research institutes, the Kaiser-Wilhelm-Institut (renamed the Max Planck Gesellschaft after the Second World War). He was emerited in 1922.

(Details on Kraepelin's scientific accomplishments may be found at **DEPRESSION: EMERGENCE: involutional melancholia** [1896]; **"depression" becomes preferred . . .** [1904]; **MANIC-DEPRESSIVE ILLNESS** [1899]; **PARANOIA**; and **SCHIZOPHRENIA: EMERGENCE: Emil Kraepelin's dementia praecox** [from 1893]; for other locations, *see* the index).

Kraepelin completely recast the way psychiatrists thought about major diagnoses, elevating such entities as depression and psychosis into diseases, a step up from syndromes, or clusters of symptoms. (*See* **PSYCHOPATHOLOGY.**) Kraepelin accomplished this feat in successive editions of his textbook, at a time when scientists influenced their colleagues by writing textbooks rather than learned articles:

- First edition (1883): *Compendium der Psychiatrie*, published by Abel in Leipzig (which was the publisher of all editions up to the fourth, after which Barth in Leipzig became Kraepelin's publisher).

- Second edition (1887): *Psychiatry: A Short Textbook for Students and Physicians, completely revised* (*Psychiatrie: ein kurzes Lehrbuch für Studierende und Ärzte*).
- Third edition (1889).
- Fourth edition (1893).
- Fifth edition (1896).
- Sixth edition (1899).
- Seventh edition (1903–1904), 2 vols.
- Eighth edition (1909–1915), 4 vols.

Kraepelin was in the act of revising the ninth edition together with Johannes Lange (1891–1938), who was shortly to become head of the clinical division of the DFA, when he died in 1926. It was published in 1927, edited by Lange.

Kraepelin also wrote in 1892 the first book of a pharmaco-psychological nature, *On the Influencing of Simple Psychic Processes through Medical Drugs* (*Über die Beeinflussung einfacher psychischer Vorgänge durch einige Arzneimittel*), although the drugs he discussed were used for research purposes rather than therapeutically. The passages on the effects of drugs upon fatigability in the performance of various intellectual functions became a point of departure for much subsequent psychological research.

American psychiatrist Clarence B. Farrar (1874–1970), who as a postdoctoral student had known Kraepelin at Heidelberg, said much later, "Research, not medical practice, was his all-absorbing interest." Kraepelin was singleminded about science. Yet, he was not dogmatic: "We're still at the very beginning."

In later years, opinions about Kraepelin and his work were highly divided. New York psychiatrist Smith Ely Jelliffe (1866–1945) called him in 1932 in the *Archives of Neurology* the "greatest synthesizer of psychiatry of the present era," in a line of systematizers going back to "Asclepiades of Bithynia." On the other hand, more recently social-psychiatrist **Michael Shepherd** at the Institute of Psychiatry in London told American schizophrenia researcher **Nancy Andreasen** that he was unable to understand her enthusiasm for Kraepelin's work: "I was very sad to see that you've turned this man into an icon. He was a monster who has done a great deal of harm" (Healy, *Psychopharmacologists*, II, pp. 247–248).

KRAFFT-EBING, RICHARD VON (1840–1902). Born in Mannheim, Germany, his father a high public official, Krafft-Ebing graduated in medicine in **Heidelberg** in 1863 and in 1864 began psychiatric training with Christian Friedrich Wilhelm Roller (1802–1878) in the Illenau asylum in Baden. Four years later, he opened a private psychiatry practice in the spa town of Baden-Baden. After military service in the 1870–1871 war against France, Krafft-Ebing resumed academic training and in 1872 was called to the (newly German) university at Strasbourg as an associate professor (ausserordentlicher Professor). In 1873, he was appointed director of the asylum in Feldhof bei Graz, Austria, simultaneously coappointed professor of psychiatry at Graz University. (He soon resigned from the asylum appointment to concentrate on the teaching of psychiatry at the university, to which was shortly added neurology.) In 1889, he was called to **Vienna** as Max Leidesdorf's replacement as professor of psychiatry in the chair in the Vienna asylum. Until 1892, Krafft-Ebing worked alongside **Theodor Meynert** (who had the professorship of psychiatry in the Vienna General Hospital), then with

Meynert's death in 1892, Krafft-Ebing switched over to the hospital chair, which had an associated neurology clinic. Krafft-Ebing retired in 1902, moving back to Graz, where he died 6 months later.

In 1872, Krafft-Ebing published an important manual, *Textbook of Psychiatry on a Clinical Basis* (*Lehrbuch der Psychiatrie auf klinischer Grundlage*), an enlarged new edition of which appeared in 1879–1880; the work took an organicist view of mental illness and was noted for its many case histories, a French quality the Germans had begun to borrow. Yet, there is no doubt that the work for which he remains historically celebrated virtually to the present was his great textbook of sexology, *Psychopathia sexualis: A Clinical-Forensic Study* (*. . . eine klinisch-forensische Studie*), the first edition of which was published in 1886; 16 subsequent German editions followed plus translations into English (1893), French (1895), and Italian (1896). In retrospect, the book established sexology as a psychiatric area of inquiry, but at the time it scandalized the Austrian academic community while making Krafft-Ebing's name worldwide a synonym for what was then considered sexual deviation. Krafft-Ebing believed that the various perversities he described in lurid detail were a result of **Morel**ian degeneration, although he later, in 1900, retracted his view that homosexuality was an activity of degenerates. (*See* **HOMOSEXUALITY AND PSYCHIATRY.**) For better or worse, this work laid the basis of the modern scientific study of sexuality. The judgment of Krafft-Ebing's life by his colleague, Viennese neurologist Moritz Benedikt (1835–1920), was that, "He was a highly gifted literary figure but in critical and scientific terms incapable to the point of feeblemindedness" (*Aus meinem Leben*, pp. 391–392).

KRETSCHMER, ERNST (1888–1964). Born into a pastor's family in a small town in Swabia, a region of southwest Germany, Kretschmer studied in church schools, then enrolled in philosophy at Tübingen University; he studied medicine at Munich and Hamburg, qualifying as a physician in 1913. He then began a residency (Assistentenstelle) at the Tübingen psychiatric clinic under Robert Gaupp (1870–1953). During the war years (1914–1918), he served as an army psychiatrist and became familiar with the combat neuroses. He received his Habilitation in 1918 under Gaupp and was a staff psychiatrist in Tübingen until becoming in 1926 Ordinarius professor in Marburg University and director of the psychiatric clinic. He returned to Tübingen as Ordinarius in 1946. Kretschmer is best known for his 1918 work on sensitive delusions of reference (*see* **PSYCHOSIS: EMERGENCE: sensitive delusions of reference**), and his 1921 book, *Body and Character* (*Körperbau und Charakter*). (*See* **PSYCHOSIS: EMERGENCE: Kretschmer's constitutional psychoses** [1921]; *see also* **PERSONALITY DISORDERS, Kretschmer's types** [1921].)

L

LACAN, JACQUES-MARIE-EMILE (1901–1981). The founder of an independent school of thought within psychoanalysis, Lacan was born in Paris into an upper-middle-class family. As an intern at the psychiatric hospitals of the Seine department (Paris), in 1928 he spent a year with Gaétan Gatian de Clérambault (1872–1934) at the Infirmérie spéciale (the Paris psychiatry emergency department) (*see* **FRENCH CHRONIC DELUSIONAL STATES** [1920]), and later referred to Clérambault as "my only teacher." In 1932, after defending an M.D. thesis on paranoid psychosis, he became chef de clinique (assistant physician) of **Henri Claude** at the **Ste.-Anne mental hospital**, in the meanwhile moving within surrealist intellectual circles. He was, according to P. Godefroy's biographical account, much influenced by Alexandre Koyré's philosophy seminar at the School for Higher Studies (École pratique des hautes études) on Hegel, and he set out to equip Freudian thought with "a philosophical set of armor."

In 1932, Lacan began a didactic (learning) analysis with the well-known Parisian psychoanalyst Rudolph Loewenstein (1898–1976) and thereafter moved exclusively within the world of psychoanalysis rather than the world of clinical psychiatry. In 1936, he gave a paper at the congress of the International Psychoanalytic Association at Marienbad on what Lacan called the "mirror phase" of infant development, initiating a long period of writing and lecturing. In 1953, Lacan, together with a band of dissidents, left the Société psychanalytique de Paris to found the Société Française de Psychanalyse (SFP). Because his controversial technique of ending analytic sessions abruptly and treating the patients unconventionally continued to cause waves (Lacan might, for example, look after his correspondence during an analytic session and then ask the patient to drop the letters in the mail), in 1963 he left the SFP to found his own society, the École Freudienne de Paris, which dissolved a year before his death. Also in 1963, he shifted his well-attended lectures from the psychiatric clinic of the Ste.-Anne mental hospital (where **Jean Delay**, in a fit of pique at Lacan's celebrity, had denied him the use of a meeting room), to the École Normale Supérieure, and thence to the Law Faculty at the Panthéon. It was an ascent to world fame as well. "One fact remains undeniable," said Paris psychiatrist Jean Thuillier (1921–) in 1996. "It is the progression of a brilliant mind going from a clear conception of psychiatry in the years before the war up to what certain people have called a 'jargonaphasia' in the last years of his life" (Thuillier, *La Folie*, pp. 601–602).

LASÈGUE, ERNEST-CHARLES (1816–1883). Originator of a crucial early differentiation in psychiatric diagnosis (that persecutory delusions without deterioration of the personality were a separate illness from madness; *see* **PARANOIA**), Lasègue was born in Paris, the son of a distinguished naturalist. He interned at the **Salpêtrière hospice** under **Jean-Pierre Falret** (having physiologist Claude Bernard [1813–1878] as a fellow intern) and defended his doctoral thesis in 1846. In 1850, he became the first medical director of the psychiatric intake service of the Paris Prefecture of Police—then called the "dêpot" rather than, as after 1872, the Infirmérie spéciale—where he continued to preside for the rest of his career while having other posts as well. This intake service functioned for Lasègue, as for a number of other clinicians over the years, as an inexhaustible source of mental pathology. In 1853, Lasègue passed his Agrégation exam, and the next year was appointed to the rank of ward chief (médecin des hôpitaux). Thereafter, he made a number of lateral moves through the Paris public hospitals, including the **Salpêtrière hospice**, Saint-Antoine hospital, and Necker hospital (where after 1862 he began lecturing on psychiatry). He lectured on psychiatry at the Salpêtrière as well, and in 1866, the final year of the series, took the students on a field trip to hear **Bénédict-Augustin Morel** discoursing on degeneration (*see* **PSYCHOSIS: EMERGENCE: mania . . . degeneration** [1857]) at the Saint-Yon asylum near Rouen. Lasègue finally landed at La Pitié hospital, where, after being promoted in 1867 to the academic rank of professor of pathology, in 1869 he received the chair in clinical medicine. He wrote widely about issues in internal medicine, but his contributions in psychiatry were his 1852 article on delusions of persecution (*see* **PARANOIA**), "hysterical anorexia" (*see* **BODY IMAGE: DISTURBANCES OF: anorexia nervosa** [1873]), and **FOLIE À DEUX**.

LEARNING DISABILITIES. *See* **AUTISM; MENTAL RETARDATION.**

LEHMANN, HEINZ EDGAR (1911–1999). A pioneer of international psychopharmacology, Lehmann was born in Berlin, his father a general surgeon and Jewish, his mother non-Jewish. After gaining his M.D. from the University of Berlin in 1935, he sensed which way the wind was blowing and in 1937 emigrated to Canada. In Montreal, he became a staff physician at the Verdun Protestant Hospital (later Douglas Hospital), a large asylum where he saw patients for the next 60 years. In 1948, he was appointed lecturer in psychiatry at **McGill University** in Montreal and remained actively involved in teaching, becoming chair in 1970. It was his scientific curiosity plus his ability to read European languages that led Lehmann to two achievements.

The first was **chlorpromazine**. Sometime in 1952 or 1953, a sales representative of the Rhône-Poulenc company left at Lehmann's office some promotional literature in French on the firm's new drug, chlorpromazine. Lehmann, perusing the pamphlets at home in his bathtub, found his curiosity arrested and conducted with his resident Gorman Edward Hanrahan (1925–) one of the first North American trials of the drug—in fact, the first to be published—appearing in the *AMA Archives of Neurology and Psychiatry* in 1954. The authors found that the drug was not just a conventional sedative but that it "selectively inhibits drive." "The drug is of unique value," they wrote, "in the symptomatic control of almost any kind of severe excitement." Lehmann's service lay in communicating the value of chlorpromazine to North American psychiatry.

His second achievement was introducing the antidepressant drug **imipramine** to North America. Able of course to read German fluently, in 1957 Lehmann discovered in the *Swiss Medical Weekly* (*Schweizer Medizinische Wochenschrift*) Roland Kuhn's report of the efficacy of **imipramine** (Tofranil) in the treatment of vital depression. He immediately requested a supply from the Geigy company and conducted a double-blind study at the hospital, together with Charles Cahn (1921–), who also had been born in Berlin, and Roger Louis de Verteuil (1919–), publishing the results in October 1958 in the *Canadian Psychiatric Association Journal*. They found that it had "definite anti-depressive properties."

During the years, Lehmann and his co-workers conducted many drug trials and developed psychometric test batteries to help lay the basis of the budding science of psychopharmacology. Yet, it is interesting that Lehmann, who had discovered Freud as a schoolboy in Berlin, remained convinced of the value of psychoanalysis and all his life adopted a deeply humanistic approach to the care of his patients, making hospital rounds for example on Christmas Day and shaking hands with all of them.

Under Lehmann, the Douglas Hospital was involved in a large number of clinical investigations of drugs, especially under the ECDEU program of the **National Institute of Mental Health.** His team of workers played an important role in the genesis of modern psychopharmacology.

LEUKOTOMY. *See* **LOBOTOMY.**

LEWIS, AUBREY (1900–1975). Called "the leading psychiatrist of his time" in Britain, Lewis was born in Adelaide, Australia, the son of a watchmaker who had emigrated from London 10 years previously. After earning his medical degree at Adelaide in 1923, he began a residency in psychiatry, then, after obtaining a Rockefeller Fellowship in 1926, he was able to study at the Boston Psychopathic Hospital, the Phipps Clinic at Johns Hopkins under **Adolf Meyer**, who had a large influence on him, and even in Berlin and **Heidelberg.**

Lewis learned to read German fluently and was fond of quoting original German passages in his papers. **Eliot Slater** later noted that Lewis had been trained by Meyer, but "much of what he passed on to us came from his earlier apprentice experiences in Heidelberg."

In 1928, Lewis joined the **Maudsley Hospital** in London, opened 5 years previously, as a researcher and in 1932 was appointed consultant. In 1936, he became clinical director of the Maudsley. During the Second World War, he accompanied the part of the hospital that was evacuated to Mill Hill School, and in 1946 was appointed professor of psychiatry in the University of London (Edward Mapother's successor) and director of the professorial unit at the Maudsley. He became emerited in 1966. In 1948, Lewis masterminded the creation of the Institute of Psychiatry which was closely affiliated with the newly merged Bethlem Royal and Maudsley Hospital, making the 500-bed facility the largest and most eminent teaching center for psychiatry in Britain. Also in 1948, he became honorary director of the first Medical Research Council Unit created with a psychiatrist in command, the Occupational Psychiatry Research Unit at the Maudsley (after 1958 it became the Social Psychiatry Research Unit). There, investigators sought to show how patients with chronic mental disease formerly kept in institutions could work and live in the community. His 1959 knighthoood was the first conferred on a psychiatrist in England.

Reflecting the influence of Meyer, Lewis took what **Michael Shepherd** called a "broad psychobiological standpoint and tried to put it into practice." He was insistent that the registrars (residents) in the 3-year course for psychiatrists-in-training take comprehensive histories and quote patients verbatim. After writing a classic paper on depression (*see* **DEPRESSION: EMERGENCE: British debate** [1934]), he became acknowledged as an expert in mood disorders. In retrospect, Lewis's main contributions were to have opened up the subject of social psychiatry in Britain and to have made the Maudsley Hospital a world-class institute for training and research.

LIBIDO. *See* NARCISSISM.

LITHIUM THERAPY: HISTORY OF (from 1949). Prehistory: On the basis of his views about excess uric acid causing depression (*see* **DEPRESSION: EMERGENCE: periodical melancholia** [1886]), Danish physician Carl Georg Lange (1834–1900) described in 1886 the systematic use of lithium in endogenous depression. His younger brother psychiatrist Frederik Lange (1842–1907), in a book published in Danish in 1894 entitled *The Most Important Groups of Insanity*, described treating acute depression with lithium carbonate alone. However, with the decline of theories about uric acid diathesis, these early attempts were forgotten.

Cade's discovery (1949). John F. J. Cade (1912–1980), who first rediscovered the therapeutic efficacy of lithium in mania, received his medical degree from Melbourne University medical school in 1934, then trained in psychiatry before going off to war in 1940 (he was a prisoner of war between 1942 and 1945). Upon returning home, in 1946 he became superintendent of the Repatriation Mental Hospital in Bundoora, Australia. Here he discovered, through a combination of serendipity in experimenting with guinea pigs and a keen observational mind, that lithium carbonate provided relief in the treatment of psychotic excitement, thus publishing an article in the *Medical Journal of Australia* in 1949. The observation about the therapeutics of mania went largely unheeded.

Mogens Schou's trial (1954). Mogens Schou (pronounced SKOW) (1918–), who confirmed the efficacy of lithium therapy in mania and argued for its prophylatic value in preventing further recurrences of depression and mania, was born in Copenhagen, the son of psychiatrist Hans Jacob Schou (who himself had manic-depressive illness). He graduated in medicine from Copenhagen University in 1944, then trained in psychiatry, in part at the Aarhus university clinic in Risskov. In 1952, **Erik Strömgren**, the head of the clinic, read Cade's paper and suggested that he and Schou look into lithium, as to have an alternative to **electroconvulsive therapy** and the **barbiturates**. Colleagues in the clinic therefore organized a double-blind trial, one of the first in psychiatry, giving one group of patients the active treatment, the other identical placebo tablets compounded by the hospital pharmacy. (The patients were randomized by the flip of a coin.) "We had accordingly established under strictly controlled circumstances that lithium exerted an antimanic action," said Schou later (in Samson, ed., *The Neurosciences: Paths of Discovery*, II, p. 153). Schou, Strömgren, and the others published their findings in 1954 in the *Journal of Neurology, Neurosurgery, and Psychiatry*. Schou was greatly helped in this work by the availability of the recently introduced Beckman flame photometer, which let him measure lithium concentrations in the patients' blood (because otherwise, lithium can be quite toxic).

In 1979, Schou determined that lithium was highly effective in treatment-refractory depression (*Archives of General Psychiatry*). Indeed, there are psychiatrists today who consider it something of a miracle drug for this indication. In 1987, Schou won a Lasker Award for "his landmark systematic clinical trials of lithim as therapy and prophylaxis for manic-depressive illness."

Lithium in the prophylaxis of depression (1963 and after). In 1959–1960, Geoffrey Philip Hartigan (M.B. 1941) at St. Augustine's Hospital in Chatham, Kent, England, and Poul Christian Baastrup (1918–2001), a staff psychiatrist at the psychiatric hospital in Glostrup, Denmark, independently of each other, both contacted Schou asking if lithium might not serve in the prevention of further episodes of depression. Schou urged them to publish their limited observations, which they did, Hartigan in the *British Journal of Psychiatry* in 1963 with a note of Schou's appearing alongside, and Baastrup in *Comprehensive Psychiatry* in 1964. All three papers went "largely unnoticed," as Schou later said. Then, Schou and Baastrup together undertook a long-term study (not double-blinded) on lithium prophylaxis of mania and depression; they presented it at an international congress in 1966 and published it in 1967 in the *Archives of General Psychiatry*. The findings in bipolar patients with mania and depression, and in unipolar depressive patients, were quite striking. (**Michael Shepherd** at the Institute of Psychiatry, however, remained unconvinced and touched off a major international controversy that interested readers may follow in interviews that David Healy did with Schou and Shepherd, published in *The Psychopharmacologists*, vol. III.)

To confound the doubters, Baastrup, Schou, and two other trialists published a double-blind study in 1970 in the *Lancet* on manic-depressive and recurrent depressive disorders, showing the efficacy of lithium prophylaxis. In 1979, Schou published in the *Archives of General Psychiatry* a trial showing the results of lithium vs. placebo and antidepressants vs. placebo in the treatment of unipolar affective illness: whereas only 22% of those on lithium relapsed within a year, 65% of the placebo patients did so. (By contrast, 35% of the patients on antidepressants relapsed vs. 68% of the placebo patients in that arm of the trial.) Schou's lifetime advocacy resulted in the general acceptance of lithium prophylaxis in many parts of the world.

LOBOTOMY (from 1935). Also called leukotomy. Although the Swiss psychiatrist and asylum-director Gottlieb Burckhardt (1836–1907) had earlier made some tentative and quite unsuccessful efforts at operating on the brain for psychiatric indications (*see* **PSYCHOSURGERY**), the modern history of psychosurgery begins in Portugal. Egas Moniz (pronounced EE-gosh Mon-ISH) (1874–1955), professor of neurology in Lisbon, had studied with the great French neurologists and in 1927 described cerebral angiography in the *Revue neurologique*. (*See* **NEUROIMAGING**.) In 1935, at an international congress of neurology in London, he heard a full-day symposium on the frontal lobes of the brain, where psychologist Carlyle Jacobsen (1902–1974) and physiologist John Fulton (1899–1960) at Yale University described the taming of a chimpanzee's behavior after the ablation of much of its frontal lobes. Thus inspired, between November 1935 and February 1936, Moniz asked Lisbon neurosurgeon Almeida Lima to resect part of the prefrontal lobes of 20 asylum patients in Lisbon once they were transferred to Moniz's neurology service. In a paper in March 1936 at the Society of Neurology in Paris, then in a book published in Paris later that year, *Operative Procedures in the Surgical Treatment of Certain Psychoses* (*Tentatives operatoires dans le traitement chirurgical de certaines psychoses*), he claimed that seven patients had been "cured," seven improved, no change in the others. This was the beginning of "frontal leukotomy," approaching the lobes of the brain through the top of the skull.

Yet, as Europe became embroiled in war, the greatest advocates of lobotomy turned out to be Americans. Walter Freeman (1895–1972), a former neuropathologist at **St. Elizabeths Hospital** in Washington who then became professor of neuropathology, neurosurgery, and neurology at George Washington University, had also attended the London conference and became an uncritical admirer of the procedure.

Together with neurosurgeon James Watts (1904–1994), in 1936 Freeman presided over the first "lobotomy"—as they called it—in the United States, at George Washington University Hospital. In 1946, they introduced the "transorbital" lobotomy, approaching the brain from the roof of the orbital cavity. Freeman first reported their results in the *Medical Annals of the District of Columbia* in 1939. By 1942, they were able to describe, in an article in *Diseases of the Nervous System*, the results of "prefrontal lobotomy" in 74 cases. Their book, *Psychosurgery: Intelligence, Emotion and Social Behavior Following Prefrontal Lobotomy in Mental Disorders*, appeared in that year. Later, Freeman went on proselytizing tours of asylums and Veterans Administration hospitals, demonstrating the procedure and seeking converts.

By the late 1940s, lobotomy had come to be widely practiced in the United States. More than 9000 operations were performed in 1949 alone. According to psychiatry historian Jack Pressman, who has written a careful history of lobotomy, "A large number of psychiatrists had found in lobotomy a tool that altered human character to an extent unmatched by any other resource in their armamentarium" (*Last Resort*, p. 10). With the marketing of **chlorpromazine** in 1954, the number of lobotomies declined sharply and the procedure, to all intents and purposes, went out of use, yet not before Moniz received a Nobel Prize for it in 1949.

LOMBROSO, EZECCHIA-MARCO ("CESARE") (1835–1909). The founder of criminal anthropology, Lombroso was born in Verona into a noble Jewish family. He graduated with an M.D. at Pavia University in 1858, served in the medical corps of the Piedmont army (where he started linking soldiers' physical types to behavior), then in 1867 became associate professor of psychiatry at Pavia, moving on in 1871 to direct the provincial asylum at Pesaro. In 1876, Lombroso received the professorship of forensic medicine at Turin University, where he would remain. In 1896, he became professor of psychiatry there, and in 1905 received the chair of criminal anthropology. He was associated with the Italian somaticist school that studied the relations between mental and physical disorders.

Although Lombroso was occupied with many different subjects during the years, the center of his life's work was **psychiatric genetics** and psychiatric anthropology. In 1864, his book *Genius and Madness* (*Genio e Follia*) appeared; *Criminal Man* (*L'Uomo delinquente*) in 1876; *Criminal Woman, the Prostitute, and the Normal Woman* (*La donna delinquente, la prostituta e la donna normale*) in 1893; and *Genius and Degeneration* (*Genio e degenerazione*) in 1898. He took a highly deterministic view of criminality and believed that such "stigmata" in physical anthropology as skull shape really did affect destiny. An avid degeneration theorist, he considered that criminals had been left a step or two behind on the phylogenetic chain. His basic finding was that criminals exhibit a greater percentage of physical and mental abnormalities than noncriminals. Lombroso may be considered one of the founders of the positivist school of criminology, along with fellow psychiatrists Jacques-Joseph Moreau (called "Moreau de Tours" [1804–1884]), and **James C. Prichard**, who in 1835 coined the term "moral insanity." It was largely Lombroso's doing that special custodial institutions for the criminal insane were established. In sum, Lombroso began the medical tradition of "seeing evil as illness." (*See also* **CONDUCT DISORDER; CRIMINALITY AND PSYCHIATRY.**)

M

MAGNAN, JACQUES-JOSEPH VALENTIN (1835–1916). Born in the Mediterranean French city of Perpignan, Magnan studied medicine at Montpellier, then interned in Lyon. In 1863, he went to Paris for a further internship, where he was taught by psychiatrist Prosper-Jean-Aimé Lucas (1808–1885) at Bicêtre Hospital and by Jules-Gabriel-François Baillarger (1809–1890) and **Jean-Pierre Falret** at the **Salpêtrière hospice**. In 1867, he joined the admissions department of the newly founded **Ste.-Anne mental hospital**, where he remained until retiring in 1912 to a private nervous clinic that he also ran. It was his work on alcoholism that steered him toward the idea of degeneration, initially conceived by Lucas in 1850 and by **Bénédict-Augustin Morel** in 1857; from 1881 on, he worked on a classification of mental illnesses based on that concept. He introduced the notion of "chronic systematized delusional disorder" in 1886 (*see* **PSYCHOSIS: EMERGENCE** [1886])—in a book of that title, *Le délire chronique à évolution systématique*, that he and Paul Sérieux (1864–1947) wrote in 1892; the two authors contrasted the "insanity of the degenerate"—for example, la bouffée délirante (**PSYCHOSIS: EMERGENCE** [1886])—with "the chronic systematic delusional disorders" of the nondegenerate but mildly predisposed. Magnan added the adjective "systematic," or better "systematized" (meaning highly structured and logical) to show that there was nothing inchoate or disorganized about it.

Psychiatrist Henri Baruk (1897–1999) (whose father Jacques Baruk [1872–1975] had interned with Magnan at Ste.-Anne) later wrote of Magnan: "[Magnan] systematized the ideas attributed to Morel, considerably inflating the concept of degeneration. Instead of limiting it, as Morel did, to a group of illnesses that were clearly hereditary, Magnan extended the concept to almost all of psychiatry." Magnan sought out physical signs of degeneration, such as the conformation of the ear. Baruk said there were really two kinds of doctors: careful clinical observers who gave to theory a subtleness that permitted them to adapt it to the complexities of nature, and system-builders, whose "rational desire to systematize everything and absolute mode of logic predominate without counterbalance and without brakes." Magnan, he said, belonged to the latter (Baruk, *French Psychiatry from Pinel to Current Times* [*La psychiatrie française de Pinel à nos jours*], 1967, p. 89). In retrospect, some observers feel that Magnan's bouffée délirante and his "délire systématique" are indeed separate disorders and are worth distinguishing from Kraepelin's schizophrenia.

MANIA. *See* **HYPOMANIA; LITHIUM; MANIC-DEPRESSIVE ILLNESS; SCHIZOPHRENIA: EMERGENCE: Kraepelin** (from 1893); **WERNICKE–KLEIST–LEONHARD PATHWAY.**

MANIC-DEPRESSIVE ILLNESS (BIPOLAR DISORDER). Before 1850, numerous physicians had commented on the alternation of mania and melancholia. In 1844, Karl Wigand Maximilian Jacobi (1775–1858), chief physician of Siegburg asylum in Germany, noted that "Exaltation and depression stand in the most intimate reciprocal relationship with each other, alternate together, and appear often mutually, if not with absolute regularity, to trigger each other" (*The Main Forms of Mental Disturbances* [*Die Hauptformen der Seelenstörungen*], I, p. xxxii). In 1844, Carl Friedrich Flemming (1799–1880) gave the alternation a name, as a separate entity, saying "[Between melancholy and mania] there is not infrequently a connection of each to the other, called Dysthymia mutabilis, in which first the one, then the other presents" (*General Journal of Psychiatry* [*Allgemeine Zeitschrift für Psychiatrie*], 1844, p. 129). Yet, Flemming's distinction was forgotten.

Circular insanity (1850). In 1850, **Jean-Pierre Falret** gave a lecture to the Paris Psychiatric Society in the course of which he mentioned "circular insanity" (la folie circulaire); the lecture was briefly summarized in 1851 in the Paris *Hospital Gazette* (*Gazette des hôpitaux*). Three years later, in 1854, Jules-Gabriel-François Baillarger (1809–1890), who taught the course on mental illness at the **Salpêtrière hospice**, gave a lecture on "madness in double form" (la folie à double forme), in which he claimed that, "There are not two diseases here but one single, that the two apparent episodes are only two phases of one sole episode" (p. 370). Upon seeing this, the outraged Falret rushed his own thoughts on the matter into print in order to claim priority. Baillarger said that the alternation of mania and melancholia represented, in fact, a distinct illness, and that Falret's description failed to recognize this novelty but rather just gave a name to the long familiar alternation of two separate illnesses. Both authors were quite gloomy about prognosis, Baillarger saying that the patients never really recovered even in apparent intervals, and Falret that the alternations occurred in an almost mechanical manner continually throughout life. *See* Falret's paper and Baillarger's heated response in the *Bulletin de l'Académie de médecine*, 1854. Baillarger's original paper, "De la folie à double forme," appeared in 1854 in the *Annales médico-psychologiques*.

In the view of **Pierre Pichot**, the priority belongs to Falret not only because he came first but he also because he highlighted the importance of clinical course ("évolution") in the description of independent disease entities. "Seen in this perspective, the birth of bipolar disorder is more than a picturesque episode illustrating the occasional smallmindedness of brilliant scientists. It can be considered as a decisive episode in the history of psychiatry" (*European Psychiatry*, 1995, p. 9).

Cyclothymia (1882). In an article on "circular insanity" in the *Friend of the Insane* (*Der Irrenfreund*), **Karl Ludwig Kahlbaum**, now owner of a private nervous clinic in the Prussian town of Görlitz, coined the term "cyclothymia" for a form of circular insanity that did not go progressively downhill, unlike "vesania typica circularis," that several earlier writers had described; cyclothymia affected mainly the emotional realm of the mind rather than intelligence and drive. "Thus we may differentiate strictly between a circular insanity that does not lead to terminal dementia and that keeps within the boundaries of the emotions, and a circular insanity that even in the stage of exaltation represents a primary impairment of all aspects of mental life and in further stages of confusion and dementia leads to complete mental degeneration." Kahlbaum suggested the term "cyclothymia" for the former (p. 155). The term stuck for many observers: **Kurt Schneider** seldom talked of manic-depressive illness but rather "cyclothymia."

Manic-depressive illness (das manisch-depressive Irresein) (1899). In the sixth edition of his textbook, **Emil Kraepelin** brought all the affective disorders—depression, mania and "mixed forms"—into the single diagnostic category of manic-depressive illness. As he wrote in *Psychiatry* (*Die Psychiatrie*), "Manic-depressive insanity . . . includes on the one hand the entire area of so-called periodic and circular forms of insanity; on the other hand it includes most of the hitherto separately treated simple manias. In the course of the years I have become increasingly convinced, that all of the above mentioned clinical pictures are only aspects of a single disease" (p. 359). Only involutional melancholia remained outside this framework. Henceforth, all cases of affective disorders would , in the Kraepelinian world, considered as constitutionally predisposed "MDI."

Manic-depressive illness arises from predisposing personality attitudes (1921). **Ernst Kretschmer** (1888–1964), then a staff psychiatrist in the department of psychiatry at Tübingen University, ventured the idea in his 1921 book, *Body Type and Character* (*Körperbau und Charakter*), that mood disorders, especially manic-depressive illness, arose from "cycloid temperaments" (zykloide Temperamente). Certain body types corresponded as well to this kind of "diathesis." "We indicate as schizoid and cycloid the abnormal personality types that fluctuate between health and illness, and that give rise to the basic psychological symptoms of the schizophrenic and the circular psychoses." The basic constitutional type, or diathesis, of the manic-depressive was "sociable, kindly, friendly, easy-going [gemütlich]." And the body type on which such a constitution rested was mainly "pyknic," meaning a big frame with a "soft, wide face on a short massive neck" (that so many of the male patients of this physical type seemed to have big stomachs as well may have been more attributable to the Swabian diet than to ancestry) (pp. 27, 115–116 of the seventh edition, published in 1929). (*See* **PSYCHOSIS: EMERGENCE: Kretschmer's constitutional psychoses** [1921].) The book went through many editions.

Manic-depressive illness seems to consist of separate diseases: bipolar and unipolar disorders (1957). On the basis of many years of longitudinal research on outcome and family history, in 1957 Karl Leonhard (1904–1988), then professor of psychiatry at Erfurt University, published *The Classification of the Endogenous Psychoses* (*Die Aufteilung der endogenen Psychosen*). (*See* **WERNICKE-KLEIST-LEONHARD PATHWAY.**) On grounds of family history and phenomenology, he demonstrated that unipolar depression and manic-depressive illness are different diseases. For Leonhard, there was a "pure melancholia" distinguished from the "pure depressions," of which latter he subdivided five forms. He borrowed Kleist's term "bipolar" illness for manic-depressive illness and revived Kleist's concept of single-polar illness for pure depressive illness and pure mania. (Kleist had used the term "unipolar," which Leonhard called "monopolar.") (On Kleist, *see* **WERNICKE-KLEIST-LEONHARD PATHWAY.**)

In 1964, writing in the *Acta Psychiatrica Scandinavica*, Carlo Perris (1928–2000), a member of the psychiatry department of Umea University in Sweden, changed Leonhard's term "monopolar" back to Kleist's term "unipolar." The first family data in this project were published by former team member Edda Neele (1910–) in 1949. (The notion that unipolar and bipolar disorders differed on grounds of family history was confirmed in 1966 in separate publications by Jules Angst at the **Burghölzli** in Zurich (*Zur Ätiologie und Nosologie endogener depressiver Psychosen* [*The Etiology and Classification of Endogenous Depressive Psychoses*]) and by Perris in an article in a supplement of the *Acta Psychiatrica Scandinavica*. Perris: "Moreover, the results of our investigation seem to indicate a specificity in the heredity of depressive psychoses. This is supported by the high morbidity risk for the same form of illness and the low for the other one within each group" (p. 41).

See **SCHIZOPHRENIA: RECENT CONCEPTS: much "schizophrenia" turns out to be manic-depressive illness** (1978).

DSM-III* renames manic-depressive illness "bipolar disorder"** (1980). The third edition of the ***DSM series said that bipolar disorder, formerly known as manic-depressive illness, was a subtype of major affective disorders, along with major depression. Within biopolar disorder, *DSM* distinguished among: "bipolar—mixed," meaning recently the full symptom picture of both mania and major depression, "intermixed or rapidly alternating every few days"; "bipolar—manic," meaning recently a manic episode; and "bipolar—depressed," meaning currently depressed with a past history of a manic episode at some point.

DSM-III also accepted "cyclothymic disorder," reviving **Karl Kahlbaum's** term, but meaning alternating periods of depression and hypomania not severe enough to meet the criteria of major depression or the manic picture.

DSM-III-R* (1987) did not change DSM-III in any important way in this area.** ***DSM-IV (1994) subdivided bipolar disorder into bipolar I disorder and bipolar II disorder. Bipolar I meant mainly mania plus mixed episodes; bipolar II meant mainly major depression plus hypomanic episodes.

MASOCHISM. (*See also* **SADISM.**) In our own time, "masochism" has taken on three meanings: (1) the voluntary acceptance of suffering; (2) in psychoanalysis, an intrapsychic mechanism for dealing with anxiety; (3) a kind of sex play among consenting adults now increasingly called "role-playing," but also referrred to as "SM" (for sadomasochism), or "BDSM" (for "bondage and domination, sadism and masochism").

The term enters psychiatry, actually, in the third sense. Although an interest in flogging and being flogged goes back for centuries—a "friend" of the fifteenth-century Italian scholar Giovanni Pico della Mirandola (1463–1494) being an example (as Pico recounts in his *Disputationes* [1495])—the taste for flogging acquired a name only after Austrian psychiatrist **Richard von Krafft-Ebing** read *Venus in Fur* (*Venus im Pelz*), the 1869 novella of Austrian nobleman Leopold von Sacher-Masoch (1836–1895) about a protagonist remarkably similar to himself who loves being flogged and humiliated by arrogant women dressed in fur. In the first edition of his 1890 book, *New Research in the Area of Psychopathia Sexualis* (*Neue Forschungen auf dem Gebiete der Psychopathia sexualis*), Krafft introduced the term "masochism" and popularized the term "sadism." The following year, in the sixth edition in 1891 of his big sex-pathology book, *Psychopathia sexualis*, he expanded the discussion, giving examples of women fantasizing about being slaves of their lovers, and also of men submitting to the control of what Krafft was calling a "domina," a woman who towered over the male sexually.

Freud borrowed Krafft's term in his own exploration of psychodynamics, but attached to it a quite different meaning. Because "masochism" was already well established, it is no surprise that Freud uses it early in his writing, noting in 1900 in the *Interpretation of Dreams* (*Die Traumdeutung*), "In the sexual constitution of so many people there is a masochistic component, which arises as a result of turning into the opposite of the aggressive, sadistic component" (*Gesammelte Werke,* II, p. 165). Yet in his 1920 book, *Beyond the Pleasure Principle* (*Jenseits des Lustprinzips*), Freud used masochism in a rather different sense: "primary" masochism as the version of the death instinct that is inwardly directed toward one's self.

In 1932, psychoanalyst Wilhelm Reich proposed in the *International Journal of Psychoanalysis* (*Internationale Zeitschrift für Psychoanalyse*) the existence of the "masochistic character," a concept he had come up with as a way of breaking with Freud's theory of the death instinct (which implied that we suffer because of a biological will to do so, or "death instinct"). The paper was incorporated into his book *Character Analysis* the following year. Reich challenged Freud's theory that "unpleasure was pleasure." "Rather," said Reich, "the masochist's specific mechanism of pleasure consisted precisely in that, while he strives after pleasure like any other person, a disturbing mechanism causes this striving to miscarry. This, in turn, causes the masochist to perceive sensations, which are experienced as pleasurable by the normal person, as unpleasurable when they exceed a certain intensity. The masochist, far from striving after unpleasure, demonstrates a strong intolerance of psychic tensions and suffers from a quantitative overproduction of unpleasure, not to be found in any other neurosis" (p. 236 of the English translation, 3rd ed.). (*See* **PERSONALITY DISORDERS: Reich's analysis of "character armor"** [1933].)

After Freud and Reich, interest within psychoanalysis shifted from masochism as a form of death instinct to "moral masochism," which psychoanalyst Theodor Reik (1888–1969) in his 1941 book, *Masochism in Modern Man,* said represented a character type. It was not that the masochist had reversed "pleasure values" and derived pleasure from pain. In a chapter called "Victory Through Defeat," Reik observed that, "The masochist aims at the same pleasure we all do, but he arrives at it by another road, by a detour. Intimidated by threatening anxiety, inhibited by the idea of punishment and later by unconscious guilt-feeling, he found his particular way of avoiding anxiety and gaining pleasure. He submits voluntarily to punishment, suffering, and humiliations, and thus has defiantly purchased the right to enjoy the gratification denied before" (p. 428). Thus, as masochism entered postwar American psychiatry, it was simultaneously a kind of character disorder and a form of sexual behavior.

DSM-I (1952) passed in silence over masochism, but ***DSM-II*** in 1968, heavily influenced by psychoanalysis, listed it among the "sexual deviations" without further specification. ***DSM-III*** in 1980 defined masochism as "sexual excitement produced in an individual by his or her own suffering." This placed the emphasis on the production of actual pain rather than the psychodrama of role-playing, and the *Manual* dwelt upon lives being "threatened." ***DSM-III-R*** had the most elaborate discussion of masochism in the series, distinguishing between "urges" that involve "being humiliated, beaten, bound, or otherwise made to suffer," and "masochistic personality disorder," a condition tentatively listed in the Appendix of *DSM-III-R* and also called "self-defeating personality disorder" in the hopes of not upsetting feminists who asserted that the masochism diagnosis implied that women enjoyed suffering.

Masochism disappeared entirely from ***DSM-IV*** in 1994.

The entirely nonpsychiatric notion of masochism as pleasureable role-playing, an activity initially psychiatrized by Krafft-Ebing, seems to have surfaced in the 1930s, with the leather-clad figure of the dominatrix whose gear asserts her authority, and has steadily increased in visibility since then. (*See* **SADISM** on sadomasochism.)

MAUDSLEY, HENRY (1835–1918). Born on a farm in the West Riding of Yorkshire, Maudsley graduated with an M.B. from University College London, in 1856. He wanted to enter the East India Company, which required of its medical officers 6 months' psychiatric experience, so he took brief posts at two asylums. Deciding to remain in the field, in 1859 he became, at 23, medical superintendent of the asylum in Manchester. In 1862, he removed to London, became editor of the *Journal of Mental Science,* and then remained in London thereafter. In London, he captured a good deal of the "carriage trade," and ultimately worked toward the establishment of the hospital (*see below*) that would be named after him. In 1867, he brought out his textbook, *The Physiology and Pathology of Mind,* which reflected the strong organicist views of **Wilhelm Griesinger**; Maudsley believed that inheritance played a large role in illness; increasingly, he would be influenced by **Morelian** notions of degeneration. "Were all madness swept from the face of the earth tomorrow, past all doubt men would breed it afresh before tomorrow's tomorrow," he once wrote (third edition, called simply *The Pathology of Mind,* 1879, p. 97).

MAUDSLEY HOSPITAL, London. In 1908, the Asylums Committee of the London County Council decided to accept a generous gift that **Henry Maudsley** was offering for the foundation of a mental hospital—not, he stressed, an "asylum"—that would incorporate an outpatient department, laboratories, and instruct medical students. It would be based on the German model of the university psychiatric clinic—yet at the same time, Maudsley had a distrust of German theoretical formulations. During the First World War, the army converted the newly finished structure into a military hospital, but in 1923 it opened its doors to psychiatric patients. Edward Mapother (1881–1940), the first medical superintendent, had simultaneously become in 1922 physician in psychological medicine to King's College Hospital and wanted to make the Maudsley the postgraduate school for the psychiatric teaching of the college.

Well before the hospital opened for psychiatric uses, in 1916 the London County Council's Pathological Laboratory, based at Claybury asylum since 1895, was transferred to the Maudsley. Frederick W. Mott (1853–1926) had been its first director (until 1923), Frederic L. Golla (1878–1968) its second until his retirement in 1938, and neurologist Samuel Nevin (1905–1979) its third from 1945. As Bethlem Royal Hospital archivist Colin Gale has remarked, "In many ways it was the precursor of the Institute of Psychiatry itself" (*see below*).

In 1924, the Maudsley Hospital was recognized by the University of London as one of its "Schools," the title "professor" being created for Mapother in 1936. Two years later, a research laboratory became funded by the Rockefeller Foundation. Thus, after the disruption of wartime, a nucleus was present for the creation of a teaching unit in psychiatry, in addition to the hospital functions. In 1946, **Aubrey Lewis** was appointed professor of psychiatry in the university (having been clinical director of the Maudsley since 1936). Under the guidance of Lewis, in 1948 the hospital school became part of the the newly founded British Postgraduate Medical Federation, and the medical school was renamed the Institute of Psychiatry (IOP); Lewis became director of the IOP, a postgraduate educational unit outside the National Health Service. As well in 1948, the Maudsley Hospital merged with the Bethlem Royal Hospital.

Starting in the late 1940s, Lewis began to beef up the research arm of the Institute by adding Medical Research Council (MRC) Units. In 1948, Lewis created the MRC Occupational Psychiatry Research Unit at the Maudsley (after 1958, it became the Social Psychiatry Research Unit); this was the first Medical Research Council Unit with a psychiatrist in command. When Lewis stepped down in 1965 as director, **John Wing** reconstituted it as a new Social Psychiatry Research Unit (director from 1965 to 1989). Julian P. Leff (1938–) was the subsequent director from 1989 to 1995. The unit closed in 1995 as it merged with the Social, Genetic and Development Psychiatric Research Centre of the Maudsley, with Sir Michael Rutter (1933–) the new director.

In 1959, **Eliot Slater** helped create the MRC Psychiatric Genetics Unit. It closed with his retirement in 1969, but a psychiatric genetics section continued on at the Maudsley under the department of psychiatry.

In 1984, Rutter helped create the MRC Child Psychiatry Unit; in 2000, it became integrated with the new Social, Genetic and Developmental Psychiatry Research Centre, of which Rutter had just become director (followed in 1998 by Peter McGuffin).

After Lewis retired in 1966, Denis Hill (1913–) became professor and director of the Maudsley, retiring in 1979. He was succeeded by Gerald F. M. Russell (1928–), who had coined the term "**bulimia**" nervosa. David Goldberg (1934–), a psychiatric epidemiologist who in 1970 developed the General Health Questionnaire, a widely used screening instrument in epidemiological psychiatry first described in the *British Medical Journal*, served as the chair holder from 1993 to 2000; Goldberg was, strictly speaking, the last professor of psychiatry at the Maudsley, because in 1999, the Institute of Psychiatry split from the Maudsley and became a school of King's College London. Robin Murray became the professor of psychiatry in 2000 and serves to date.

MAYER-GROSS, WILHELM (William, "Willy," 1889–1961). Importer of German scientific rigor and psychopathological thinking to British psychiatry, Willy Mayer was born in Bingen, Germany, into a merchant's family. Gross was his mother's maiden name, which he adopted around the time of his marriage in 1919. He took his final exams in medicine at Heidelberg in 1912 and in 1913 began training at the psychiatry clinic under **Franz Nissl**. Yet, Mayer-Gross had much more interest in **Jaspers's psychopathology** than in Nissl's research in brain histology and wrote his doctoral thesis on "the phenomenology of abnormal feelings of happiness" (later published as an article in 1914 in the *Journal of Pathopsychology* (*Zeitschrift für Pathopsychologie*). As Karl Wilmanns (1873–1945) took over the clinic in 1918, Mayer-Gross continued as an assistant, becoming associate professor of psychiatry (extraordinarius) in 1929. Here, he was part of a nucleus interested in psychopathology known as the "**Heidelberg school**," including Jaspers, Hans Walther Gruhle (1880–1958), and Kurt Beringer (1893–1949). His 1924 Habilitation on *Self-descriptions of Confusional States: the Oneiroid Form of Experience* (*Selbstschilderungen der Verwirrtheit: die Oneiroide Erlebnisform*) is considered the first monograph to use the psychopathological method (what German psychiatrists called the "phenomenological" method); Mayer-Gross highlighted a special dream-like state (oneiroid) in psychosis and dissected its psychology; it was a form of psychosis neighboring on schizophrenia yet not schizophrenic. In the chapters on clinical aspects of schizophrenia that he wrote in 1932 for Wilmanns' schizophrenia volume in the series *Handbook of Mental Illnesses* (*Handbuch der Geisteskrankheiten*—edited by Munich psychiatry professor Oswald Bumke [1877–1950]), the distinctive German approach to the illness received its most articulate expression. As Mayer-Gross's biographer, U. H. Peters, notes rather poignantly, "Weeks after the appearance of this volume, the Heidelberg school was destroyed."

As life for Jews in Germany started to become intolerable after 1933, a Commonwealth Fund of America grant together with the encouragement of Edward Mapother made it possible for Mayer-Gross, Erich Guttmann (1896–1948), and Alfred Meyer (1895–1990) to emigrate to England. Mayer-Gross was able to stay on thanks to a Rockefeller Foundation grant. Thus, together with Guttmann (who was to lead the Maudsley's research on mescaline), Mayer-Gross brought what was possibly the most exciting orientation in psychiatry of the day to the **Maudsley Hospital**, where they influenced the next generation of British psychiatrists already attuned by Aubrey Lewis and Edward Mapother to the importance of research. **Eliot Slater** later said, "I think the effect of these Germans upon me and some others was to promote enthusiasm. You really become enthusiastic about the subject in which you spend your every day" (in Wilkinson, *Talking about Psychiatry*, p. 8).

Mayer-Gross also brought clear ideas about how to do systematic research in psychiatry. After passing his qualifying exams for medicine in Britain, in 1939 he went up to Dumfries in Scotland as clinical research director of the Crichton Royal Mental Hospital, where he organized an **insulin coma** unit, staying at Dumfries until he retired in 1954. Then in 1955, Mayer-Gross came down to **Joel Elkes's** department of experimental psychiatry at Birmingham and helped to start the Uffculme Clinic. As *Munk's Roll* reports, "The psychiatry he had helped to forge out of German system and British empiricism had now come to be recognised as having a leading status" (*Munk's Roll*, V, p. 277). Mayer-Gross's final achievement was the textbook of psychiatry, *Clinical Psychiatry*, that he, Slater, and Martin Roth brought out in 1954. Mayer-Gross wrote most of the first draft, Slater's task being "to turn his Germanic English into English." Interestingly, despite Mayer-Gross's background, the textbook does not really represent the phenomenological school at all, but rather, with its emphasis on constitution and genetics, is a precursor of the biological approach. Mayer-Gross called himself, even in several of his German publications, "Willy."

McGILL UNIVERSITY, Montreal, Canada, history of psychiatry and neurosciences at (from 1940). From the 1940s through the 1960s, McGill University was, alongside Washington University in **St. Louis**, arguably the premier North American institution for training in biological psychiatry.

In 1940, Sir Hugh Allan's son donated the family's historic mansion to Royal Victoria Hospital and to McGill, to be called the "Allan Memorial Institute." The backers of the new department were Dean Jonathan Meakins and the neurosurgery pioneer Wilder Penfield (1891–1976). They chose D. Ewen Cameron (1901–1967), a Scotsman then teaching at the Albany Medical School, as director and first chair of the department. Cameron arrived in 1943 with a grant from the Rockefeller Foundation "and money from Mr. J. D. McConnell, owner of the *Montreal Star*," as one historian of the institute said. The first patients were admitted in 1943. The Allan Memorial became the psychiatric wing of the "Royal Vic."

Among Cameron's and Penfield's recruits to the Allan were:

Psychoanalyst Miguel Prados (1894–), who arrived in 1944 after fleeing Fascist Spain. (Prados was a student of the Spanish histologist Santiago Ramón y Cajal [1852–1934], of **Emil Kraepelin**, and of British neurologist Frederick Walker Mott [1859–1926].)

The neuropathologist Karl Stern (1906–1975), who had come to the Verdun Protestant Hospital ("VPH," a Montreal mental hospital) in 1940; he also lectured in neuropathology and established a gerontological unit in 1944 at the Allan, the first in the world.

The neuropathologist Vojtech Adalbert Kral (1903–1988), a graduate of Charles University in Prague, who had studied in Zurich, Munich, and Vienna. He came to the VPH in 1949 (after spending 3 years in a concentration camp), then moved to the Allan in 1953 as director of the gerontology division. (*See* **DEMENTIA: separating . . .** [1958].)

Robert Cleghorn (1904–1995), a neurophysiologist, came to the Allan from Toronto in 1946 and organized a neuroendocrine unit and an experimental therapeutics laboratory.

Charles Shagass (1920–), himself a Montrealer, trained at the Allan, studied stress under the physiologist Hans Selye (1907–1982), and then stayed on for the years 1952–1958 in the electrophysiology department. Shagass determined, notably in an article on "The Sedation Threshold" in *Electroencephalography and Clinical Neurophysiology* in 1954, that different people respond differentially to the same drug. This is the premise of psychopharmacology, and it may be demonstrated qualitatively or quantitatively, Shagass doing so quantitatively with the electroencephalogram. (*See* **BARBITURATES: sedation threshold** [1954]).

Eric Wittkower (1899–1983), who had graduated in medicine in Berlin in 1924, had gone to the United Kingdom in 1932, then to the Allan and the Montreal General Hospital in 1951; Wittkower was one of the founders of psychosomatic medicine and in 1955 set up the section of transcultural psychiatric studies as a cooperative venture between the departments of psychiatry and anthropology at McGill. Wittkower recruited Henry B. M. Murphy (1915–1987), who became head of the section after Wittkower retired in 1965.

Heinz Lehmann (1911–1999), a member of the founding generation of psychopharmacology, had left Germany for Canada in 1937, becoming the clinical director of VPH in 1947; he was cross-appointed to psychiatry at McGill and later had an office at the Allan. (*See* **CHLORPROMAZINE; ANTIDEPRESSANT: imipramine.**)

This founding period came to an end when Cameron left in 1964 to return to Albany under something of a cloud because of internal political conflicts. He had founded what was to become the largest single training program in the world.

McLEAN HOSPITAL (Waverley, Massachusetts), from 1818. The Board of Trustees of the Massachusetts General Hospital opened an asylum for the insane at Charlestown in 1818, christening it The McLean Asylum after receiving a legacy in 1823 from Boston merchant John McLean. One of the earliest asylums in the United States, the McLean Asylum became synonymous with scientific care in American psychiatry and was among the mental institutions affiliated (via the parent organization the Massachusetts General Hospital) with the department of psychiatry of Harvard University. In 1895, the institution, now renamed McLean Hospital, removed from Charlestown to Waverley (Belmont). It was **Adolf Meyer's** opinion that the scientific breakthrough in American psychiatry took place first at McLean at the end of the nineteenth century: a pathology department was organized in 1888, a chemical laboratory in 1900, and a psychological laboratory in 1904. The staff at McLean were mindful of the scientific advances in European psychiatry and attempted to keep abreast: Swiss-born August Hoch (1868–1919), an early McLean pathologist and leader of the laboratories, had studied in Germany with **Franz Nissl** and **Kraepelin**. (*See* **DEPRESSION: EMERGENCE: benign stupor** [1921].) After 1955, under the influence of psychiatrist-in-chief Alfred H. Stanton (1912–1983), the hospital pioneered concepts of the therapeutic community in the United States (*See* **PSYCHOTHERAPY: "therapeutic community."**) In 1978, with the opening of the Mailman Research Center, the hospital acquired leading-edge research facilities in the neurosciences; Seymour Kety (1915–2000) was director of psychiatric research laboratories until his retirement in 1983. It was at McLean that neuropathologist Philip S. Holzman (1922–2004) (who had been recruited by Kety) and co-workers continued their research on abnormal eye-tracking dysfunction (ETD) in many schizophrenics and family members. The work first appeared in *Science* in 1973.

MELANCHOLIA. As a term used in medicine since the ancient Greeks, "melancholia" had two core elements of meaning, neither specifically referring to sad forms of depression: (1) All mental affections in which mood, drive, and intellectual function were somehow down ("mania" meant the opposite); (2) Melancholia as a synonym for madness, in the sense of fixed delusional ideas (mania involved false perceptions, or hallucinations). For example, in 1809 John Haslam (1764–1844), the "apothecary" of **Bethlem Hospital** ("Bedlam") in London, wrote, "As the terms Mania and Melancholia are in general use, and serve to distinguish the forms under which insanity is exhibited, there can be no objection to retain them; but I would strongly oppose their being considered as opposite diseases. In both there is an equal derangement" (*Observations on Madness and Melancholy*, 2nd ed., pp. 36–37).

Breaking with centuries of humoral theory, in which melancholia was linked to an excess of "black bile," in his *First Lines of the Practice of Physic* (1777), **William Cullen**, professor of the institutes of medicine at Edinburgh University, attempted to rearrange the classification of diseases on a more modern basis. He was not the first to break with the past on this, but he was the most important. He identified the "Vesaniae," or disorders of intellectual function, and among the Vesaniae he singled out melancholia, by which he meant "partial insanity," and mania, which meant "universal insanity." Cullen's system, of great influence upon his successors, thus paid little attention to mood disorders as such (though he did mention "despondence" and "weariness of life," and considered "depressed spirits" elsewhere in the volume, among the "adynamiae").

Many pre-1850 accounts of melancholia make clear that depression of mood was often at the core, though the authors highlight other features of "madness." Timothy Bright (1551–1615), a physician to St. Bartholomew's Hospital in London, wrote in his 1586 book, *A Treatise of Melancholie*, that one kind of melancholia—"natural" he called it—results from "the mind's apprehension" (later, reactive depression), the other "unnatural" kind being a more somatic illness of the humors of the body (later, endogenous depression). Bright is discussing here not undifferentiated madness but more what we would recognize as depression.

In his great work on melancholia, *The Anatomy of Melancholy* (1621), Oxford cleric Robert Burton (1577–1640) said, "I think I may truly conclude that they are not always sad and fearful, but usually so. . . . Some are afraid that heaven will fall on their heads; some afraid they are damned, or shall be" (p. 328). Melancholic patients, Burton continued, are "most part sad: pleasant thoughts depart soon, sorrow sticks by them still continually, gnawing as the vulture did Tityus' bowels, and they cannot avoid it. [After terrible dreams] their heavy hearts begin to sigh: they are still fretting, chafing, sighing, grieving, complaining, finding faults, repining, grudging, weeping . . . Aretaeus well calls it a vexation of the mind, a perpetual agony" (p. 331). In fact, Burton seems to have been describing a mixture of depression and anxiety, which is more common in community psychiatry than either pure depression or pure anxiety. Burton was himself a sufferer.

In 1801, **Philippe Pinel** in his book, *Medical-Philosophical Treatise on Mental Alienation* (*Traité médico-philosophique sur l'aliénation mentale*), contrasted "the gay and expansive passions that may lead reason astray" with "a melancholic constitution, frequent cause of the most extreme estrangements and the most exaggerated ideas" (from the second ed., 1809, pp. 34, 59). Thus, even though traditionally "melancholia" did serve as a kind of catch-all for insanity, there always has been an understanding that at its core lay what we would call "depression."

Starting late in the nineteenth century, the diagnosis depression began to displace melancholia, and the term went out of style in the understanding of mood disorders.

Then in 1957, in his *Classification of Endogenous Psychoses* (*Die Aufteilung der endogenen Psychosen*), German psychiatrist Karl Leonhard (1904–1988), who had only just moved from the University of Erfurt to the Charité teaching hospital in Berlin, began the rehabilitation of melancholia with his notion of "pure melancholia" as one of the "phasic" (bipolar) psychoses. (*See* **WERNICKE–KLEIST–LEONHARD PATHWAY**.)

Melancholia entered the ***DSM*** system in the second edition in 1968 in the form of "involutional melancholia" (a Kraepelinian diagnosis that Kraepelin had later abandoned). (*See* **DEPRESSION: EMERGENCE: involutional melancholia** [1896].) The third edition in 1980 made melancholia a subtype of "major depression," and specified as operational criteria a loss of pleasure in life; a lack of reactivity to pleasurable things; and at least three of a list of six symptoms, including feeling worse in the morning than the afternoon, marked motor retardation or agitation, and inappropriate guilt feelings. ***DSM-III-R*** in 1987 changed this hierarchy of symptoms a bit by simply calling for five out of a list of nine potentially melancholic symptoms. ***DSM-IV*** returned to the style of the 1980 by insisting that the patient have loss of pleasure or lack of reactivity in addition to three out of a list of six other symptoms. (Readers will understand the impatience of many observers at the failure of *DSM*-style psychiatry to isolate homogeneous, treatment-responsive subgroups.)

For other developments in the melancholia diagnosis, *see* **DEPRESSION: EMERGENCE** and **DEPRESSION: RECENT CONCEPTS: psychotic depression.**

MENNINGER FAMILY

Charles Frederick Menninger (1862–1953). Founder of the psychoanalytically oriented Menninger Clinic in Topeka, Kansas, C. F. M. was born in a small town in Indiana, into the family of a miller. Graduating with an M.D. from the Kansas Medical College in Topeka in 1908 (after a previous homeopathy M.D. from Chicago), he visited the Mayo Clinic in Rochester, Minnesota, and wanted to reproduce that achievement in Topeka. In 1919, together with his son Karl, he established the Menninger Diagnostic Clinic. Yet as another son, William, joined the clinic, its orientation became increasingly psychiatric. In 1941, C. F. M. created the Menninger Foundation to encourage psychiatric training; in 1945, the Menninger Sanitarium joined the Foundation, and in 1954 the Charles Frederick Menninger Memorial Hospital opened, 1 year after C. F. M.'s death.

Karl Augustus Menninger (1893–1990). Born in Topeka, Kansas, he graduated with an M.D. from Harvard University in 1917. After training in neuropathology at Harvard from 1918 to 1920, he returned to Topeka to help his father found the family clinic in 1919 (*see above*), where he served as the Foundation's director of education. In 1931, under Franz Alexander's (1891–1964) leadership, K. A. M. was one of the founding members of the Chicago Psychoanalytic Society. He was active in the world of American psychoanalysis and is remembered for *Man Against Himself* (1938) and *The Vital Balance* (1963). Among other achievements, in 1934 in the *Psychoanalytic Quarterly*, he coined the term "polysurgery addiction," a form of hysteria. (*See* **HYSTERIA.**)

William Claire Menninger (1899–1966). Born in Topeka, he graduated with an M.D. from Cornell University Medical College in 1924 and the following year joined the staff of the family clinic. In 1927, he trained in psychiatry for a year at **St. Elizabeths Hospital** in Washington, D.C., returned to Topeka to the family clinic, then studied psychoanalysis between 1934 and 1935 at the Chicago Psychoanalytic Institute. For the rest of his career, he held various positions at the clinic, including general secretary after 1946. In 1948–1949, he was president of the American Psychiatric Association and between 1947 and 1949 president as well of the American Psychoanalytic Association. During the Second World War, in the United States Army Medical Corps he was director of neuropsychiatry, where he promoted the expansion of psychiatry in the public. In 1946, he became the founding chairman of the Group for the Advancement of Psychiatry (GAP), a ginger group within psychiatry encouraging psychoanalysis.

MENTAL RETARDATION. (*See also* **AUTISM.**) Mental retardation (MR) was once in the province of psychiatry, but even though the diagnosis continues to be included in ***DSM***, the condition has now largely passed into the hands of pediatrics. MR is defined by three criteria: (1) an intelligence quotient (IQ) of less than 70–75; (2) a significant limitation in meeting the challenges of life ("two or more adaptive skill areas," according to the American Association on Mental Retardation); (3) the condition having been present from childhood. There follow some landmarks in the understanding of MR, which is considered to be a developmental disability rather than a medical disease.

Before the nineteenth century, children with MR were seen as objects of demonic possession. The modern history of encouraging their development begins with the work of Onésime-Édouard Séguin (1812–1880), a Parisian educator who in 1839 founded a school for the training of "idiot children." Séguin had highly prescient ideas about their education: in his 1846 book, *Psychological Therapy, Hygiene and Training of Idiot Children* (*Traitement moral, hygiène et éducation des idiots*), he believed that with training, MR could partially be overcome, and advocated a system of drills and physical exercises. In 1850, Séguin emigrated to the United States, where in 1852 he established in South Boston a special school, then another in Syracuse, New York, in 1854, collaborating in founding a number of such schools in the 1850s in other states. Finally, after gaining an American medical degree in 1861, he settled in New York, and in Orange, New Jersey, opened the doors of the Séguin Physiological School for Feeble-Minded Children. In 1866, he wrote *Idiocy and Its Treatment by the Physiological Method*, becoming in 1876 the founding president of the Association of Medical Officers of American Institutions for Idiotic and Feeble-Minded Persons.

The "degeneration" period in the history of MR sounded notes quite different from Séguin's: viewing retarded children as objects of poisoned heredity and as potential threats to society. In 1871, the Elwyn Training School in Pennsylvania added a custodial department for mentally retarded people of all ages. Psychologist Henry Goddard (1866–1957), director of the psychological laboratory of the Vineland Training School in New Jersey (who in 1909 introduced Alfred Binet's [1857–1911] and Théodore Simon's [1873–1961] IQ test to the United States), described in his 1911 book on *The Kallikak Family: A Study in the Heredity of Feeble-Mindedness*, a stream of "degeneracy" flowing from the Piney Woods. In 1927, Justice Oliver Wendell Holmes of the U.S. Supreme Court, upholding a sterilization law for the mentally retarded, declared, "Three generations of idiots are enough."

In terms of the diagnosis and treatment of MR, there has been some progress. (*See* **PHENYLKETONURIA [PKU]**.) A major step forward has entailed rescuing people with MR from the often horrifying institutions to which they had been consigned and giving them the opportunity to develop in the community to their maximum ability. The seminal figure in the United States is Wolf Wolfensberger (1934–), professor in the school of education at Syracuse University, who as early as 1969 in a volume of essays edited by Robert Kugel, later in a book on the *Principle of Normalization* (1972), advocated the "normalization" of MR, which previously had been considered deviant behavior. Inspired by what he had seen in an earlier trip to Scandinavia, Wolfensberger campaigned for conditions in which people with MR could lead "culturally valued lives."

Beginning in 1968 at the Special Olympics in Chicago, Eunice Shriver (1921–), her husband Sargent Shriver (1915–), and the Joseph P. Kennedy, Jr. Foundation, led efforts to reactivate children with MR by getting them involved in competitive athletics. Special Olympics turned into a worldwide program that has realized many of the principles of Séguin.

METRAZOL SHOCK THERAPY. *See* **CONVULSIVE THERAPY: CHEMICAL.**

MEYER, ADOLF (1866–1950). Meyer, who was German-Swiss, introduced to the United States a number of European concepts and helped train the leadership of American psychiatry in the interwar years.

Born in Niederweningen, Switzerland, into the family of a Protestant minister, Meyer earned his M.D. from the University of Zurich in 1892, immediately immigrating to the United States. After teaching briefly in the neurology department of the University of Chicago, Meyer served as pathologist at a number of mental hospitals: the Illinois Eastern Hospital for the Insane at Kankakee (1893–1895); the Worcester, Massachusetts, Insane Hospital (1895–1902); and as director of the Pathological (later Psychiatric) Institute of the New York State Hospitals. After teaching psychiatry at Cornell University Medical School in New York City from 1904 to 1909, in 1909 he became professor of psychiatry at Johns Hopkins University, then the most prestigious American medical school, and director of the newly opened Henry Phipps Psychiatric Clinic, from which posts he retired in 1941.

Meyer played an influential role in psychiatry for several reasons: he helped train a number of prominent U.S. psychiatrists; he also brought over as postdoctoral fellows on Rockefeller Foundation money some rising British psychiatrists, such as **Aubrey Lewis**. From 1913 to 1915, David K. Henderson (1884–1965), later professor of psychiatry at Edinburgh, was Meyer's first chief resident. (Meyer was close friends with Alan Gregg [1890–1957], the director of the medical sciences program at Rockefeller, and it was evidently at Gregg's behest that bright overseas fellows were channeled to Baltimore.) As part of his "psychobiological" orientation, Meyer preached that the entire patient had to be addressed; he called psychobiology "ergasiology" and derived his own nosology, including such terms as "merergasias" and "kakergasias." After an initial flirtation with the Kraepelinian system, Meyer insisted that the illnesses of patients had to be understood in terms of distinctive "reactions" to their own personal problems. For Meyer, all psychiatric problems were reactions, or unsuccessful adjustment patterns, and this language surfaced again in ***DSM-I*** (1952). Meyer later became enthusiastic about psychoanalysis and was one of the founders in 1911 of the American Psychoanalytic Association.

Leo Alexander (1905–1985), an early American biological psychiatrist then at Duke University, said somewhat wryly in 1958, "I believe that Adolf Meyer cut the Gordian knot a bit prematurely when he denied altogether that mental illnesses are diseases and instead visualized all of them as 'reactions'" (*Objective Approaches to Treatment in Psychiatry*, p. 4).

MEYNERT, THEODOR (pronounced MY-Nert) (1833–1892). Remembered for having placed the structure and function of the central nervous system on a scientific basis, Meynert was born in Dresden, Germany, his father a writer and historian and his mother a singer at the Court Opera. In 1841, the family moved to **Vienna**, where Meynert studied medicine, obtaining in 1865 under the great Vienna pathologist Karl von Rokitansky (1804–1878) his Habilitation as private docent for neuroanatomy. In 1865, he also became a staff psychiatrist at the Lower Austrian Insane Asylum in Vienna and was placed in charge of the pathology department. After visiting a series of asylums abroad, in 1868 Meynert was made lecturer in psychiatry and 2 years later, in 1870, became professor of psychiatry in the clinic of the Vienna Asylum. (It was only in 1872 that he got the university chair of psychiatry.) Interestingly, he became professor of psychiatry with professional training only in neuroanatomy.

Owing to personal conflicts, in 1875 a second chair of psychiatry was created in Vienna expressly for Meynert, this one at the General Hospital (in addition to the chair at the Vienna asylum). Meynert shifted to this new chair, which he occupied until his death. (*See also* **VIENNA** for the academic politics of these moves.)

Among Meynert's students were some of the most distinguished psychiatrists of the day, including Carl Wernicke (1848–1905) (*see* **WERNICKE–KLEIST–LEONHARD PATHWAY**); **Auguste Forel** (1848–1931); Arnold Pick (1851–1924, *see* **DEMENTIA: Pick's disease** [1892]); and Josef Berze (1866–1958), for many years director of the Vienna city asylum "Am Steinhof." **Sigmund Freud** also studied with Meynert for a period, though he detested Meynert's organicism, as psychiatry historian Albrecht Hirschmüller has noted.

Meynert is remembered for his great treatises on neuroanatomy, *The Architecture of the Cerebral Cortex and Its Regional Variations* (*Der Bau der Gross-Hirnrinde und seine örtlichen Verschiedenheiten*) published in 1869, and *Psychiatric Clinic: Illnesses Involving the Forebrain, on the Basis of Its Architecture, Function and Physiology* (*Psychiatrie. Klinik der Erkrankungen des Vorderhirns, begründet auf dessen Bau, Leistungen und Ernährung*), published in 1884–1885 and translated into a number of languages. Although much mocked by the psychoanalytically oriented Viennese (and by later generations of psychoanalyst-historians), Meynert's interest in brain biology turned out to be prescient. In retrospect, Meynert stands with **Kraepelin** and **Freud** among the great psychiatrists of the nineteenth century.

MILIEU THERAPY. *See* **PSYCHOTHERAPY: "therapeutic community"** (from 1939).

MINKOWSKI, EUGENE (1885–1972). One of the cofounders of the movement "Évolution psychiatrique" in France, Minkowski was born in St. Petersburg, Russia, of Jewish-Lithuanian parents. The family moved to Warsaw when he was 7, and he began medical school there, finishing his studies in philosophy and medicine in Munich in 1909. At the outbreak of the First World War, Minkowski moved to Zurich to study with **Eugen Bleuler** and became interested in schizophrenia, which he interpreted as "a loss of vital contact with reality." Migrating then to France in 1915 in the middle of the war, he enlisted in the French army and saw combat at the Somme and Verdun. Rewarded with French citizenship , as well as a Croix de Guerre and membership in the Legion of Honor, he decided to settle in Paris. There, he served as staff physician at the Rothschild hospital and was in charge of the psychotherapy service at the Henri-Rousselle hospital (part of **Ste.-Anne mental hospital** complex).

In 1925, Minkowski became one of the founders of the journal *L'Évolution psychiatrique*, the organ of the vaguely pro-psychoanalytic group of the same title, that had as its philosophical underpinnings the writings of Henri Bergson (1859–1941), as well as Edmund Husserl's (1859–1938) doctrine of phenomenology. Minkowski's was one of the branches of phenomenological analysis, dedicated to understanding phenomena through immediate experience. In psychiatry, this pointed toward psychoanalysis and toward spending much time interviewing patients and endeavoring to achieve empathy. When **Aubrey Lewis** visited Paris in 1937, he said of the Évolution psychiatrique group: "Most of the more progressive people now seem to be associated with this group. . . . They take a broad psychiatric view. Minkowski himself seems still to be the most potent influence in maintaining this desirable emphasis on the broader medical aspects of psychopathology, and his strong philosophic bent gives depth to the general studies carried on by the group" (Angel, *Report*, p. 80). Minkowski's own phenomenological analysis of schizophrenia appeared as a book in 1923 (*Étude psychologique et analyse phénoménologique d'un cas de mélancholie schizophrénique*). Minkowski wore the yellow armband of the Jews during the Second World War but was not deported, and after the war, he resumed his activity in the group.

MITCHELL, S[ILAS] WEIR (1829–1914). Proponent of the "rest cure" for neurasthenia, Mitchell was born in Philadelphia into a doctor's family. He graduated with an M.D. from Jefferson Medical College in 1850, began general practice, then served as a Union army surgeon in the U.S. Civil War. Returning to Philadelphia, he took up private practice as a neurologist and consulted for a private nervous clinic, the Infirmary for Diseases of the Nervous System. Although he is widely considered the founder of neurology in the United States, his large practice included many patients with psychiatric illnesses, and, because neurologists were responsible for "nerves," the books for which he is best known are of a psychiatric nature.

In 1875, in *A Series of American Clinical Lectures*, edited by the neurologist Edward C. Seguin (1843–1898),* Mitchell first described his "rest cure" for neurasthenia, which involved admitting the patient (usually a woman) to a private nervous clinic, where she would be isolated under the supervision of a private nurse, and given electrotherapy, massage, and a milk diet. The technique emphasized "childlike obedience," and its success was based on the authority of the physician. His 1877 book, *Fat and Blood: And How to Make Them*, enjoyed great popularity in translation in Europe, even more so his *Lectures on Diseases of the Nervous System, Especially in Women* (1881). Mitchell's "rest cure" became internationally known as one of the most popular treatments of the late-nineteenth century for community psychiatric disorders among the well-to-do. (*See also* **BODY IMAGE: DISTURBANCES OF: phantom-limb** [1871].) He was highly critical of the asylum psychiatry of his day.

MONOAMINES. *See* **NEUROTRANSMITTERS.**

MOOD DISORDER. *See* **DEPRESSION: EMERGENCE; DEPRESSION: RECENT CONCEPTS; HYPOMANIA AND MANIA; MANIC-DEPRESSIVE ILLNESS; WERNICKE–KLEIST–LEONHARD PATHWAY.**

"MORAL TREATMENT" IN THE SENSE OF PSYCHOLOGICAL TREATMENT. The phrase "moral treatment" came into vogue late in the eighteenth century and was used by **Vincenzo Chiarugi** and by **Philippe Pinel** in their respective textbooks. In his 1801 work, Pinel explained, "the general precepts to follow in psychological treatment" (le traitement moral). "In the well-founded hope of returning to society individuals who seemed lost," Pinel recommended gaining the confidence of patients by talking to them and treating them fairly, organizing fixed daily schedules of asylum life, involving patients in work of various kinds, giving them timely and appetizing meals, and other steps directed toward a well-run and orderly mental hospital. Given that

* The son of Édouard Séguin; *see* **MENTAL RETARDATION.**

many of the patients suffered from "a lesion of their psychological faculties" (lésion des facultés morales; p. 211), a psychological approach rather than sheer physical confinement seemed the best way of imposing "energetic and long-lasting impressions on all of their external senses" (1809, 2nd ed., pp. 251, 258). In the words of Pinel's biographer, Dora Weiner, "The reserved but well-meaning attitude of [Pinel] encouraged the patients to confide in him their worries and to recall their vicissitudes. The daily presence of this inhabitant of the Salpêtrière reassured them. Thus took wing the popular image of 'the good Monsieur Pinel'" (*Pinel*, p. 244).

The private mental hospital "York Retreat," founded in 1791 by York merchant **William Tuke** (1732–1822), practiced "moral treatment" in addition to "medical treatment." As Quaker philanthropist and merchant **Samuel Tuke** (1784–1857), William's grandson, explained in his 1813 book, *Description of the Retreat, an Institution near York, for Insane Persons*, "If we adopt the opinion, that the disease originates in the mind, applications made immediately to it are obviously the most natural." Learning from the experience of the Retreat, "much may be done towards the cure and alleviation of insanity, by judicious modes of management, and moral treatment." "Take, for example, the unhappy manic . . . frequently unconscious of his own disease. . . . He is unable to account for the change in the conduct of his wife, his children, and his surrounding friends. They appear to him cruel, disobedient, and ingrateful." "In such cases, the judicious kindness of others appears generally to excite the gratitude and affection of the patient" (pp. 131–136). Thus, by moral treatment the Tukes seem to have understood a general kind of extension of Quaker principles.

MOREL, BÉNÉDICT-AUGUSTIN (1809–1873). Popularizer of the doctrine of degeneration in psychiatry and among the first to describe schizophrenia, Morel was born in Vienna during the French campaign against Austria. His father was a French military provisioner; nothing is known of his mother. After drifting about in adolescence, he arrived in Paris in 1831, attempted a career in journalism, and in 1839 began medical studies. He roomed with the young scientist Claude Bernard (1813–1878), and both were said to be so poor that they shared between them the only dress suit they had, the one wearing it while the other slept; it was Bernard who introduced Morel to his teacher, psychiatrist **Jean-Pierre Falret**. Thus, Morel began his own career of psychiatric research, publishing papers early on and involving himself in medical journalism. In 1856, Morel was appointed chief physician of the Saint-Yon asylum near Rouen in the Seine-Inférieure department, remaining thereafter. Morel was an enlightened asylum administrator, abolishing restraints, encouraging early discharge, and boarding patients out with local families. He is, however, best known for his *Treatise on Degeneracy* (*Traité des dégénérescences*) published in 1857, which some observers view as the origin of **psychiatric genetics** (*see* **PSYCHOSIS: EMERGENCE: mania . . . degeneration** [1857]), and his *Treatise on Mental Illness* (*Traité des maladies mentales*) in 1860. (*See* **SCHIZOPHRENIA: EMERGENCE: dementia praecox** [1860].) In 1866, the fecund Morel published an article in the *General Archives of Medicine* (*Archives générales de médecine*) on "emotional delusions" (le délire émotif) that represented the beginning of medical writing on anxiety disorders and phobias. (*See* **ANXIETY: Morel's délire émotif** [1866].)

Morel was operating under popular theories of the day that said acquired characteristics could be inherited. These theories were widely influential in psychiatry until the end of the 1920s, indeed in Russia to the 1950s, and were crucial in merging the physical and the psychological elements of the discipline of psychiatry.

MORSELLI, ENRICO (1852–1929). Morselli is known outside of Italy for having coined the term "**dysmorphophobia.**" In Italy, he is known for a big psychiatry textbook, *A Guide to the Semiotics of Mental Illness* (*Manuale di semeiotica delle malattie mentali,* 1885–1894), and for cofounding with his teacher Carlo Livi (1823–1877) and Augusto Tamburini (1848–1919) in 1874 *The Journal of Experimental Psychiatry and Legal Medicine* (*Rivista sperimentale di freniatria e medicina legale*). In 1889, Morselli was appointed professor of psychiatry and neuropathology in Genoa, but psychiatry historian German Berrios notes that in the 1880s, when he was still professor of psychiatry in Turin, "he built up a rich private practice, probably his main source of dysmorphophobic patients (in general, these complaints were very rare in asylums for the insane)" (*History of Mental Symptoms,* p. 279).

MULTIPLE PERSONALITY DISORDER (from 1886). Modern interest in multiple personality disorder may be dated from **Pierre Janet's** article on "the doubling of the personality under hypnotism" ("le dédoublement de la personnalité pendant le somnambulisme provoqué") in the *Revue philosophique* in 1886. Lively interest in the subject continued for about a decade, at which point the theme subsided.

In 1957, two psychiatrists at the Medical College of Georgia in Augusta, Corbett H. Thigpen (1919–1999) and Hervey M. Cleckley (1914–1984), described a challenging case of a female patient with supposed "multiple personalities." Although this phenomenon had been occasionally discussed in previous medical literature, it was their book *The Three Faces of Eve* (1957) that caused an epidemic of "MPD" to emerge. The epidemic is of interest as a moment in the destigmatization of psychiatric illness, representing the first time that a psychiatric diagnosis has ever been widely coveted. "Multiple personality disorder" entered ***DSM-III*** in 1980, remained in ***DSM-III-R*** in 1987, then was replaced by "dissociative identity disorder"—together with the comment that "the syndrome has been overdiagnosed in individuals who are highly suggestible"—in ***DSM-IV*** (1994).

MUNCHAUSEN SYNDROME. Deliberately simulating medical or surgical illness in order to be admitted to hospital for an operation is a form of malingering, unlike involuntary addiction to surgery. (*See* **HYSTERIA: Karl Menninger describes "polysurgical addiction"** [1934].) The faking of illness is called Munchausen syndrome, after an anonymous pamphlet that appeared in 1785 in London, *The Adventures of Baron Munchausen,* which was partly based on the adventures of the real Hieronymus, Count von Münchhausen, who in the service of the Russian army before 1760 achieved fantastic military and athletic feats. In 1951, Richard A. J. Asher (1912–1969),* a London internist affiliated with the Central Middlesex Hospital who had a special interest in mental disorder, suggested the term "Munchausen syndrome" in the *Lancet* for

* Asher is also remembered for a 1947 paper in the *British Medical Journal* on "the dangers of going to bed," a warning to physicians against overprescribing bed rest.

patients with fantastical medical stories who simulated illness in order to gain an operation: "The patient . . . is admitted to hospital with apparent acute illness supported by a plausible and dramatic history. Usually his story is largely made up of falsehoods; he is found to have attended, and deceived, an astounding number of other hospitals; and he nearly always discharges himself against advice, after quarrelling violently with both doctors and nurses. A large number of abdominal scars is particularly characteristic of this condition" (p. 339).

In 1977 in the *Lancet*, (Samuel) Roy Meadow (1933–), a pediatrician at a child hospital in Leeds, proposed "Munchausen syndrome by proxy" for parents who falsely reported that their children had a variety of fantastical illnesses. He assigned it to "the hinterland of child abuse." Sir Roy, as he later was knighted in 1997, achieved national prominence for the observation that, "one sudden infant death is a tragedy, two is suspicious and three is murder, unless proven otherwise." This gained him a reputation for being particularly severe in assessing multiple crib deaths in one family.

N

NARCISSISM. The Greek myth of Narcissus, the god who destroyed himself by gazing continuously at his own image reflected in the pool, speaks so powerfully to the human condition that the concept of "narcissism" lay easily available for discovery. And during the years, various psychiatrists have commented on the elements of self-love, self-involvement, and self-destruction in their patients that doomed Narcissus. The introduction of the term "narcissism" into psychiatry, however, comes by a rather indirect route. It was French psychologist Alfred Binet (1857–1911) who, in the *Revue philosophique* in 1887, first applied the "fable of the beautiful Narcissus" to a "sad perversion," in this case fetishism (p. 264). Then, in April 1898, in an article in the *Alienist and Neurologist,* English sexologist Havelock Ellis (1859–1939) described as "Narcissus-like" the activities of a woman who often masturbated. Ellis later remarked in his *Psychology of Sex* on "the Narcissus-like tendency sometimes found, more especially perhaps in women, for the sexual emotions to be absorbed, and often entirely lost, in self-admiration" (1933, quote from 2nd ed., p. 134). In 1898, Ellis had sent a copy of his article to German psychiatrist Paul Näcke (1851–1913), who referred to the concept in an article in the *Archiv für Psychiatrie und Nervenkrankheiten* in 1899, using the term "Narcismus," meaning self-love (Selbstverliebtheit).

It was this article that **Sigmund Freud** saw. Freud uses the term for the first time in 1905 in his *Three Essays on Sexuality* (*Drei Abhandlungen zur Sexualtheorie*), where he coins the phrase "narcissistic libido." (For Freud, libido meant the quantitative amount of sexual energy that the body and psyche working together could produce.) Freud employed narcissistic libido as a synonym for "ego-libido" (die Ichlibido), meaning the psychic representation of the quantity of libidinal energy, as well as how all this energy was directed.

Freud returned to the subject again in 1911 in his essay, "Psychoanalytic Remarks on an Autobiographically-Described Case of Paranoia (Dementia Paranoides)" ("Psychoanalytische Bemerkungen über einen autobiographisch beschriebenen Fall von Paranoia ([Dementia paranoides])," in the *Yearbook for Psychoanalytic and Psychopathological Research* (*Jahrbuch für psychoanalytische und psychopathologische Forschungen*), often known as the "Schreber case." Here, he made "narcissism" a fundamental stage of infant sexual development: "What happens is that the developing individual is trying to focus his autoerotically-oriented sex drive in order to gain a love object; he now chooses himself, his own body, as a love object" (Freud rendered the term in German as Narzismus, instead of the customary Narzissismus) (*Gesammelte Werke*, VIII, p. 297). This kind of choice characterized homosexuality, Freud thought. (On Freud's analysis of Schreber, *see* **PARANOIA: Freud's view** [1911].)

Freud next ruminated about narcissism in 1914, again in the *Yearbook*, as he attempted to refute an argument of **Carl Jung's** (who was now in the enemy camp) about the supposed inapplicability of libido theory to schizophrenia. Freud said he had been made mindful by Otto Rank's (1884–1939) recent work that the notion of narcissism actually might have a wider application than merely the understanding of homosexuality: It gives us some insight into what happens to the sexual energy of schizophrenics (*Gessammelte Werke*, X).

After the First World War, Freud's interest in narcissism dimmed as he became preoccupied with structuring the psyche around ego, superego, and **id**. The next important theoretical contribution to narcissism within psychoanalysis was made many years later by Heinz Kohut (*See* **FREUDIAN PSYCHOTHERAPY: TECHNIQUE: Kohut's "self-psychology"** [1971].)

NARCOLEPSY. Narcolepsy means sudden, irresistible sleep attacks, often accompanied by cataplexy (sudden loss of muscle tone), "hypnagogic" hallucinations (just before falling asleep), and sleep paralysis (sensation of being figuratively nailed to the bed). Although physicians going back to the seventeenth century had described the phenomenon, the first modern characterization of it comes from Berlin psychiatry professor Carl Westphal (1833–1890) in 1877, as he lectured the Berlin Medical Society—in an article subsequently published in the *Archiv für Psychiatrie und Nervenkrankheiten*—about "Singular Seizures Associated with Falling Asleep" ("Eigenthümliche mit Einschlafen verbundene Anfälle"). "I myself have had repeated occasions to observe the attacks of this patient [a bookbinder named Ehlert]. He experienced one while I was talking to him. While he was still speaking . . . one sees that his eyelids are gradually drooping. . . . Then the patient stops speaking after mumbling something incomprehensible; his head sinks to his chest . . . and the patient now offers the picture of someone who has fallen asleep while seated" (p. 632). Three years later, in 1880, Jean-Baptiste-Édouard Gélineau (1859–1906), in two articles in the Parisian *Gazette des hôpitaux*, coined the term "narcolepsie": "I propose to give the name narcolepsy . . . to a rare, or at least little-known, neurosis characterized by an imperious, sudden and transitory need to sleep, occurring at more or less close intervals. This name will recall the double analogy of narcolepsy to somnolence and to catalepsy [cataplexy is meant*]" (p. 626).

As for treatment, in 1930 John Benedict Doyle (1894–1971), an associate consultant in neurology at the Mayo Foundation in Rochester, Minnesota, and Luman E. Daniels (1895–1971), a resident in neurology there, proposed ephedrine for the treatment of narcolepsy; *see* the *Proceedings of the Staff Meetings of the Mayo Clinic* (1930). (This was 4 months after a similar report, in Czech, by Prague university psychiatrist Otakar Janota [1898–1969] in the Purkyne Society. So Janota had the priority but nobody knew it until he wrote about his discovery again in 1931 in German in the *Medizinische Klinik*.)

In 1935, Myron Prinzmetal (1908–1987), a Los Angeles cardiologist (who described in 1955 a distinctive kind of angina named after him), and Wilfred Bloomberg (1905–1987), a Harvard psychiatrist, in the *Journal of the American Medical Association* suggested the newly introduced drug Benzedrine (racemic amphetamine sulfate) for

---

* Catalepsy means wax-like postures; cataplexy, the sudden loss of muscle force, occurs in narcolepsy. As Gélineau himself said, "Moreover, even popular language in a manner of speaking has consecrated the usage in speaking of someone exhausted by late nights and work, 'He's falling down with sleep.' [Il tombe de sommeil]" (p. 636). If Gélineau had not confused the two, the coinage would have been "narcoplexy."

narcolepsy. They had done a controlled trial, one of the first in psychiatry. The amphetamines remained the treatments of choice in narcolepsy for many years.

Narcolepsy is not primarily a psychiatric diagnosis, and its representation in ***DSM*** has been rather haphazard. Among the sleep disorders, ***DSM "One"*** (1952) and ***DSM-II*** (1968) discussed only somnambulism, or sleepwalking. ***DSM-III*** (1980) mentioned the term "narcolepsy" as one of the "disorders of excessive somnolence," without any discussion of it. ***DSM-III-R*** (1987) had a fuller account without making narcolepsy a separate diagnosis (still a form of hypersomnia). However, in ***DSM-IV*** in 1994, narcolepsy took wing as a disease of its own alongside other "sleep disorders."

NATIONAL INSTITUTE OF MENTAL HEALTH (NIMH) in the United States (from 1949). The Narcotics Division of the Public Health Service (PHS) was established in 1929 and was renamed in 1930 the Division of Mental Hygiene. (*See also* **WIKLER, ABRAHAM.**) This division constituted the nucleus of the later NIMH. In 1934, Lawrence Kolb (1881–1972), a PHS officer, was appointed its chief medical officer, becoming in 1938 assistant surgeon general in charge of the Division of Mental Hygiene. Kolb retired in 1944, but he had wanted to set up a national neuropsychiatric institute within the National Institutes of Health (NIH) modeled on the recently founded cancer and heart institutes.

After the Second World War, the large number of veterans with mental-health problems focused federal attention on this area. The National Mental Health Act of 1946 called for the creation of a National Institute of Mental Health with an in-house research program, and in 1949 the new institute got its first congressional appropriation. Robert Felix (1904–1990), who had succeeded Kolb as the director of mental hygiene, was the new institute's director; after 1951, Seymour Kety (1915–2000) was in charge of research. During the years, billions of federal dollars would go into "intramural" mental-health research (done at NIMH) and "extramural" research (grants to outside investigators).

In 1963, NIMH received a new role in the provision of services with the Community Mental Health Centers Construction Act.

Spooked by fears of psychiatry becoming just another medical discipline, in 1967 director Stanley Yolles (1919–2001) moved the NIMH outside the NIH structure, leaving the intramural research program attached to NIH. (NIMH definitively rejoined NIH only in 1989.) In 1973, research on addiction at the newly established National Institute on Drug Abuse (NIDA) was moved outside the NIMH into a new federal agency (the Alcohol, Drug Abuse, and Mental Health Administration, or ADAMHA*) that also housed the National Institute on Alcohol Abuse and Alcoholism, or NIAAA (created in 1970), as well as NIMH itself.†

* Administratively established by the Department of Health, Education and Welfare (DHEW) in 1973; officially recognized in Public Law 93–282 in 1974.

† In 1989, when ADAMHA was abolished and the research components of NIMH returned to NIH, the research programs of NIAAA and NIDA came into NIH as well. The services components of the three institutes became part of a new PHS agency, the Substance Abuse and Mental Health Services Administration (SAMHSA).

The NIMH has played a distinctive role in the development of psychopharmacology in the United States. In 1955, Felix set up an Ad Hoc Committee on Psychopharmacology, jointly chaired by Kety, then chief of the laboratory of clinical science of NIMH, and by Robert Cohen (1909–), the clinical director. The following year, 1956, NIMH created the Psychopharmacology Service Center (PSC), generously funded by Congress after testimony by **Nathan Kline** and lobbyist Mike Gorman (1913–1989). Jonathan Cole (1925–) became the director of the PSC, with **Gerald Klerman** his assistant (Klerman traveled to the United Kingdom to see how clinical trials were done). Cole was replaced in 1967 by Jerome Levine (1934–). The drug trials arm of the PSC was the Early Clinical Drug Evaluation Unit program (the "ECDEU"), which began in 1960 and was funded until the mid-1970s. By 1969, some 35 ECDE units had studied 177 investigational drugs. In 1966, the PSC became the Psychopharmacology Research Branch of NIMH.

As well, in 1957 **Joel Elkes** created the Clinical Neuropharmacology Research Center of NIMH in the William A. White building of **St. Elizabeths Hospital** in Washington, D.C. (NIMH would retain control of these facilities and their successors even as St. Elizabeths Hospital was transferred in 1987 from NIMH to the District of Columbia; the labs were moved to the NIH main "campus" only in 1996.)

The changing directors of NIMH reflect the changes in the research orientation of American psychiatry. Robert H. Felix (1904–1990) (director 1949–1964) was a psychoanalyst; Stanley Yolles (1919–2001) (in office 1964–1970), and Bertram Brown (1931–) (in office 1970–1977) were both interested in community psychiatry and drug abuse; Herbert Pardes (1934–) (in office 1978–1984) and Shervert Frazier (1921–) (in office 1984–1986) were psychoanalysts who had switched to biological psychiatry. Subsequent directors had really spent their lives in biological research, including Lewis Judd (1930–) (in office 1988–1992), Frederick Goodwin (1936–) (in office 1992–1994), and Steven Hyman (1952–) (in office 1996–2002), who conducted research on synaptic transmission and genetics. (Rex W. Cowdry was acting director between 1994 and 1996.)

NEURASTHENIA AND GEORGE MILLER BEARD (from 1869). Although New York electrotherapist George Beard (1839–1883) did not coin the term "neurasthenia"—meaning literally tired nerves—he launched it on its century-long worldwide trajectory. A graduate of the College of Physicians and Surgeons in New York in 1866, 2 years later Beard began lecturing on nervous diseases at New York University; between 1870 and his death in 1883 he was on staff at the Demilt Dispensary there. In an 1869 article in the *Boston Medical and Surgical Journal* (the forerunner of the *New England Journal of Medicine*), Beard published an article on "Neurasthenia, or Nervous Exhaustion." For Beard, the key characteristic of the disorder was not that the patients were chronically tired, or had a psychiatric illness, but rather that "the central nervous system becomes dephosphorized, or, perhaps, loses somewhat of its solid constituents; probably undergoes slight, undetectable, morbid changes in its chemical structure, and, as a consequence, becomes more or less impoverished in the quantity of its nervous force" (p. 218). The symptoms of the disorder were manifold: "If a patient complains of general malaise, debility of all the functions, poor appetite, abiding weakness in the back and spine, fugitive neuralgic pains, hysteria, insomnia, hypochondriasis, disinclination for consecutive mental labor, severe and weakening attacks of sick headache . . . we have reason to suspect that . . . we are dealing with a typical case of neurasthenia" (p. 218).

By the time Beard brought out his big book, *A Practical Treatise on Nervous Exhaustion (Neurasthenia)* in 1880, the symptoms had become even more protean, including such frank psychiatric phenomena as anxiety, phobias, and "hopelessness." The following year, Beard brought forth yet another hit: *American Nervousness: Its Causes and Consequences, a Supplement to Nervous Exhaustion (Neurasthenia)*. *Sexual Neurasthenia* followed posthumously in 1884. Beard's *Practical Treatise* reached a fifth U.S. edition in 1905; his *Sexual Neurasthenia*, a six edition in that year. Moreover, his numerous writings on electrotherapy stayed long in print. (It is actually inexact to call him a neurologist because he wrote little of a neurological nature: He was a specialist in the electrotherapy of neurasthenia.)

No previous American medical writer had enjoyed the international prominence that Beard attained with his three volumes on neurasthenia. His book on sexual neurasthenia appeared in French in 1895; his *Practical Treatise* was translated at once (in 1881) into German and enjoyed three German editions; *Sexual Neurasthenia* had reached a second German edition by 1890. The reasons for this extraordinary literary success can only remain speculative. Yet, the concept of neurasthenia fitted perfectly the notion of the "rest cure" that **Silas Weir Mitchell** was simultaneously propagating; and the large number of private nervous clinics avid for the business of wealthy "neurasthenia" patients caused an international boomlet in electrotherapy, bed-rest, milk cures, massage, and the other appurtenances of "rest" for neurasthenia. As well, a middle-class that liked to believe it was continually tired from workaday urban occupations gratefully responded to the suggestion that their storage batteries were depleted and unable to recharge themselves by a night's sleep. In any event, by the turn of the century an organic-sounding "neurasthenia" had trumped all competing "nervous" diagnoses, such as hysteria and hypochondria, to become illness-attribution number one in Western society.

Neurasthenia began to lose favor as it became psychiatrized. It turned into a mental diagnosis rather than an organic-seeming one, as the brain and mind became its locus rather than those "exhausted spinal centers." Such influential papers as that of Kiel psychiatry professor Georg Stertz (1878–1959) on "exogenous neurasthenic reactions" (that appeared in Oswald Bumke's [1877–1950] massive *Handbook of Psychiatric Illnesses [Handbuch der Geisteskrankheiten]* in 1928) were really the kiss of death for it as a popular diagnosis. Neurasthenia retained, however, a place in ***DSM-II***, and the drafters of ***DSM-III*** saw it as the equivalent of "chronic depressive disorder," although that latter diagnosis did not make it into the published *DSM-III* in 1980. Yet, in the World Health Organization's *ICD-10 Classification of Mental and Behavioural Disorders*, "neurasthenia" retained a prominent place, meaning either unusual fatigability or "feelings of bodily or physical weakness and exhaustion after only minimal effort" (p. 170). (*See also* **ANXIETY AND PHOBIAS: Beard's neurasthenia** [1880].)

NEUROIMAGING. The radiological imaging of the brain is important because it occasionally permits the linking of psychiatric symptoms to underlying brain lesions.

Neuroradiology: plain film studies of the skull and spine (from 1896). This story begins with the earliest days of x-ray as young Harvey Cushing (1869–1939), later pioneer neurosurgeon but at the time a house officer at Johns Hopkins University, produced in 1896 a radiograph of the cervical spine of a patient who had just been shot in the neck. Yet, the major figure of the "plain film" era was the Viennese physician Arthur Schüller (1874–1957), who coined the term "Neuro-Roentgenologie" and in 1912 wrote the standard text, *Röntgendiagnostik der Erkrankungen des Kopfes*, translated into English in 1918 as *Roentgen Diagnosis of Diseases of the Head*.

Air encephalography, or ventriculography (from 1918). Because air casts a different radiographic shadow than either bone or soft tissue, injecting air as a contrast medium into the space around the spinal cord—and thence into the ventricles of the brain—may be used to illuminate lesions in the central nervous system. The Johns Hopkins neurosurgeon Walter Edward Dandy (1886–1946) first described this procedure in 1918 in the *Annals of Surgery*, useful as a means of spotting brain cancer. (In 1919, in the same journal, Dandy used air actually to outline the shape of the brain [encephalography].)

In psychiatry, pneumoencephalography in the investigation of chronic schizophrenic patients was initiated by two psychiatrists—Walter Jacobi (1889–1937) and H. Winkler—at Stadtroda mental hospital near the university town of Jena; it was **Hans Berger**, professor of psychiatry in Jena (the inventor of electroencephalography), who instigated the investigation. In an article in 1927 in the *Archive of Psychiatry and Nervous Diseases* (*Archiv für Psychiatrie und Nervenkrankheiten*), the authors found the patients' ventricle systems somewhat enlarged. During the years, pneumoencephalography produced many such hints of the organicity of major psychiatric illness, especially of cerebral atrophy in chronic schizophrenia (but because the studies were uncontrolled, one could not say for sure). A landmark study was Gerd Huber's (1921–) 1957 monograph, *Pneumoencephalography and Psychopathology in the Endogenous Psychoses* (*Pneumencephalographische und psychopathologische Bilder bei endogenen Psychosen*). In 1966, Peter Brett Storey (M.B. 1953) at St. George's Hospital in London carried out the first controlled study of chronic schizophrenia using lumbar air encephalography. Reported in the *British Journal of Psychiatry*, he was unable to settle the question whether schizophrenics had atrophy or not. (*See* **SCHIZOPHRENIA: RECENT CONCEPTS**.)

Carotid arteriography (1927). Concerned at the risks to the patient of introducing air into the brain, as well as the inexactness of the air images, in 1927 Lisbon neurologist Egas Moniz (1874–1955), known also for having begun the practice of leukotomy (*see* **LOBOTOMY**) a few years later, proposed in the *Revue neurologique* the injection of a contrast medium (sodium iodide) directly into the internal carotid arteries (which pass up through the neck to become the brain's main blood supply). As neuroradiology historian Ronald Eisenberg explains, "The procedure involved making two permanent scars, one on each side of the neck, unpleasant stigmata particularly for an attractive woman to carry for the rest of her life, especially if the investigation proved negative" (*Radiology*, p. 338).

Radionuclide brain scanning (1948). As part of a continuous effort to localize brain tumors more precisely, George E. Moore (1920–), a young surgeon serving in Minneapolis a fellowship in the Public Health Service, conceived the idea of tagging a radioactive substance to the compound fluorescein (which seemed to show a certain affinity for tumors), injecting it into the brain, then using a Geiger counter to see if it was taken up selectively by brain tumors. It worked, and the research, published in

Science in 1948, represented the beginning of the kind of radioactive neuroimaging that would later prove a boon to psychiatry.

Measurement of cerebral blood flow (1948). If psychiatric illnesses might be localized to various areas of the brain, one way to identify those metabolically more (or less) active areas would be to measure regional differences in cerebral blood flow (CBF). This entire concept of measuring CBF was initiated by two physiologists who later stood quite close to psychiatry, Seymour Kety (1915–2000) and Carl Frederic Schmidt (1893–1988), who in an article in 1945 in the *American Journal of Physiology* used nitrous oxide to evaluate overall CBF. In 1948 in the *American Journal of Psychiatry*, these two researchers, together with others, discussed their use of the nitrous oxide technique to ascertain if schizophrenic patients' overall CBF differed from that of controls: It did not. (*See* **BARBITURATES: restorative effects in schizophrenia** [1948].) Later technology for measuring CBF improved upon the Kety–Schmidt technique mainly in using radioactive xenon gas.

The availability of computers, plus the ability to produce nuclides with a cyclotron, transformed neuroimaging in the 1960s and after. The new technology may be divided between devices that illuminated brain structure as opposed to function. (*See* **SCHIZOPHRENIA: RECENT CONCEPTS: Weinberger** [1986].)

Computed tomography (CT) (from 1972). Tomography means visualizing different layers of the body, or body section imaging. The term was coined by Berlin x-ray engineer Gustav Grossmann (1878–?), who in 1935 described "lung tomography" in the *British Journal of Radiology*. Yet, the first efforts to undertake the radiography of body layers go back to the 1920s. Although the mathematics of converting a series of two-dimensional projections of a given layer of the body into a three-dimensional image had been worked out early in the century, only in 1972 did the availability of a computer make it possible to convert these calculations into actual body images. This was the work of Geoffrey Hounsfield (1919–2004), a scientist at EMI Limited in London, who, in a study of a woman with a brain lesion at Atkinson Morley's Hospital in London, was able to produce a serviceable CT image of the "cyst." The EMI scanner was limited to the head. (He received a Nobel Prize for this in 1979, and the image was published in 1980 in the *Journal of Computer Assisted Tomography*.) In 1976, Eve Johnstone (*see* **WOMEN IN PSYCHIATRY**), leading a team of researchers that included **Timothy J. Crow** at the Clinical Research Centre in Harrow, England, introduced CT into psychiatry with a controlled study of ventricular size in schizophrenia patients. Publishing in the *Lancet*, they found that schizophrenics did indeed have enlarged ventricles. The basic difference between CT and air encephalography lay in making possible density measurements of tissues, to see for example if cell death had taken place, as opposed merely to identifying abnormal bulges in the ventricles.

Magnetic resonance imaging (MRI). MRI entered medicine in the late 1970s, after the theoretical groundwork for it had been laid beginning in 1971.* The

* The 2003 Nobel Prize in Physiology or Medicine went to Paul Lauterbur (1933–) at the University of Illinois in Urbana and Peter Mansfield (1933–) at the University of Nottingham for their development of MRI. Raymond Damadian (1936–), who had made an important contribution, beginning with an article in *Science* in 1971, felt he had been wrongly overlooked.

technique involved subjecting tissues to strong magnetic fields, in a way that differentiates among the density of protons in various tissues. MRI has nothing to do with x-rays and owes its development to the physics of nuclear magnetic resonance (NMR) that began in the mid-1940s. (The term "nuclear magnetic resonance" gave way to "magnetic resonance imaging" because of patient fears about anything "nuclear.") The earliest clinical application of this technology in neuroimaging came in 1981 as Ian R. Young (1932–) at the Thorn-EMI company's Central Research Laboratories at Hayes in Middlesex, together with four physician collaborators at Hammersmith Hospital, published in the *Lancet* comparable NMR and CT scans of the brain in multiple sclerosis: Whereas the CT scans identified only 19 lesions in one patient, the MRI (called "NMR") scans identified 131.

In psychiatry, the first controlled study using MRI was led by **Nancy Andreasen** and published in *Archives of General Psychiatry* in 1986: in a population of schizophrenic males, nearly 40% of the patients had "markedly smaller frontal lobes" (p. 142). Beginning in the 1990s, "functional" MRI was used to study metabolic abnormalities in psychiatric illness.

MRI distinguishes between gray and white matter better than CT. For example, the characteristic lesions of multiple sclerosis (MS) appear in an MRI of the gray matter as "black holes," because MS causes demyelination of the axons (the long tail ends of the neurons). This is of importance in psychiatry in determining whether one's patient suffers from "hysteria" or a demyelinating disease of the nervous system.

Functional studies in tomography (PET and SPECT). The anatomy can be normal in mental illness yet brain function seriously disturbed. This led to a search for ways of studying metabolism, as distinct from structure. In the 1980s, such work focused on cerebral blood flow and glucose uptake, as well as on brain receptors for neurotransmitters. (For example, in Alzheimer's disease, glucose uptake in the temporal-parietal cortex is greatly reduced and is visible in a positron emission tomography, or PET, scan.)

In PET scans, positron-emitting isotopes are attached to such natural substances as glucose, then put into the body; as the positrons collide with electrons, they give off gamma rays, and a gamma camera records these rays, a computer then constructing a three-dimensional image of these signals. In SPECT (single-photon emission computed tomography) scans, radionuclides that emit gamma rays are given to subjects, and gamma cameras around the patient record these gamma photons; a computer then translates these records into images. Unlike PET scans, a cyclotron is not required for SPECT scans. Michel Ter-Pogossian (1925–1996), professor of radiation sciences at Washington University in St. Louis, and co-workers initiated PET scanning in 1975, with an article on the subject in *Radiology*. (He called it "PETT," for positron-emission transaxial tomograph; the research had first been presented at a radiology meeting in 1974.)

PET scanning was first used in psychiatry in 1982 as a team of scientists led by Monte Stuart Buchsbaum (1940–), professor of psychiatry at the University of California at Irvine, published in the *Archives of General Psychiatry* a PET study of regional blood flow in schizophrenia: The finding was lower glucose use in the frontal cortex of patients with schizophrenia. SPECT scanning was introduced into neurology and psychiatry in 1984 by B. Leonard Holman (1941–), professor of radiology at Harvard, and Thomas C. Hill (1945–), chief of nuclear medicine at New England Deaconess Hospital in Boston, who used the isotope ^{123}I-iodoamphetamine to study cerebral blood flow. In research published in *Applied Radiology*, the authors showed how the technique could be used to contrast ictal (epileptic seizure) and interictal images of the brain.

NEUROLEPTIC. The term "neuroleptic" was coined by **Jean Delay** and **Pierre Deniker** in 1952 at a French-language psychiatry conference in Paris for the kind of drug that reduces the symptoms of psychosis; neuroleptics are called "**antipsychotics**" in the United States. (*See also* **CHLORPROMAZINE.**)

NEUROSIS. In his *First Lines of the Practice of Physic*, the first volume in the English translation of which was published in 1777, **William Cullen** introduced the term "neuroses" to mean diseases of the nervous system in which there was no obvious physical lesion. Mental illnesses (the "Vesaniae") were a subcategory of neuroses. Of the "neuroses" he wrote, "I propose to comprehend . . . all those preternatural affections of sense or motion which are without pyrexia [fever] as a part of the primary disease; and all those which do not depend upon a topical affection of the organs, but upon a more general affection of the nervous system" (p. 122 of vol. III of the 1799 edition).

Thus launched, the term "neurosis" was taken up by a number of authors, notably Vienna's Ernst von Feuchtersleben (1806–1849), who in a series of lectures on psychiatry in 1845 (*see* **PSYCHOSIS: EMERGENCE**), distinguished between "psychosis" and "neurosis": "Every psychosis [disorder of the psyche] is at the same time a neurosis [disorder of the brain], because without the mediation of the nervous system no mental change is able to become manifest; but every neurosis is not simultaneously a psychosis" (p. 265).

Yet, subsequent authors would reverse the meaning of the two terms, making psychosis the major form of psychiatric illness and neurosis a lesser disturbance.

In his 1872 *Textbook of Psychiatry* (*Lehrbuch der Psychiatrie*), **Richard von Krafft-Ebing** distinguished between "psychoneuroses," meaning "mental illnesses that affect individuals with normal brains," and "psychic degeneration." "For those mental disorders that affect individuals with healthy brains let us use the designation psychoneuroses; for those that arise on the basis of predisposition the expression psychic degeneration will serve" (2nd ed., 1879, vol. II, p. 3).

For **Sigmund Freud**, psychoneurosis meant symptoms arising from unconscious conflict as opposed to current life issues (which latter category he called "actual neuroses"). The first time he used the term "psychoneurosis" was in his essay on "Sexuality in the Etiology of the Neuroses," published in the *Vienna Clinical Review* (*Wiener Klinische Rundschau*) in 1898: "The significant differentiation, one that in each case may be made through careful evaluation of the symptoms, is whether the case has the character of a neurasthenia or a psychoneurosis (hysteria, obsessive thoughts)" (*Gessammelte Werke*, I, p. 496). The term "neurosis" as such, however, had long entered medical discourse, and Freud employed it from the very beginning to mean "disorder." See, for his example, his essay on the distinction between neurasthenia and "anxiety neurosis" (Angstneurose) in 1895 in the *Central Journal of Neurology* (*Neurologisches Zentralblatt*). (*See* **ANXIETY: Freud differentiates . . .** [1895].)

The Freudian psychoneuroses embraced much of the range of psychopathology. In 1913, in an essay on "The Disposition to Obsessive Neurosis" ("Die Disposition zur Zwangsneurose") in the *International Journal of Medical Psychoanalysis* (*Internationale Zeitschrift für ärztliche Psychoanalyse*), Freud argued that, "The order in which the psychoneuroses are conventionally discussed—hysteria, obsessive neurosis, paranoia, dementia praecox—corresponds to (if not exactly) the order in which they appear in life. Hysterical forms of illness may be observed as early as infancy; obsessive neurosis reveals its first symptoms in the second stage of childhood (from 6 to 8 years old); the two other psychoneuroses, which I have brought together under the term 'paraphrenia,' manifest themselves only after puberty and in young adulthood" (*Gesammelte Werke*, VIII, pp. 443–444).

After Freud, the term "neurosis" remained largely in the domain of psychoanalytic speculation, although it retained some currency in neurology as a synonym for "functional," or symptoms without lesions. As London neurologist Samuel Alexander Kinnier Wilson (1874–1937) pointed out in his posthumous textbook *Neurology* (1940), "Current neurological opinion takes the word [neurosis] to signify a disorder of nervous function for which as yet no underlying basis has been found" (p. 1626). "Neurosis" was banned from psychiatry officially by ***DSM-IV*** in 1994 (the two previous editions, ***DSM-III*** [1980] and ***DSM-III-R*** [1987] having used it in parentheses as a synonym for disorder).

NEUROSYPHILIS. The syphilitic infiltration of the central nervous system, though today belonging to internal medicine or neurology, was once treated by psychiatrists. The patients themselves frequently landed in asylums because the illness first becomes manifest in the form of psychiatric symptoms; paralysis and convulsions are later symptoms. But because neurosyphilis progresses from psychiatric symptoms such as the compulsive shopping of mania to the frank neurological symptoms accompanying lesions in central nervous tissue, it was formerly called "progressive paralysis," or "general paralysis of the insane" (also known as "GPI"). In some asylums, up to half of all patients in the men's wards had neurosyphilis, and so the history of the diagnosis and treatment of the condition is highly germane to the history of psychiatry.

Although careful clinical descriptions of the spinal form of neurosyphilis, called "tabes dorsalis" (wasting of the posterior columns of the spinal cord), or "locomotor ataxia," go back to Sigismund Loewenhardt's (1796–1875) Latin treatise *De myelophthisi chronica* in 1817, it was only in 1822 that the young Paris physician Antoine Laurent Jessé Bayle (1799–1858) described in his medical thesis what turned out to be the cerebral form of syphilis. (*See* **UNITARY PSYCHOSIS**.) Not until 1894 did Jean-Alfred Fournier (1832–1914), a distinguished Parisian syphilologist, link statistically a primary syphilis infection to the later appearance of paresis and tabes (in *Les affections parasyphilitiques*). (Paresis means paralytic symptoms.) Indeed, in the real world of medical practice, before 1905 there was great confusion about the difference between syphilis and gonorrhea and about whether progressive paralysis was caused by an infectious organism at all, but was not rather the result of masturbation or overwork. Then in 1905, the Berlin parasitologist Fritz Schaudinn (1871–1906), in serum that Erich Hoffmann (1868–1959), an associate professor (Privatdozent) at the Berlin university clinic for syphilis and dermatology, had obtained from a genital lesion, identified the spiral organism that causes syphilis, the "Spirochaeta pallida." Schaudinn later renamed the organism "Treponema pallidum." Their classic discovery appeared in the *Studies of the Imperial Health Office* (*Arbeiten des kaiserlichen Gesundheitsamtes*) in Berlin, where Schaudinn was employed.

In terms of the diagnosis of neurosyphilis, a vexatious issue for physicians dealing with previously healthy middle-aged men acutely presenting with the symptoms of mania, it had long been known that there was some kind of relationship between syphilis and the symptom of paresis (paralysis). Yet, many writers considered cerebral syphilis and progressive paralysis separate diseases. Then in 1905, August Wassermann (1866–1925), a staff physician at Robert Koch's Institute for Infectious Diseases at the Charité Hospital in Berlin, described in the *German Medical Weekly* (*Deutsche Medizinische Wochenschrift*) a diagnostic test for syphilis based on the cerebrospinal fluid; later that year in the same journal he and Felix Plaut (1877–1940), a young assistant physician at **Emil Kraepelin's** psychiatric clinic in Munich, showed that the test obtained positive results in the great majority of paresis patients.

In 1913, Hideyo Noguchi (1876–1928) at the Rockefeller Institute for Medical Research in New York and Joseph W. Moore (1879–?) at the Central Islip State Hospital on Long Island reported in the *Journal of Experimental Medicine* that out of 70 "paretic" brains, Noguchi had succeeded in obtaining a culture of *T. pallidum* in 12; Moore then confirmed the finding. This strongly suggested that general paralysis of the insane was a form of late syphilis.

As for therapy, a specific treatment for primary syphilis had been discovered in 1909, as Frankfurt internist Paul Ehrlich (1854–1915) established the efficacy of an organic arsenical that became marketed as Salvarsan (generically arsenobenzol; arsphenamine in the United States). Yet, Salvarsan does not cross the blood–brain barrier well and was less effective in neurosyphilis; it was also quite toxic and difficult to administer. In 1917, **Julius Wagner von Jauregg** initiated the malarial-fever cure of neurosyphilis, which involved giving neurosyphilis patients injections of the blood of malarial patients, then, several weeks later, after the neurosyphilis patients had started spiking malarial fevers, curing them with quinine. (The spirochaete that causes syphilis is heat-sensitive.) In 1944, the penicillin panel of the subcommittee on venereal diseases of the United States National Research Council, led by John H. Stokes (1885–1961), a Philadelphia dermatologist, announced in the *Journal of the American Medical Association* that penicillin was effective in neurosyphilis. This represented the definitive treatment, and the prevalence of the condition declined sharply.

NEUROTRANSMITTER. Neurotransmitters are the chemicals involved in communication between nerve cells ("neurons"). Substances released from the end bulb of an upstream ("presynaptic") neuron into the synaptic space in order to excite or inhibit the downstream ("postsynaptic") neuron are called neurotransmitters. Although more than 100 chemicals have been identified as neurotransmitters, most research has been done on (1) acetylcholine (an ester of choline); (2) the "monoamine" neurotransmitters dopamine and norepinephrine; a monoamine contains one amino (NH) group; dopamine and norepinephrine are also called "catecholamines" because they have a "catechol" portion; (3) the monoamine neurotransmitters serotonin and melatonin, which are also called "indolamines" because of their "indole" portion; (4) the amino acid neurotransmitters such as gamma-aminobutyric acid, or GABA. (*See* **CATECHOLAMINE HYPOTHESIS OF DEPRESSION; DOPAMINE; SYNAPSE.**)

The chemicals that transmit the nerve impulse in the central nervous system were previously called "neurohormones," or "neurohumors," in a usage going back to Otto Loewi's (1873–1961) expression "humoral transmission" in *Pflügers Archiv* in 1921. The term "neurotransmitter" became current in psychiatry in the 1960s, a foreshadowing of which is Ulf von Euler's 1959 article on "Neurotransmission in the adrenergic nervous system" in the *Harvey Lectures*. (In the article, however, he refers to "nerve transmitter" rather than "neurotransmitter.")

The substance Loewi discovered in 1921 was later identified as acetylcholine, the first neurotransmitter. (*See* **SYNAPSE.**) In 1946, Ulf von Euler (1905–1983), professor of physiology at the Karolinska Institute in Stockholm, identified noradrenaline as the adrenergic neurotransmitter; he won a Nobel Prize for this in 1970.

In 1957, Bernard B. Brodie (1909–1989) and Parkhurst A. Shore (1924–), in the Laboratory of Chemical Pharmacology of the National Heart Institute, part of the National Institutes of Health in Bethesda, Maryland, suggested that serotonin, or 5-hydroxytryptamine (5-HT) as it is also called, and norepinephrine functioned alike as "chemical mediators of mutually antagonistic centers in the brain." This proposal, in research published in the *Annals of the New York Academy of Sciences*, was tantamount to calling serotonin a neurotransmitter, although the authors used the phrase "central neurohumoral agent" (p. 631). Referring to the antagonism between serotonin and LSD, Brodie said, "It is probable that subtle biochemical events, peculiar to the brain, will ultimately explain normal brain function and the changes responsible for mental illnesses" (p. 641). (On LSD, *see* **HALLUCINOGEN**; on serotonin *see* **SELECTIVE SEROTONIN REUPTAKE INHIBITORS**; on these events, *see also* **IPRONIAZID.**)

In 1957, Swedish neuroscientist Arvid Carlsson (1923–) discovered the role of **dopamine** as a neurotransmitter, and published his work in *Science* in 1958 (the research had been submitted for publication in 1957, the true year of the discovery).

Amino acids also function as neurotransmitters, in addition to the monoamine neurotransmitters and acetylcholine. The first amino acid to be identified as having a role in neurotransmission was gamma-aminobutyric acid (GABA), isolated in 1963 by Edward Arthur Kravitz (1932–) and co-workers at the National Institute of Neurological Disorders, in research published in the *Journal of Neurophysiology*. (In 1974, **Solomon Snyder** discovered the receptor for it.)

In his Nobel Lecture in 2000, Carlsson observed, "During the past half-century brain research has been dominated by biochemical approaches. . . . [This] is understandable in view of the entrance of the neurohumoral transmission concept into brain research in conjunction with the spectacular progress of molecular biology. However, it must be recognized that the brain is not a chemical factory but an extremely complicated survival machine." Carlsson ventured that further progress in such areas as **neuroimaging** and pattern recognition "will help to reveal the enormous width of our present ignorance of the human brain" (*Bioscience Reports*, 2002, p. 707).

NIMH. *See* **NATIONAL INSTITUTE OF MENTAL HEALTH.**

NISSL, FRANZ (1860–1919). Pioneer of neurohistology, Nissl was born in a small town in the Palatinate (Bavaria), into a schoolteacher's family. In 1885, he wrote his doctoral dissertation in medicine at Munich University, then began training in psychiatry as an assistant to Professor Bernhard von Gudden (1824–1886), an important brain anatomist. In 1889, Nissl became a staff psychiatrist at the Frankfurt City Aslyum, the direction of which Emil Sioli (1852–1922) had just taken over. Sioli had a strong bent toward biological research and just a few months previously had recruited **Alois Alzheimer** as well. The scene changed from Frankfurt to Heidelberg in 1895, as **Emil Kraepelin** persuaded Nissl to come to the university psychiatric clinic for an academic career (Alzheimer would follow in 1902); in 1896, Nissl received his Habilitation at Heidelberg with a study on cell biology. As Kraepelin left Heidelberg for Munich in 1903, Nissl became acting head of the clinic and was appointed director and professor of psychiatry in 1904. In 1918, Nissl finally followed Kraepelin to Munich, to the new German Psychiatric Research Institute (Deutsche Forschungsanstalt für Psychiatrie, or DFA) that Kraepelin had founded in 1917, where Nissl was to lead the histopathology division until his death from a kidney disorder in 1919.

"Nissl is the founder and creator of the anatomy of mental illness," wrote DFA colleague Walther Spielmeyer (1879–1935) in a biography of Nissl in 1924 (Kirchhoff, II, p. 288). As a medical student, Nissl discovered a procedure for visualizing the cells of the central nervous system that involved, first, fixing the tissues in alcohol, then, staining them with aniline dyes—magenta red and later methylene blue. This caused the nuclei of individual cells to stand out clearly, thus making their study possible in a manner that disclosed internal cell detail. The concept "nerve cell" comes from Nissl, and in contradiction to **Theodor Meynert** in **Vienna**, Nissl realized there were different kinds of nerve cells. In 1904, he undertook with Alzheimer the first of an intended series of volumes on the histopathology of the cerebral cortex, the first volume clarifying the pathological changes that take place in **neurosyphilis** and differentiating it from other kinds of **dementias**. Nissl had the misfortune to be on the wrong side in the debate over the doctrine of the neuron (opposing the Spanish histologist Santiago Ramón y Cajal [1852–1934], he doubted its existence), and so historically he is remembered mainly for his stains.

O

OBSESSIVE-COMPULSIVE DISORDER. Physicians and non-physicians alike have always recognized the existence of obsessive thoughts and compulsive behavior. Across the ages, examples are common in religion of praying compulsively or dwelling obsessively on salvation or damnation, but religious practices are customarily exempted from psychiatric diagnosis. James Boswell (1740–1795) spoke in 1791 of "the anxious care" of his friend the famous English lexicographer Samuel Johnson (1709–1784) "to go out or in at a door . . . by a certain number of steps from a certain point . . . so that either his right or his left foot (I am not certain which) should constantly make the first actual movement when he came close to the door." When Johnson had miscounted, "I have seen him go back again, put himself in a proper posture to begin the ceremony, and, having gone through it . . . walk briskly on and join his companion" (*Life of Johnson*, pp. 127–128).

Similarly, physicians during the years have been well familiar with patients who had obsessions and compulsions. Buried within Pinel's amorphous category of "mania without madness," for example, were patients with obsessive thoughts. Yet, in the nineteenth and twentieth centuries, psychiatry has broken into ever smaller descriptive units these great phenomena of obsession and compulsion. For the sake of convenience, this *Dictionary* distinguishes between **anxiety-phobic**-type illness, **panic**, and obsessive-compulsive illness. Yet in reality, the three kinds of disorders interblend and tend to occur in the same patients.

Esquirol's "instinctual monomania" (monomanie instinctive, or monomanie sans délire) (1838). "Sometimes there is a lesion of volition," **Étienne Esquirol** said in volume two of his work *On Mental Illness* (*Des maladies mentales*). Esquirol noted that intelligence was preserved. "Acting abnormally, the patient is led to actions dictated by neither reason nor sentiment, that his conscience says is wrong but that his willpower no longer has the force to suppress. The actions are involuntary, instinctive and irresistible. It is monomania without madness (monomanie sans délire), or instinctual monomania" (p. 2). (Note that Esquirol's monomania in general [**PSYCHOSIS: EMERGENCE: monomania** (1816, 1838)] permitted the existence of delusions and hallucinations.)

Morel's "emotional delusions" (délire émotif) (1866). **Bénédict-Augustin Morel** described in the *General Archives of Medicine* (*Archives générales de médecine*) in 1866 "emotional delusions" (délire émotif), a category for patients with anxiety as well as with obsessions and compulsions. (*See* **ANXIETY: Morel** [1866].) One of Morel's patients, for example, had "reduced his life to habits of stereotypical silliness and was known for his ridiculous tics. . . . This man did not dare touch copper coins, and when he went out alone in a taxi coach, his friends had to pay the coachman in advance or else wrap the money in a piece of paper. He never dared open a door or window without wrapping a cloth about his hand." The patient was led to these "stupid automatic acts of which I have seen so many in 'emotive' patients, such as stopping fixedly in front of a door without daring to open it, hovering over a piece of paper without putting pen upon it, stopping in front of a carriage without stepping on the running board, etc." (p. 400). Morel believed that these patients suffered from a "heightened affective state."

Falret *fils'* "fearfulness disorder" (maladie du doute) (1866). This is the first full-blown description of obsessive-compulsive disorder in the literature, yet Jules Falret (1824–1902), **Jean-Pierre Falret**'s son, has never really been credited properly for it because he buried the disease label amidst a rambling account of "intelligent insanity" (la folie raisonnante) and defined it as "partial insanity with a fear of contact with external objects" (l'aliénation partielle avec prédominance de la crainte du contact des objets extérieurs) (p. 413). Nonetheless, in an article in the *Annales médico-psychologiques* (1866), he clearly describes compulsive actions and obsessive thoughts, the pathological nature of which the patient is fully aware, and yet from which he is unable to refrain. Falret singled out as an example touching doorknobs only with a handkerchief for fear of contamination. He noted of the multiplicity of phobic "fears," "These patients have a perfect awareness of their state; they recognize the absurdity of their fears and they seek to distance themselves from them, but they are unable to and are, despite themselves, always constrained to come back to the same ideas and to repeat the same actions." Falret also said that "this variety of mental affection is more frequent than one might think," merely that these patients rarely come to the attention of asylum physicians. It was because of the state of "perpetual internal hesitation," Falret said, that his father, Falret *père*, had proposed the term "fearfulness disorder" (maladie du doute; douter in French means among other things "to fear") (p. 414).

Krafft-Ebing's "obsessive thoughts" (Zwangsvorstellungen) (1867). In his psychiatry textbook *Contributions to the Recognition of Pathological States of Mind* (*Beiträge zur Erkennung . . . krankhafter Gemüthszustände*) published in 1867, **Richard von Krafft-Ebing**, then a staff psychiatrist in the Illenau asylum, coined the term "obsessive thoughts" from the German "Zwang-", meaning compel. "To the degree that an idea [eine Vorstellung] imposes itself ever more strongly and frequently, it enforces its influence upon the will, a matter that even in healthy individuals essentially constricts the action of free choice, but in illness must turn the patient into a pure automaton" (p. 19). In his 1872 *Textbook of Psychiatry*, Krafft-Ebing amplified his concept: obsessions and compulsions were "primary," meaning not a secondary effect of some other illness; and they had a powerful constitutional component, arising from the same soil as neurasthenia. "Compared to delusions, where the content of thought is pathological, in obsessive thoughts it is merely the form of thought that is pathological. The justification for classifying this form of disturbance under delusions [die Verrücktheit] is that the illness is genuinely constitutional, thus long-lasting and relatively unchanging, and is not part of the conditions that progress to psychic deterioration. Here as well, obsessive thoughts are primary, meaning that they do not have an affective basis, and spring from the depths of unconscious mental life" (quote from 1879 edition, vol. II, p. 95). (For these writers, an "affective basis" meant derived from melancholy or mania.)

Griesinger's "obsessional brooding" (Grübelsucht) (1868). In one of his last papers, **Wilhelm Griesinger** described a small number of patients who kept brooding about nonsensical questions. He had never encountered this in an asylum, but had recently seen several cases in the community. Acknowledging that it was similar to Falret *père et fils'* "maladie du doute" (*see above*), Griesinger baptized it "Grübelsucht" (grübeln, meaning brooding about something, plus sucht, or addictive) after one patient himself put a finger on the diagnosis: "I cannot free myself from my eternal brooding [Grübeleien]; the thoughts persecute me constantly and give me not a minute's rest."* The article "On a Little-Known Psychopathic State" ("Über einen wenig bekannten psychopathischen Zustand") appeared in the first volume of Griesinger's new journal, the *Archive of Psychiatry and Nervous Diseases* (*Archiv für Psychiatrie und Nervenkrankheiten*).

Legrand du Saulle's "fearful insanity and the psychosis about touching things" (la folie du doute et du délire du toucher) (1873). Here it is "fearful insanity" rather than the Falrets' "fearfulness disorder" (*see above*). Henri Legrand du Saulle (1830–1886) was previously an assistant of **Bénédict-Augustin Morel** at the St. Yon asylum; by 1873, he had become an assistant physician in **Ernest Lasègue's** psychiatric emergency ward of the Paris Prefecture of Police. In 1873, he described in a series of articles in the Paris *Hospital Gazette* (*Gazette des hôpitaux*) (a series that 2 years later, in 1875, appeared as a book) patients subject to irresistible thoughts with psychotic feelings of uncertainty about whether one has performed some specific act (maladie du doute) and fear of touching objects (délire du toucher). "Many of those with partial madness," he noted in his monograph, "are in fact very curious to study, having a quite profound personal awareness of their condition and not being any less unhappy for it; they drift about without an apparent diagnosis and navigate with some inquietude on the fragile ground of circumscribed sanity" (p. 5).

As for the course of the illness: "Uncertainty opens the scene," he wrote. "Much later, eccentricities about touching things close it" (p. 7). He saw the disorder evolving in three stages, whereby the third "is characterized by a serious and permanent state of illness. The patient's symptoms become daily more intolerable: all social contacts tend to disappear; many routines of daily living are impossible; leaving the house becomes a matter of severe distaste, then absolute refusal; the patient's activities become slower and slower, and a number of hours become taken up in the act of dressing or for each of the day's meals" (p. 8). The patients who Legrand saw in the emergency department were largely psychotic, and so, unlike Falret *fils* (*see above*), he interpreted this as a formal variety of insanity (folie, délire). This began the French tradition of seeing obsessive-compulsive disorders as delusional.

"Obsessive ideas" (Zwangsvorstellungen) as a disorder of intellect, not emotion (1877). Carl Westphal (1833–1890), by now professor of psychiatry in Berlin, defined obsessive ideas in 1877 as "ideas which, in the presence of intact intelligence and with no disorder of the emotional life or affect, intrude into the foreground of consciousness against the will of the concerned individual; they do not allow themselves to be banished, and they obstruct and divert the normal course of ideas. The patient sees them as abnormal and alien as he contemplates them with his healthy consciousness."

* In 1903, **Pierre Janet**, recognizing Griesinger's priority (though misdating it as "1848"), called this "la manie d'interrogation," or "la manie de la recherche," patients who endlessly tortured themselves with senseless questions (*Les Obsessions*, vol. II, pp. 291–292).

Westphal did not mention Krafft-Ebing but acknowledged that Legrand had already described the same illness as folie du doute. He said that Griesinger's 1868 description of "Grübelsucht" represented a subform of this larger concept of obsessive ideas. Unlike the relatively unknown publication of Krafft-Ebing in 1867, Westphal's article, published in the *Berlin Medical Weekly* (*Berliner Medizinische Wochenschrift*), reached a huge international public and sufficed, incorrectly, to give him for a long time the priority for first description of obsessive-compulsive disorder. Westphal is remembered for having fully characterized the disorder.

Kaan's differentiation of treatable neurasthenia and obsessive thoughts (1892). Some authors described obsession as a hereditary trait that could turn into madness, others as a form of acquired neurasthenia that was quite treatable. In 1892, Hanns Kaan (1861–?), a former assistant of **Richard von Krafft-Ebing** at the university clinic in Graz and now a staff psychiatrist at a private nervous clinic in Vienna, said that the two forms were distinct. To understand the neurasthenic variety, Kann reached back to **Morel's** 1866 notion of obsessions as a disturbance of the visceral (sympathetic) "ganglia." Kaan suggested that the pathological anxiety of neurasthenia provided a kind of somatic platform for cerebral obsessiveness that went via the sympathetic nervous system. In his book *The Affect of Neurasthenic Anxiety in Obsessive Thoughts and in Primary Obsessional Brooding* (*Der neurasthenische Angstaffect bei Zwangsvorstellungen und der primordiale Grübelzwang*), Kaan downplayed the inborn elements and said that obsessive ideas arise from the general fearfulness created by neurasthenia-driven disorders of the sympathetic nervous system. Distinguishing among phobias, obsessive impulses (Zwangsimpulse), and formal thought disturbances, Kaan hypothesized that the mechanism of obsessions was "irritability of the motor centers" of the brain. "The feeling of lessened cortical inhibition produces fear of one's self, through mistrust of one's ability to resist this toxic feeling." These contrasting psychological "associations" result in "obscene and sacrilegious obsessive thoughts" (p. 49).

As for the second form, Kaan said there existed also "primary obsessional brooding" (primordialer Grübelzwang) that **Krafft-Ebing** had described in 1868 alongside obsessive thoughts (Zwangsvorstellungen); this was not the same thing as obsessive impulses. Primary brooding represented a hereditary condition that Krafft-Ebing believed frequently turned into insanity; Kaan added that this primary form of obsession could also turn into Legrand's psychotic "folie du doute." This distinction between good-outcome and bad-outcome obsessions was important for therapists. Also, Kaan pointed out that obsessions had an affective component, which Westphal had denied. Kaan's views on the pathophysiology were highly speculative and were not taken up.

Psychoanalytic interpretations of obsession and compulsion (from 1896). *See* **FREUDIAN INTERPRETATIONS OF OBSESSION AND COMPULSION; NEUROSIS.**

The "obsessive ideas" of Janet's "psychasthenia" (1903). In the context of a theory about psychiatric illness that emphasized "lowered psychic tension" and "abulia" or loss of will, **Pierre Janet**, director of the psychology laboratory at the **Salpêtrière hospice**, argued that obsessive ideas were core symptoms. In his two-volume work *Obsessions and Psychasthenia* (*Les Obsessions et la psychasthénie*), the second volume written with Fulgence Raymond (1844–1910) who was the professor of nervous diseases in the **Charcot** chair at the **Salpêtrière**, Janet said obsessive ideas that involuntarily invaded one's consciousness represented an advanced stage of psychasthenia. Illness, shame, crime, and sacrilege, he said, were the main content of obsessive ideas. He had a separate analysis of the "form" of obsessions. Janet laid out a whole treatment program involving simplifying one's life, hypnosis and other forms of suggestion, and the increasing of "psychological tension."

DSM-I* on "obsessive compulsive reaction"** (1952). The first edition of the ***DSM series accepted the by now familiar usage of calling the symptoms "obsessive compulsive" and applied the **Meyerian** term "reaction" to them. The disorder, said the *Manual*, "is associated with the persistence of unwanted ideas and of repetitive impulses to perform acts which may be considered morbid by the patient" (p. 33). The *Manual* also accepted the existence of a "compulsive personality" (p. 37).

Mayer-Gross et al. distinguish between "obsessional" (constitutional) states and "compulsive" (minor neurotic) symptoms (1954). In their influential textbook *Clinical Psychiatry*, **Willi Mayer-Gross**, **Eliot Slater**, and Martin Roth distinguished between "compulsive symptoms," widespread in persons suffering from various illnesses and among normal people, and patients with inborn "obsessional" traits subject to a variety of psychiatric syndromes ("states"). On compulsive personality traits they wrote: "The outstanding features of this type of personality are its rigidity, inflexibility and lack of adaptability; its conscientiousness and love of order and discipline; and its persistence and endurance even in the face of obstacles" (p. 143). As for the more severely ill patients with obsessional personalities in the grip of major obsessions: "There may be a history of actual nervous breakdown, an anxiety state, a mild depression or an obsessional state, earlier in life" (p. 146).

***DSM-II* on "obsessive compulsive neurosis"** (1968). The gist was the same as in *DSM-I*, except for calling it a "neurosis." The section on "obsessive compulsive personality" also called it "anankastic personality" (after the term "Anancasmus—psychic compulsions" [Zwangszustände]) coined in 1897 by Budapest psychiatry lecturer, later professor, Gyula (Julius) Donath [1849–1945] in the *Archiv für Psychiatrie*).

DSM-III* on "obsessive compulsive disorder"** (1980). Except for the term "disorder," the essence remained the same as in previous editions. This applied also to the section on "compulsive personality disorder." There were no important changes in ***DSM-III-R (1987) or ***DSM-IV*** (1994).

Scientific study of obsessive-compulsive disorder (OCD) with brain imaging begins; an animal model (ca. 1989). Judith Rapoport, chief of pediatric psychiatry at the **National Institute of Mental Health**, is associated with use of modern **neuroimaging** techniques such as magnetic resonance imaging in the study of OCD. (*See* **WOMEN IN PSYCHIATRY**.) She and her group developed the first animal model for studying OCD. This work put the study of OCD on a scientific basis and raised awareness of the disorder, so that currently there are about 500 treatment clinics specifically for OCD across the United States. In 1989, she wrote a best-selling book, *The Boy Who Couldn't Stop Washing*. (*See* **WOMEN IN PSYCHIATRY: Rapoport.**)

The cerebral localization of obsessive-compulsive disorder (1994). A group of researchers led by Scott L. Rauch (1960–) and Michael A. Jenike (1945–) of the psychiatry department of the Massachusetts General Hospital, using a short half-life tracer oxygen 15-labeled carbon dioxide, first measured the cerebral blood flow of OCD patients while giving them a clean towel, then measured blood flow again after the towel had been "contaminated by touching after defecating." Such challenge stimuli provoked contamination obsessions in the patients, and the tracer localized the increased blood flow of those obsessions in several sites in the brain, including the right caudate nucleus. This work, published in the *Archives of General Psychiatry*, provided strong circumstantial evidence that these areas of the brain were part of a "loop" mediating the symptoms of OCD.

P

PANIC DISORDER. Panic has always been considered a symptom of larger psychiatric illnesses. Yet, only recently has it come to be considered a disorder of its own. The whole panic story is interesting as an example of how symptoms wax and wane in the history of psychiatry, treated as one among many at one point, and the focus of all nosology at the next. There may be good scientific reasons for the fluctuating historical courses of such symptoms, yet commerce plays a role as well, for if industry needs a symptom for a compound it has developed, one may be sure that entities such as panic will stand in good service. The following subentries represent the major steps in the panic story. (*See also* **ANXIETY AND PHOBIAS: Westphal's agoraphobia-panic** [1872].)

Paroxysmic attacks of panic (1873). Maurice Krishaber (1836–1883), a Hungarian physician practicing in Paris, described patients who "are taken out of the blue . . . with a peculiar sensation in the head, 'like a flush [bouffée] or a rising wave'; instantly there occurs a clouding of the senses, ringing in the ears, and the seeing of sparks at the same time as a sense of anguish in the area of the heart accompanied by palpitations, a sense of nausea. . . . [There follow] vertigo, staggering around [titubation]." Krishaber said the attacks may occur episodically during the months ahead and may or may not be accompanied by insomnia (pp. 158–159). He attributed them to misadventures on the cerebro-cardiac axis and called the disorder, in a book of that title published in 1873, "la névropathie cérébro-cardiaque." This is generally thought the first description in the French literature of paroxysmic anxiety, later called "panic attacks."

This priority may hold true for France but not for Germany. In 1872, German psychiatrist Rudolph Gottfried Arndt (1835–1900), associate professor at Greifswald University, gave a paper at a psychiatry meeting in Leipzig on "melancholic anxiety attacks" ("der melancholischer Angstanfall," published in the *General Journal of Psychiatry* (*Allgemeine Zeitschrift für Psychiatrie*) in 1874, in which he took for granted that the phenomenon had long been described in the German literature. For Arndt, "melancholic" meant general nervous and mental illness rather than depression. He associated such attacks with disorders of the nerves of the heart.

Entry of term "panic" into psychiatry as part of melancholia (1879). In his *The Pathology of Mind,** **Henry Maudsley** offered a careful description of panic attacks: "These paroxysms of anguish or panic, which are a notable feature of melancholia—paroxysms of melancholic panic they might be called—deserve careful notice. They often come on quite suddenly; the patient has perhaps been lying down to rest [then] starts up in great agitation, his heart beating tumultuously, his senses distraught, and rushes wildly to the window to throw himself out of it. . . . In some cases the

---

* *The Pathology of Mind* was considered the "third edition," extensively reworked, of his *Physiology and Pathology of Mind* (1867). Yet, the earlier volume does not use the term "panic."

convulsive panic is preceded by an anomalous and alarming sensation of distress about the region of the stomach or of the heart, a sensation which, appearing to rise thence to the head, is accompanied by an indescribable terror and a dreadful feeling of helplessness. . . . The whole affair is suggestive of the onset of mental epilepsy" (p. 365). Yet, Maudsley's term "panic" was not taken up in the literature.

Differentiating somatic "anguish" (later "panic") and mental "anxiety" (1890). Édouard Brissaud (1853–1909), a neurologist at St.-Antoine hospital in Paris who had an organicist view of psychiatry, differentiated in an article in the Parisian *Medical Weekly* (*la Semaine médicale*) between "anguish" (l'angoisse), and "anxiety" (l'anxiété). Anguish represented the sensation of somatic distress, as for example in precordial (heart–stomach region) pain. Anxiety was "angoisse intellectuelle," a mental phenomenon, the mind's processing of the somatic sensation of anguish. In heart pain, "anxiety is attached less to the physical sensation of thoracic constriction and a sense of suffocation than to the mental state accompanying this situation. It announces the disturbance, the disquiet and the terror that arise as the immediate consequences of this [chest] oppression." Paroxysmic anxiety, said Brissaud, is found not just in cardiac problems but in hysteria, neurasthenia and hypochondria. "It is common to see anxious melancholia begin with paroxysms of this nature." By contrast, somatic anguish in paroxysmic form would be the core of what was later called panic attacks, though some authorities believed somatic "angoisse" and psychic "anxiété" were so closely intermingled that in attacks they occurred together. (See Francis Heckel, *La névrose d'angoisse et les états d'émotivité* [1917].)

Reentry of term "panic" into psychiatry (1932). Oskar Diethelm (1897–1993), then an associate professor of psychiatry at Johns Hopkins University, suggested in an article in 1932 in the *A.M.A. Archives of Neurology and Psychiatry* that panic represented an independent illness entity, "characterized by fear, extreme insecurity [and] suspiciousness." Making no reference to **Henry Maudsley's** previous usage (*see above*), Diethelm described a patient who, fearing a forthcoming operation, "had to rush out of bed. She felt a tightening in her throat, palpitation, nausea, and . . . fear of 'mental disease'" (p. 1154). Diethelm said that another author had described the rather limited case of "homosexual panic," but added, "I also find masturbation panics and panics due to unmanageable heterosexual desires, as well as many other situations that are unbearable to certain make-ups and from which the subjects see no escape either by mastery or flight" (p. 1156). He distinguished panic from anxiety neuroses, which usually lacked the element of fear; also from Wernicke's anxiety psychoses (*see* **ANXIETY: Wernicke . . .** [1895]) and from extreme fright reactions, for which the Swiss-born Diethelm (who was highly familiar with the German literature) also used the German term "Schreckneurosen."

Cohen describes precipitating "anxiety" (panic) attacks in patients with anxiety neurosis (1940). Mandel Cohen (1907–2000) and Stanley Cobb (1887–1968), psychiatrists at Harvard University, described in 1940 in the *Journal of Clinical Investigation* how giving carbon dioxide to patients with anxiety neurosis could precipitate an anxiety attack. (Far fewer controls experienced such attacks in rebreathing CO_2.) Cohen is thus seen as the immediate father of the concept of "panic attack," although he himself did not use that term. Cohen later said of this work, "We have shown that a number of things became abnormal during the anxiety attack, such as blood lactate levels, even though nothing appeared to be abnormal at baseline. . . . Since then there has been a whole field of lactogenic anxiety attacks" (Healy interview, in the journal *History of Psychiatry*, 2002, p. 212).

Roth's phobic anxiety-depersonalization syndrome (1959). In the *Proceedings of the Royal Society of Medicine* in 1959, Martin Roth (1917–), professor of psychiatry in Newcastle-on-Tyne, described a recurring combination of symptoms involving anxiety attacks, phobic avoidance of crowds, and a feeling of depersonalization. "There was a fearful aversion to leaving familiar surroundings, to walking in the street and to entering shops, travelling in vehicles or visiting cinemas or theatres. Waiting or sitting still in such settings was prone to evoke a sense of impending disaster, acute agitation and flight in panic" (p. 590). The patients, typically women in their late twenties, displayed familiar symptoms in this syndrome: "the syncopal attacks with fear of losing consciousness, the anxiety about falling asleep, the terrified starts from slumber. . . . The cases also have in common the transient stage of clouding of consciousness after the impact of stress" (p. 594). Some observers see Roth's syndrome as an early description of panic attacks.

Differentiation of panic from anxiety on the basis of drug response (1962, 1964). In 1962, **Donald Klein** and **Max Fink** at Hillside Hospital, in a clinical trial of **imipramine** that was published in the *American Journal of Psychiatry*, discovered that anxious patients with panic disorders responded to the drug but that anxious patients with phobias did not. Klein then received a grant from the **National Institute of Mental Health** and did a second, controlled trial on his own. Published in 1964 in *Psychopharmacologia*, his paper confirmed that imipramine was effective for panic but not for other kinds of anxiety. This set the stage for discriminating panic on a pharmacological basis as a disease separate from anxiety. (For details, *see* **KLEIN, DONALD F.**)

The Research Diagnostic Criteria included panic (1978). **Robert Spitzer**, Columbia University psychologist Jean Endicott (1936–), and **Eli Robins**, building on the work of the **St. Louis school**, proposed in the *Archives of General Psychiatry* a revised list of diagnoses to be used in research. Called the "Research Diagnostic Criteria," the RDC system included "panic disorder," described as similar to anxiety neurosis.

Panic in *DSM-III* (1980). This edition continued the RDC (1978) category of panic disorder, which would become a huge diagnosis in the coming years. "The panic attacks," the *Manual* explained, "are manifested by the sudden onset of intense apprehension, fear, or terror, often associated with feelings of impending doom" (p. 230). Twelve symptoms were mentioned, such as chest pain, dizziness, feelings of unreality, and fear of "going crazy or doing something uncontrolled during an attack," and to qualify for a diagnosis of panic disorder the patient had to exhibit four of them. There were some kinds of attacks in which the diagnosis agoraphobia with panic would be more suitable, it said.

DSM-III-R in 1987 introduced the formal distinction between panic with and without agoraphobia. And ***DSM-IV*** in 1994 further distinguished among "panic attack," "agoraphobia," and "panic disorder," the latter meaning recurrent panic attacks plus worry about having them.

Anxiety, panic, and phobic disorders in *ICD-10* (1992). The tenth edition of the World Health Organization's *International Classification of Diseases* (ICD) distinguished between "phobic anxiety disorders" and "other anxiety disorders" including panic. British psychiatrist Simon Wessely comments, in a personal communication to me, as follows on these international differences: "*DSM* is not the bible as far as we are concerned. [Shorter] seems to have missed the vital US/Europe difference here, that we regard avoidance/phobia as the prime mover, hence agoraphobia sits at the top of our system, with panic just a symptom of it, while the US, partly because of the success of **[Donald] Klein/imipramine**, puts it in reverse order."

PARANOIA. (*See also* **EROTOMANIA; FOLIE À DEUX; FRENCH CHRONIC DELUSIONAL STATES; PSYCHOSIS: EMERGENCE.**) Paranoia means a fixed false belief formed via logical reasoning (making it distinct from schizophrenia); aside from his delusional system, the patient is perfectly normal in every other respect. In the eighteenth and early nineteenth centuries, the Greek term "paranoia" had surfaced occasionally in psychiatric discussions, to become common by the late-nineteenth century. The term "delusion" is a synonym for it.

Heinroth calls paranoia a disorder of intellect (1818). Johann C. A. Heinroth (1773–1843) began to chisel the modern meaning into the term "paranoia" in his 1818 *Textbook of Disturbances of Mental Life* (*Lehrbuch der Störungen des Seelenlebens*) as a disorder of intellect with preserved feeling and volition. (*See* **GERMAN "ROMANTIC" PSYCHIATRY: Heinroth.**) He said of "insanity with dementia (ecstasis paranoia)": "The symptoms of pure insanity are associated with perversion of concepts and judgment. . . . The disease has gained sway over both the intellect and the imagination of the patient. . . . The field of insanity is narrowed down and reduced, and as a result its form is altogether altered. . . . The intervention of the intellect results in partial consciousness" (p. 155 of George Mora's English translation).

Yet, throughout much of the nineteenth century, as the outlines of the syndrome were being hammered in place, the term "paranoia" was not used. (The preferred expressions for delusional psychosis had been delusion in English, délire in French, and Verrücktheit in German.)

Esquirol's "intellectual monomania" (1838). Among major landmarks in the formation of the modern doctrine of paranoia is Étienne Esquirol's "intellectual monomania" (monomanie raisonnante) as discussed in 1838 in his textbook *Des maladies mentales*. For Esquirol, patients with this kind of monomania seem to have derived their delusional systems via logical reasoning; they seem otherwise normal. "There are monomaniacs who do not appear insane, whose ideas retain their natural associations and whose reasoning is logical and their speech coherent [suivis], often lively and full of spirit. But the actions of these patients are contrary to their emotions, to their self-interest and to social mores. . . . However irrational their actions might be, these monomaniacs always have more or less plausible arguments to justify them, in the manner that one might say of them they are rational madmen (des fous raisonnables)" (*Des maladies mentales*, II, pp. 49–50). Esquirol's definition is really the fundamental paving stone in the modern doctrine of paranoia.

Griesinger's notion that delusions represent "partial" remnants of insanity (1845). **Wilhelm Griesinger** suggested in his 1845 textbook, *The Pathology and Therapy of Mental Diseases* (*Die Pathologie und Therapie der psychischen Krankheiten*), the concept of delusional "partial insanity" ("die partielle Verrücktheit") as a sequel of total insanity. "We understand here those secondary forms of insanity, where even after a significant reduction . . . of the original pathological affect the patient has not recovered, but remains ill, exhibiting most conspicuously fixed delusional ideas that he carefully cultivates and repeats again and again; this is always a secondary form of illness, arising from melancholia or mania" (p. 258). Griesinger gave as an example of such fixed delusional thinking, "The patients believe themselves persecuted, surrounded by plots, tortured with electricity by secret enemies, menaced by Freemasons, possessed by the devil and damned to eternal torment, robbed of their dearest possession etc." (p. 262).

Delusions of persection (1852). **Ernest-Charles Lasègue** introduced into the French literature—in *General Archives of Medicine* (*Archives générales de la médecine*)—the idea that paranoid delusions (délires de persécutions) constituted an illness separate from undifferentiated madness. (The French term "délire" may be translated as delusion, delirium, or psychosis depending on the context.) As Lasègue complained of his predecessors (neglecting to cite Griesinger), "Under this common label of madness (aliénation), the most dissimilar forms of pathology have been grouped together if not confused in a false unity" (p. 129). He applauded efforts to separate "generalized insanity" (délires généraux), affecting all mental functions, from "partial insanity" (délires partiels), leaving much of the intellectual realm intact; he proposed as an entity in partial insanity the delusion of persecution (le délire de persécutions) (p. 133). This use of "délire" to mean fixed delusional beliefs became a keystone of French psychiatry for the next 100 years.

Kahlbaum: In paranoia the personality does not deteriorate (1863). A major contribution to the growing understanding of paranoia as a syndrome was that of **Karl Kahlbaum**. If his views were often overlooked by his successors perhaps it was because he chose such an ungainly word for delusions: "diastrephia." ("Paranoia" he reserved for "disturbances in the sphere of intelligence, *Gruppirung*," p. 96.) Kahlbaum observed in his *Classification of Mental Diseases* (*Die Gruppirung der psychischen Krankheiten*) in 1863 that in the diastrephias, the patients' personalities did not deteriorate, as in the Vesaniae (full madness), and that they could go through life otherwise perfectly normal except for the "exquisitely partial nature" of their mental disorder. "The pathological abnormalities of their intellectual life will long be considered moral perversities, their bizarre enterprises, their insults and injuries to man and beast will be endured by their friends and family or willingly accepted, until the conflict affects some outsider, or otherwise comes to the attention of the authorities" (pp. 102–103). Unlike Griesinger, he did not consider it secondary to some other deeper illness.

Mendel restores the term "paranoia" (1883). In a lecture to the Berlin Psychiatric Society on "secondary paranoia" in 1883 (published in the *Archiv für Psychiatrie* in 1884, pp. 289–290), Berlin psychiatrist Emanuel Mendel (1839–1907) proposed a revival of the older term "paranoia." As a "secondary" complication of melancholia, the paranoid patient attributed the fault to the surrounding world rather than, as in melancholia, to himself. At a professional meeting in 1890, Mendel rather indignantly called attention to his priority as Karl Wilhelm Werner (1858–1934), an asylum psychiatrist in (Stadt-) Roda, announced that he himself had just authored the distinction between what he proposed to call "paranoia" and madness (Wahnsinn) (*Allgemeine Zeitschrift für Psychiatrie*, 1890, p. 531). Werner said that patients often found the term "Verrücktheit" (in common speech "craziness") offensive.

Magnan's "chronic systematized delusional disorder" (le délire chronique à évolution systématique) (1886). **Valentin Magnan** introduced the notion of "chronic systematized delusional disorder" in 1886 in a lecture at the Medical-Psychological Society, a chronic kind of well-circumscribed delusional disorder that went through four stages after a period of incubation: inquietude-hallucinations, persecution, manic-grandeur, dementia. The delusions were highly structured, hence the adjective "systematic," or "systematized." In 1888, Magnan published a series of articles on it in *Le Progrès médical*, then in 1892 together with his colleague Paul Sérieux (1864–1947) he described the illness in a monograph entitled *Le délire chronique à évolution systématique*. The two authors contrasted the "insanity of the degenerate"—for example la bouffée délirante (*see* **PSYCHOSIS: EMERGENCE** [1886])—with "the chronic systematized delusional disorders" of the nondegenerate but mildly predisposed. Henceforth in the French tradition, Magnan's "great discovery," as it was often called, was preferred to the term "paranoia."

Chronic nonhallucinatory delusional states (Le délire d'interprétation) (delusional thinking) (1909). Around 1900, Magnan's views about degeneration started to go out of style. This occasioned a new bout of Parisian thinking about delusional disorder. In 1909, psychiatrists Sérieux and Capgras in their book, *Intelligent Insanity: Delusional Thinking* (*Les folies raisonnantes: le délire d'interprétation*), hived these off from the larger block of psychotic illness on the grounds that the absence of hallucinations and the failure to progress to dementia were important diagnostic features. At the time, Paul Sérieux (1864–1947) was the chief psychiatrist at a private nervous clinic, and Jean-Marie-Joseph Capgras (1873–1950) was about to become chief psychiatrist at the Maison-Blanche asylum. Both were pupils of Magnan. The authors defined "delusional thinking" (délire d'interprétation) as "false reasoning having as its point of departure a real sensation, a precise fact which . . . driven by erroneous deductions or inductions, takes on personal significance for the patient, who ineluctably is compelled to relate everything to himself" (p. 3). The various delusions were in turn subject to elaborate subclassification on the basis of their object and whether they were tightly focused on a given notion or not. Le délire d'interprétation was asserted to be different from **Kraepelin's** paranoia because the French diagnosis did not include individuals with querulancy. (For Kraepelin, Querulantenwahn was a part of paranoia.)

The délire'd'interprétation, in its turn, was part of a larger group of chronic delusional states that the authors called "intelligent insanity" (les folies raisonnantes). (*See* **FRENCH CHRONIC DELUSIONAL DISORDERS**.) Its characteristics: "With the exception of their well-circumscribed delusions [délire partiel], the patients retain all of their liveliness of intellect, often with a remarkable propensity to argue about and defend their convictions. The interprétateurs do not qualify for the epithet insane [aliénés] . . . remaining in contact with their milieu and appearing normal; some succeed in living in liberty up to the end of life. . . . The majority become institutionalized, not because of their delusional notions but because their violent and impulsive character makes them dangerous" (p. 5).

Jaspers's "pathological jealousy" as development not process (1910). In a fundamental article in the *Journal of Combined Neurology and Psychiatry* (*Zeitschrift für die* *gesamte Neurologie und Psychiatrie*) in 1910, **Karl Jaspers** called delusional jealousy (Eifersuchtswahn) the result of a slow development within the patient's personality rather than the sudden inexplicable eruption of psychosis, a "process." This clearly separated developmental kinds of delusional systems from "process" illnesses such as schizophrenia. Paranoia thus became more a kind of personality disorder than a pathological brain disease. "You can reconstruct a patient's entire life on the basis of a personality trait," Jaspers said (p. 612).

Freud's view of paranoia (1911). For **Freud**, the distinction between psychosis and neurosis was never watertight. Paranoid thinking could also be neurotic in nature, a defense against homosexual desires. In his analysis of the case of Daniel Paul Schreber (1842–1911), a high official in Leipzig who had become psychotic and was admitted to the psychiatric clinic of Professor Paul Flechsig (1847–1929), Freud articulated a theory of paranoia as the withdrawal of libido from the outside world. Based on Schreber's published autobiography, *Memoirs of a Nervous Patient* (*Denkwürdigkeiten eines Nervenkranken*, 1903), Freud argued in "Psychoanalytic Remarks on an Autobiographically-Described Case of Paranoia (Dementia Paranoides)" ("Psychoanalytische Bemerkungen über einen autobiographisch beschriebenen Fall von Paranoia ([Dementia paranoides])" in the *Yearbook for Psychoanalytic and Psychopathological Research* (*Jahrbuch für psychoanalytische und psychopathologische Forschungen*) that when libido is withdrawn from external objects and has further inflated the ego, paranoia—an overweening kind of grandiosity—eventuates. In paranoia, the child's sexual development undergoes a "fixation" somewhere between autoeroticism and **narcissism**. Freud concluded the essay by pointing out that "neuroses basically arise from the conflict of the ego with the sex drive, and that their various forms retain the print marks of the developmental history of the libido and of the ego" (*Gesammelte Werke*, VIII, p. 316). (Some observers believe, however, that Schreber was suffering from **neurosyphilis** rather than intrapsychic conflict.)

Paranoia in Kraepelin's work (from 1893). It was with the fourth edition of his textbook *Psychiatry* (*Psychiatrie*), published in 1893, that **Emil Kraepelin's** innovative thinking about diagnosis began, soon after his arrival in **Heidelberg**. In this edition, he distinguished two forms of paranoia: (1) "die Verrücktheit (Paranoia)," which he understood as a "durable delusional system in the presence of an intact personality" (dauerndes Wahnsystem bei vollkommener Erhaltung der Besonnenheit) having a relatively unfavorable prognosis. (Verrücktheit translates into English as "craziness" but Kraepelin meant it more in the sense of dislocation of a patient's life as a result of crazy ideas.) The discussion makes clear that he is trying to filter delusions from the larger soup of "madness," because he includes affective disorders and hallucinations in the psychopathology of paranoia. (2) Kraepelin coined the term "dementia paranoides" and classed it among the "psychic processes of degeneration," to characterize patients with confused ideas, rather than tidy delusional systems, who sink rapidly into dementia; Freud thought Daniel Paul Schreber was one (*see above*).

The fifth edition in 1896 did not change these two diagnoses themselves but shifted them to larger disease categories: Dementia paranoides had become a dementing process under the larger rubric of "metabolic diseases"; and Verrücktheit-Paranoia had been assigned to the class of "hereditary illnesses" (Geistesstörungen aus krankhafter Veranlagung).

The sixth edition in 1899—famous for its creation of "manic-depressive illness"—(1) shifted "dementia paranoides" to a subform of dementia praecox (**Bleuler's** schizophrenia) (*see* **SCHIZOPHRENIA: EMERGENCE**); (2) retained Verrücktheit-Paranoia; and (3) added as a special illness, paranoia in the pre-senile elderly (der praesenile Beeinträchtigungswahn).

The seventh edition in 1904 made no changes to the above.

In the eighth edition, a sprawling document published in multiple volumes during the years 1909–1915, Kraepelin (1) retained Verrücktheit-Paranoia; (2) discussed paranoid forms of dementia praecox; (3) dissolved pre-senile paranoia into the larger picture of presenile "insanity"; and (4) set up "paranoid dementia," also called "paraphrenias,"* as a separate category of "endogenous dementias" (endogene Verblödungen) alongside dementia praecox (*see* **PARAPHRENIA**); by paranoid dementia he meant maintenance of the personality as semi-intact, heavily paranoid pathology, yet downhill course.

In sum, despite the several meanders in Kraepelin's thinking, his version of paranoia differs from the Freudian in being profoundly organic, hereditary, and nonpsychogenic. As well, Kraepelin maintains a clear boundary between the major psychiatric illnesses, such as paranoia and dementia praecox, and the "psychogenic" ones (he uses the term in the eighth edition in 1915), such as "nervous exhaustion" and the traumatic neuroses; also as distinct from "hysteria." It was one of Kraepelin's main contributions to have isolated the notion of paranoia from schizophrenia and other psychoses.

Gaupp's reactive paranoia (abortiva paranoia) (1909). At a meeting that year, Robert Gaupp (1870–1953), professor of psychiatry in Tübingen, proposed reactive paranoia as an independent illness entity, distinct from manic-depressive illness and from obsessive-compulsive disorder. Occurring typically in middle-aged individuals with previously healthy personalities (but with an inborn disposition to paranoia or depression), the paranoid ideation tended to be well-circumscribed (usually not involving the physician, for example); the patients did not deteriorate and often recovered completely with full insight. The paper was published in 1910 in the *General Journal of Psychiatry* (*Allgemeine Zeitschrift für Psychiatrie*). (Gaupp did not use this precise diagnosis in analyzing what was probably the most famous case of paranoia in pre–First World War Germany: the schoolteacher Ernst Wagner, who in 1913 committed mass murder in a Swabian village and was referred by the court to Gaupp for a psychiatric opinion. *See* Gaupp's article in the *Munich Medical Weekly* [*Münchener Medizinische Wochenschrift*] of March 24, 1914. In Gaupp's view, the case demonstrated the "purely affective" nature of paranoia.)

Kretschmer's "sensitive delusions of reference" (1918). Kretschmer's book *Sensitive Delusions of Reference: A Contribution to the Question of Paranoia and to the Doctrine of Character in Psychiatry* (*Der sensitive Beziehungswahn: ein Beitrag zur Panaroiafrage und*

---

* In the ninth edition of the Kraepelin textbook (published posthumously in 1927), editor Johannes Lange (1891–1938), a staff psychiatrist at Kraepelin's German Psychiatric Research Institute in Munich (known as the DFA), made paraphrenia part of paranoid schizophrenia, after Wilhelm Mayer's research published in the *Zentralblatt für Neurologie* in 1921 on the poor outcomes of these patients. (Mayer practiced psychiatry in Munich and was affiliated with the DFA.)

zur psychiatrischen Charakterlehre) was inspired by Gaupp's teaching at Tübingen, where **Ernst Kretschmer** was on staff. (*See* **PSYCHOSIS: EMERGENCE: sensitive delusions of reference** [1918].)

Paranoia in the *Diagnostic and Statistical Manual (DSM)* of the American Psychiatric Association (after 1952). The first volume of ***DSM*** in 1952 was notable for making many psychiatric illnesses into "reactions" of various types. Among the "psychotic disorders," there were "schizophrenic reaction: paranoid type," as well as "paranoid reactions," subdivided into "paranoia" and "paranoid state." This distinction between schizophrenic paranoia and nonschizophrenic paranoia corresponds roughly to Kraepelin's distinction between "paranoid dementia" and "Verrücktheit-Paranoia." It also upheld the Kraepelinian distinction between major, often "endogenous," illnesses and psychoneuroses. ***DSM "One"*** also included "paranoid personality." (*See* **PERSONALITY DISORDERS**.)

DSM-II in 1968 maintained the paranoid schizophrenia of ***DSM-I*** and the paranoid reactions, but called them "paranoid states": "paranoia" was one such state (said to be an "extremely rare condition"); "involutional paranoid state" (also called "involutional **paraphrenia**") was another. "Paranoid personality" of *DSM-I* was retained.

In ***DSM-III*** (1980), notable for bone-wrenching change in much psychiatric diagnosis, little was changed in paranoia. There was the schizophrenia: "paranoid type," and then the "paranoid disorders." One such disorder was "paranoia," with its insidious development and unshakable delusional system; another was "shared paranoid disorder" (once known as **folie à deux**); a third was "acute paranoid disorder" of rapid onset often under stress. This edition admitted, as before, "paranoid personality disorder."

DSM-III-R in 1987 saw considerable innovation. (1) Shared paranoid disorder became "induced psychotic disorder." (2) Although schizophrenia: paranoid type was kept, paranoia as such was renamed "delusional disorder." "The essential feature of this disorder," according to the *Manual*, "is the presence of a persistent, nonbizarre delusion that is not due to any other mental disorder" (p. 199). One compares that with the definition in *DSM-III* that said paranoia meant basically delusions of persecution or jealousy. Delusional disorder was divided into subtypes: **erotomanic**, grandiose, jealous, persecutory, and somatic. (3) Paranoid personality was unchanged in essence.

DSM-IV (1994) changed little.

PARAPHRENIA. Karl Kahlbaum coined the term in his *Classification of Psychiatric Diseases* (*Die Gruppirung der psychischen Krankheiten*, 1863), to mean both hebephrenia in the young (*see* **SCHIZOPHRENIA: EMERGENCE**) and the dementia of the elderly; his idea was that people undergoing physiological change at both ends of the life cycle are subject to mental illness, hence "para-" (p. 129).

Kraepelin took up the term "paraphrenia" in the eighth edition of his *Psychiatry* (*die Psychiatrie*) textbook, in the volume published in 1913, to mean a downhill form of **paranoia** close to dementia praecox. Yet, paraphrenia vanished from the next, posthumous edition in 1927.

In 1954, Martin Roth, (1917–), then director of research at Graylingwell Hospital in Chichester, revived the Kraepelinian concept of late paraphrenia. Paranoia in the elderly had first surfaced as an independent disease in the sixth edition (1899) of the Kraepelin textbook as presenile delusional insanity (praeseniler Beeinträchtigungswahn). It remained in the Kraepelinian system as part of "presenile and senile insanity." But did this category have subdivisions?

As early as 1952, in an effort to differentiate separate illnesses in the elderly aside from dementia, Roth called attention to "paraphrenia"; yet the emphasis in his article in the *Journal of Mental Science* was on depression in the elderly. It was only in the 1954 textbook of psychiatry, which Roth cowrote with **Eliot Slater** and **Willi Mayer-Gross**, that he gave a full description of the disorder: "There is . . . a group of cases with firmly systematized paranoid delusions occurring in the setting of a well-preserved personality which are likewise sharply defined from the organic diseases." The presentation: "The patient usually becomes quieter and more solitary, and avoids her friends. Her suspicions may fasten on one of them or a neighbour or relative, and she may then pester the police with complaints, or bombard others with anonymous letters. She sees her enemies communicating with one another by shining lights from the windows. . . . Finally, her behaviour becomes so bizarre, noisy or aggressive, that the attention of public authorities is attracted, and she is removed to hospital" (pp. 474, 501). As the treatment of choice, the authors recommended leukotomy (*see* **LOBOTOMY**).

Paraphrenia in the elderly surfaced in the ***DSM*** series only once: in *DSM-II* in 1968 as "involutional paranoid state (involutional paraphrenia)," evolving from "involutional psychotic reaction" in *DSM-I* (1952). (*See also* **WERNICKE–KLEIST–LEONHARD PATHWAY.**)

Roth's concept of paraphrenia in the elderly was officially abandoned after a consensus conference led by Robert Howard (1961–) of the Institute of Psychiatry in London on Late Onset Schizophrenia [LOS], the results of which were published in the *American Journal of Psychiatry* in 2000. It is interesting that once again the Kraepelinian urge to swallow up rivals with the diagnosis dementia praecox had prevailed. (*See* **SCHIZOPHRENIA: RECENT CONCEPTS: late onset schizophrenia** [1997].)

PARKINSONISM: NEUROLEPTIC-INDUCED. Parkinsonism is a movement disorder involving muscle rigidity, akinesia, and tremor first described in 1817 by the English physician James Parkinson (1755–1824) in his *Essay on the Shaking Palsy.* In 1954, two Swiss psychiatrists at different institutions noted simultaneously that the new **antipsychotic** drugs caused Parkinson-like movement disorders: Hans Steck (1891–1980), professor of psychiatry at the university clinic at Céry-Lausanne, called attention in the *Annales médico-psychologiques* to an "extrapyramidal syndrome," later also referred to as "**extrapyramidal side effects,**" or EPS, in patients on **chlorpromazine** and serpasil. (*See* **RESERPINE**). As well, Hans-Joachim Haase (1922–), then a staff psychiatrist at the mental hospital in Oberwil-Zug, reported in the *Nervenarzt* that chlorpromazine patients were developing a "Parkinsonian" syndrome. The symptoms of EPS are thought related to the blockade of the dopamine receptors in the basal ganglia, just as Parkinson's disease itself is caused by a deficiency of dopamine. (*See also* **AKATHISIA: neuroleptic-induced; EXTRAPYRAMIDAL SIDE EFFECTS; TARDIVE DYSKINESIA.**)

PASSIVE-AGGRESSIVE. *See* **PERSONALITY DISORDERS: *DSM* series.**

PERSONALITY DISORDERS. Even though upsetting behavior is as old as the human condition, systematic attention to disorders of the personality appears relatively late in the development of psychiatry. On the whole, the asylum generation of psychiatrists had little to say about character disorders, unless they occurred in conjunction with psychoses, because patients with such traits did not end up in the asylum.

The oldest of the personality disorders by far is "**hysteria**," understood classically as a convulsive disorder combined with such somatic symptoms as a lump in the throat ("globus hystericus") or blinding headache ("clavus hystericus"). In the nineteenth century, it became interpreted also as a personality type.

The beginning of the inclusion of personality disorders in psychiatric nosology: Pinel's "emotional insanity" (1801). In his textbook, **Philippe Pinel** differentiated madness with psychosis (manie avec délire) from madness without psychosis (manie sans délire), or emotional insanity, a form of insanity that did not involve loss of reasoning (l'entendement) but rather was characterized "by a sort of instinctual fury, as though only the affective faculties had been impaired." (*See* the discussion of Pinel's "emotional insanity" at **PSYCHOSIS: EMERGENCE: Pinel** [1801].) He then gave several examples of patients quite unable to bridle unruly tempers or violent impulses, including one gentleman farmer who had thrown a woman down a well (pp. 155–157 of second edition, 1809).

Hysteria as a character type (1845). Hysteria becomes understood in part as a personality type, found principally in the female sex. References to a hysterical type of character peculiar to women go well back into the history of psychiatry. But a landmark is Viennese psychiatry professor Ernst von Feuchtersleben's (1806–1849) *Textbook of Medical Psychology* (*Lehrbuch der ärztlichen Seelenkunde*), published in 1845: "[The causes of hysteria] include everything that increases sensitivity, weakens spontaneity, gives predominance to the sexual sphere, and validates the feelings and drives associated with sexuality" (p. 245).

Koch introduces the first classification of "psychopathic inferiorities" (1888). Inspired by French accounts of degeneration, Julius Ludwig August Koch (1841–1908), director of the state asylum at Zwiefalten in Württemberg, compiled in his *Brief Guide to Psychiatry* (*Kurzgefasster Leitfaden der Psychiatrie*, 1888) a list of what he called "psychopathic inferiorities" (psychopathische Minderwertigkeiten). Some of the patients were born psychopathically laden, others acquired their psychopathic inferiority (for Koch, a further subpopulation of both of these groups counted as "degenerate"). Those whose inferiority was constitutional in nature would have certain personality characteristics, such as obsessiveness; those with degenerate weakness were worse off, suffering from a lack of forcefulness or a "pathological lack of reproductive drive" (p. 45). None of the entities represented actual mental illnesses, he said, although the degenerate group could easily tip over into mental illness. Koch's own observations extended back over his experiences in private nervous clinics, one in Swabia owned by his family, another in Göppingen where he had worked before joining the civil service.

Janet profiles "hysterical" personality (1893). Even though **Pierre Janet** considered hysteria a constitutional disease, hysterical personality was something one acquired, he said, a response to developing hysterical physical symptoms such as cutaneous anesthesia. As he wrote in his 1893 book on the psychology of hysteria, "The mental state of the hysteric patient, overwhelmed and much reduced by the illness, becomes definitively reorganized along certain lines." "[Such symptoms] represent a mental illness, a psychological illness; [the anesthesia] does not exist in the limbs, nor the spinal cord, nor in the nuclei of the brain, but in the mind." For Janet, the essence of the hysterical personality was dissociation: "[Hysteria] is based on a very special kind of mental operation: on the personal perception that permits someone at any moment of one's life to assimilate the ensemble of new sensations to one's personality. Hysteria is due to a weakness of this synthesis of psychological elements that I have called elsewhere psychological disaggregation. Hysterical anesthesia is an illness of the personality" (*L'état mental des hystériques*, 1893, pp. 48–50).

Kraepelin classifies the "psychopathic personalities" (1904). In the seventh edition of his book *Psychiatry*, **Emil Kraepelin** said that "among those forms of mental illness that arise from a pathological constitution, there is a broad borderland between those frankly pathological conditions and those personal eccentricities that we find in healthy people as well" (*Psychiatrie*, 7th ed., II, p. 815). Among the "pathological personal deviations" in this borderland were (1) "the born criminal" (here he cited **Cesare Lombroso**, as well as **Eugen Bleuler's** 1896 book on the born criminal) (*see* **CONDUCT DISORDER; CRIMINALITY AND PSYCHIATRY**); (2) the "irresolute," suffering from lack of will power (die Haltlosen, with Willenschwäche, or weak will); (3) "the pathological liars and swindlers"; (4) the "pseudo-querulants" (the real querulants had a delusional illness classified elsewhere in his book *Psychiatry*). By "pseudo-" is meant people who become excitable about petty matters without actually becoming psychotic.

By the eighth edition of his *Psychiatry*, published in 1915, the list had expanded to seven types of "psychopathic personalities": (1) the excitable (die Erregbaren); (2) the irresolute; (3) those suffering from "driven" behavior (die Triebmenschen), including wastrels, drifters, periodic drinkers, and pleasure-lovers; (4) the eccentric (die Verschrobenen); (5) the liars and swindlers; (6) "the enemies of society (the antisocial)"; (7) the quarrelsome (die Streitsüchtigen), a label that had now replaced the "pseudo-querulants."

Inevitably, a list of this nature represents as much the compiler's pet-peeves as it does scientifically validated disorders. Kraepelin himself led a highly ascetic lifestyle and was completely teetotal; it is unsurprising that he would pathologize social drinking and "pleasure-seeking."

Freud and the "anal character" (1908). Freud, generally speaking, was not terribly interested in the issue of differing personality types. Yet, his main contribution to the subject was his essay on "Character and Anal Eroticism" ("Charakter und Analerotik") in the *Psychiatric-Neurological Weekly* (*Psychiatrisch-Neurologische Wochenschrift*). He wrote, "Among the people whom one attempts to help through psychoanalytic treatments, there is quite frequently a certain type characterized by the coincidence of certain character qualities. . . . I can no longer recall on which specific occasions I started to get the impression that there was a relationship between that kind of character and behavior surrounding a certain body organ." The patients who caught his attention were distinguished by three character qualities: they were orderly, in the sense of being clean, but also tidy and meticulous about the conduct of business; they were parsimonious, sometimes to the point of miserliness; and they could be stubborn. As Freud quizzed them about their childhood, their memories of toilet training caught his attention. "There was a very clear emphasis on the anal region in the sexual constitutions that they subsequently developed." Freud speculated that this triad of character qualities had arisen as these patients attempted later in life to shuck off their anal fixations (*Gesammelte Werke*, VII, pp. 203–204).

Jaspers distinguishes between "abnormal" and "pathological" types of personalities (1913). In his *General Psychopathology*, Jaspers distinguished between abnormal character variations that represented just extreme versions of normal personalities—such as neurasthenic and hysteric personalities—and pathological changes in personality arising from a "process," such as schizophrenia, in which the dissolution of the personality in disease bears little in common with the premorbid personality. He did not attempt a systematic classification of personality types. (*See also* **JASPERS, KARL; PSYCHOPATHOLOGY: Jaspers** [1913]; **PARANOIA: "pathological jealousy"** [1910]; **PSYCHOSIS: EMERGENCE.**)

Kretschmer's constitutionally based character types (1921). (*See* **KRETSCHMER, ERNST;** *see also* **PSYCHOSIS: EMERGENCE: Kretschmer's constitutional psychoses** [1921].) In his book *Body Structure and Character* (*Körperbau und Charakter,* 1921), Kretschmer classified the temperaments on the basis of the body types producing them (and according to the psychiatric illnesses for which the temperaments furnished a substrate). Thus he differentiated between:

- The "cycloid" temperament (fluctuating in and out of circular psychosis) as being "almost childishly good-hearted, trusting and tractable" (p. 116).
- The "schizoid" temperament that lapses into schizophrenia in episodes (rather than in "waves" as the cycloid); Kretschmer denoted them as individuals whom one could never really know, having the quality Bleuler had called **"autism"**: "That of living inside themselves. You can never know what they feel; sometimes they don't know it themselves, or only uncertainly. . . . What they feel, whether it is a banality, a whim [eine Schrulle], a commonplace or a magical notion, nobody else will know—they keep it for themselves" (p. 131) (quotes from seventh ed., 1929).

Jung's "extraverted" vs. "introverted" personalities (1921). *See* **JUNG, CARL GUSTAV.**

A comprehensive schema of psychopathic personalities: Schneider (1923). **Kurt Schneider** set out to construct a comprehensive scheme of all character traits and their opposites as an exercise in the study of character, not psychiatric pathology. His character chart was based on psychologist Ludwig Klages's (1872–1956) book *Principles of Characterology* (*Prinzipien der Charakterologie,* 1910). Schneider denied that any of these traits represented illness: Just as previous observers such as Paul Julius Möbius (1853–1907) had claimed that, "The degenerate individual is not mentally ill in the sense of the law, and he must bear the consequences of his actions as any other person," so Schneider did not see psychopathic personalities as "ill individuals" but rather as "characterological varieties." In his 1923 book, *Psychopathic Personalities* (*Die psychopathischen Persönlichkeiten*), Schneider said, "Psychopathic personalities are those abnormal personalities who suffer from their abnormality or from whose abnormality others suffer" (p. 16). Although he saw character as constitutional in nature—one has the personality one is born with—he rejected previous notions of "degeneracy" in understanding character abnormality.

Schneider devised the following types, supporting each with an extensive review of the literature: (1) hyperthymic psychopaths, psychopathic only when they—people with basically happy dispositions—spill over into hypomania; (2) depressive psychopaths, individuals who are continually gloomy; (3) insecure psychopaths, of whom he distinguished the subtypes: highly sensitive individuals and those prone to obsessive thoughts (anancastic); (4) fanatical psychopaths, people who struggle on behalf of overvalued ideas; (5) psychopaths with labile moods, highly reactive one day, tolerant and easy-going the next; (6) recognition-seeking psychopaths (Geltungsbedürftige) (Schneider said that **Karl Jaspers** seized the core of this: "To appear to be more than one is"); (7) emotionally-blunted psychopaths (Gemütlose): Schneider would have accepted antisocial as a synonym, he said, were the latter term not a sociological rather than a characterological construct; (8) weak-willed psychopaths, shallow people with little resolve; (9) asthenic psychopaths, meaning people who are "nervous" and "neurasthenic" (Schneider said of the decades-long speculation about the purported neurophysiology of neurasthenia, "That is all mythology"); (10) explosive psychopaths, people who "blow a fuse" at the slightest occasion (Schneider said "affective epilepsy" was a close neurological neighbor). The list was revised somewhat in subsequent editions.

Abraham links child-development phases to character types (1924). Berlin psychiatrist Karl Abraham (1877–1925), one of Freud's closest lieutenants, said in 1924 that a separate character type was associated with disruptions in each of the three phases of psychosexual development that Freud believed children passed through. An arrest at the oral stage could produce a dependent type of character; at the anal stage, obsessive-compulsive character; at the phallic stage, hysterical character. Abraham's essay "A Short History of the Development of the Libido" ("Versuch einer Entwicklungsgeschichte der Libido auf Grund der Psychoanalyse seelischer Störungen") appeared in the volume *New Studies in Medical Psychoanalysis* (*Neue Arbeiten in der ärztlichen Psychoanalyse*, 1924). This codified many of Freud's previous thoughts about the development of the libido. (*See* **ID; NARCISSISM; PARANOIA.**)

Wittels' "hysterical character" (1930). Siegfried ("Fritz") Wittels (1880–1950) acquired most of his psychiatric experience in the private sector, as consulting internist and psychiatrist to Vienna's "Cottage Sanatorium," an exclusive clinic for often female nervous patients. Yet in the late 1920s, Wittels was in the United States a good deal, definitively settling in New York in 1932. In 1951 his last book, *Sex Habits of American Women*, appeared posthumously, and it was doubtless out of the crossruff between Vienna and New York that his influential but misogynistic sketch of the "hysterical character"—later called the "hysterical" or "histrionic personality"—appeared in the *Medical Review of Reviews*. "As an actress," he said, "the hysteric is capable of achievements that cannot be surpassed. But she is unreliable, and at times will prove to be unsupportably bad in the same or some other role. . . . As a loving woman she represents a veritable martyrdom for the serious, compulsive male who, enwrapped in love and enjoyment in an hour of happiness, sees himself betrayed the following day."

The cause of hysterical character, according to Wittels, was the fixation of character development at the "infantile level." "Hence [the character] cannot attain its actuality as a grown-up human being; it plays the part of a child, and also of the woman" (p. 187).

Partridge introduces "sociopathic personality" (1930). Differentiating "sociopaths" from the general pool of "psychopathic personality" in an article in the *American Journal of Psychiatry*, psychologist George Everett Partridge (1870–1953) at the Sheppard and Enoch Pratt Hospital in Baltimore identified sociopathy as an almost constitutional trait that "produces persistent anti-social or socially futile behavior." Characteristic of the sociopathic personality were "emotional excesses and instability, [they are] generally unstable, have difficulty in acquiring permanent moods or sentiments in their social relations, are egocentric and show . . . decided lack of good sense and judgment, have the child's impractical attitude towards values . . . and have the child's irresponsibility and attitudes toward authority" (p. 97).

Reich's analysis of "character armor" (1933). Among early psychoanalysts, it was Vienna's Wilhelm Reich (1897–1957) who developed most fully the concept of character disorders. Reich saw "the character of the ego . . . as an armor protecting the id against the stimuli of the outer world" as well as against repressed inner drives. Various kinds of character types, all flying against "the original contrary tendencies," performed this function: (1) The "hysterical character," which Reich called "the simplest, most transparent type of character armor," was the result of a genital fixation in childhood. To deal with anxiety surrounding this fixation, the bearers of this particular set of armor, in this case usually but not necessarily women, developed an "importunate sexual attitude, yet backed away or became frigid when it was time to close the deal. (2) The "compulsive character," hallmarked by a "pedantic sense of order," parsimony, and a mix of hostility and aggression, served as a reaction against the fixation of ego development at the anal-sadistic stage. (3) The "phallic-narcissistic character," which Reich himself had first described in 1926, bore armor that was "predominantly inhibited, reserved, depressive." Filled with aggression, people of this type displayed their **narcissism** by going on the offensive. Just at the cusp of mature sexual development, their psychosexual growth had been arrested at the "proud, self-confident concentration on one's own penis," a way of defending oneself against backsliding to earlier stages. (4) The "masochistic character," a concept Reich had developed in 1932 as a way of breaking with Freud's theory of the death instinct (which implied that we suffer because of a biological will to do so, or "death instinct"). (*See* **MASOCHISM: Reich** [1932].) Reich said that masochists have "a chronic, subjective feeling of suffering which is manifested objectively . . . as a tendency to complain. Additional traits of the masochistic character are chronic tendencies to inflict pain upon and debase oneself . . . and an intense passion for tormenting others" (pp. 237–238). The character armor function here was a "fantasized or actual non-fulfillment of a quantitatively inordinate demand for love." This demand creates anxiety. The psyche tries to bind the anxiety by "courting love through provocation and defiance" (quotes from the English translation, 3rd ed., p. 246).

Beginning of "borderline personality disorder" (1938). *See* **BORDERLINE PERSONALITY DISORDER.**

Eysenck's dimensions of personality (1948). In his book *Dimensions of Personality*, **Hans Jürgen Eysenck**, then director of the psychological department of the **Maudsley Hospital**, began to elaborate his lifelong interest in pathological personality types. He distinguished between neuroticism and introversion–extraversion. In 1952 in *The Scientific Study of Personality*, he added psychoticism, arguing that these qualities were entrenched deep in the nervous system and body type: "The introverted neurotic shows symptoms of anxiety, depression, and irritability; he has overly high levels of aspiration . . . and tends to be of the leptomorph [asthenic] body build." "The extraverted neurotic is characterized by hysterical conversion symptoms; he has unduly low levels of aspiration . . . and tends to be of the eurymorph [short, heavy] type of body build" (*Scientific Study of Personality*, p. 122). In general, Eysenck (and others) argued for a dimensional approach to personality disorders, seeing them as maladaptive variants of normal personality.

See **SCHIZOID PERSONALITY DISORDER** (1952).

"Personality disorders" in DSM "One" (1952). Personality disorders in the first edition of the ***DSM*** series were understood as "developmental defects" in indivudals who had little anxiety or distress. They were subdivided into (A) Personality pattern disturbances that were almost constitutional in nature and inaccessible to basic change through psychotherapy; these included: "inadequate personality," "**schizoid personality**," "cyclothymic personality," and "paranoid personality"; (B) Personality trait disturbances that were potentially less serious than the above, and included: "emotionally unstable personality" (formerly psychopathic personality), "passive-aggressive personality," and "compulsive personality"; (C) Sociopathic personality disturbances whose bearers were defined largely as rule-breakers, including: "antisocial reaction," "dyssocial reaction," and "sexual deviation" (homosexuality, fetishism, and the like).

Sociopathic personality: the diagnosis validated (1966). On the basis of a follow-up study of 500 children brought to child guidance clinics in St. Louis and then tracked down 30 years later, Lee Nelken Robins (1922–) in the department of sociology of Washington University in **St. Louis** found that **conduct-disordered** children often became sociopathic adults. Her book *Deviant Children Grown Up: A Sociological and Psychiatric Study of Sociopathic Personality* (1966) again focused light on a disorder to which **Emil Kraepelin** (*see above*) had called attention in 1915 as "the antisocial" personality and that became in ***DSM-II*** in 1968 (*see below*) "antisocial personality disorder."

"Personality disorders" in *DSM-II* (1968). This part of *DSM-II* deviated from *DSM-I* in two ways: first, it abolished the subdivisions of the personality disorders (PDs) and simply gave a straight list; second, now under psychoanalytic guidance, it was insisted in the *Manual* that the personality "disorder" be differentiated from the "neurosis" of the same name, distinguishing in other words between brain-malfunction-style "maladaptive behavior" (as in a PD) and "neurotic symptoms" explicable in psychodynamic terms. The disorders included "paranoid personality," "cyclothymic personality," "**schizoid personality**," "explosive personality (epileptoid personality disorder)," "obsessive compulsive personality (anankastic personality)," "hysterical personality (histrionic personality disorder)," "asthenic personality" (which had to be differentiated from "neurasthenic neurosis"), "antisocial personality," "passive-aggressive personality," and "inadequate personality." "Sexual deviations" went into another category.

Chodoff attacks the "hysterical personality" disorder as pejorative (1974). Recognizing as pejorative many descriptions of the supposedly "hysterical" female—accounts that made her labile, egocentric, seductive, frigid, and childish—Washington, D.C., psychoanalyst Paul Chodoff (1914–) proposed in the *American Journal of Psychiatry* that classic "hysterical" PD be scrapped. "I have had the impression," he wrote, "that susceptible male residents may classify as a hysterical personality any reasonably attractive woman with whom they come into therapeutic contact" (p. 1076). Chodoff proposed that the concept of "histrionic" PD, already foreshadowed in ***DSM-II***, be adopted instead. These recommendations were partly acted on in ***DSM-III*** (1980; *see below*), and more fully in *DSM-III-R* (1987), when Chodoff was on the subcommittee for personality disorders.

"Personality disorders" in *DSM-III* (1980). The third edition of the *DSM* series broke from the second edition in assigning all of the personality disorders (along with the developmental disorders) to a separate axis, called "axis II." (All other psychiatric illnesses went on "axis I.") It defined PDs as "personality traits" that cause dysfunction and distress. The PDs were grouped into "clusters."

One cluster included paranoid, schizoid, and schizotypal PDs, the latter being new. (*See* **SCHIZOID PERSONALITY.**) This cluster embraced individuals who "often appear 'odd' or eccentric."

The second cluster included histrionic, antisocial, narcissistic, and borderline personality disorders (BPD). (*See* **BORDERLINE PERSONALITY DISORDER.**) The latter two were new in the *DSM* series: psychoanalytic categories now operationalized by developing observable criteria; by the end of the twentieth century, "BPD" would be by far the most commonly diagnosed PD.* A portion of what had formerly been considered borderline personality disorder became classified in this edition as schizotypal PD. As for **narcissism**, Reich in 1933 (*see above*) had developed the concept of narcissistic personality disorder, and New York psychoanalyst, Heinz Kohut (1913–1981), in his book *The Analysis of the Self* (1971), had seen to it that it retained a high place in psychoanalysis even after Reich was excommunicated from the temple. Typically, individuals in this second cluster "often appear dramatic, emotional, or erratic."

In the third cluster were avoidant, dependent, compulsive (in later editions "obsessive-compulsive"), and passive-aggressive PDs, whereby avoidant and dependent were new. Common to this cluster were individuals who "appear anxious or fearful."

In this edition, the distinction between PD and neurosis, so central to the second edition, was abolished. This classification was arrived at after extensively querrying practitioners in the field and represented a consensus, rather than being derived from any particular theoretical system.

DSM-III-R (1987) made no changes in the basic structure of the PD section of *DSM-III*.

DSM-IV (1994) removed "passive-aggressive" PD from the main list and, under the alternative title "negativistic personality disorder," made it a candidate for "further study" in the nonofficial diagnoses at the end of the book (along with "depressive personality disorder").

***ICD-10* Classification of personality disorders** (1992). The tenth edition of the World Health Organization's nosology did not diverge sharply from the personality disorder classification of the *DSM*, except for making the PDs just an additional group

---

* The deliberations of the advisory committee on personality disorders of the task force were evidently influenced by the work of Harvard psychoanalyst John Gunderson. (*See* **BORDERLINE PERSONALITY DISORDER: Gunderson defines** [1978].)

of disorders rather than a separate axis. Among the PDs listed in *The ICD-10 Classification of Mental and Behavioural Disorders* (1992) were paranoid, schizoid (schizotypal disorder was classed elsewhere), dissocial, emotionally unstable (subdivided into impulsive type and borderline type), histrionic, anankastic, anxious (avoidant), dependent, and a grab-bag category that mentioned the following as acceptable PD diagnoses without specifying their characteristics: eccentric, "haltlose" type, immature, narcissistic, passive-aggressive, and psychoneurotic.

PHANTOM LIMB. *See* **BODY IMAGE: DISTURBANCES OF.**

PHENYLKETONURIA (PKU). In 1934, Norwegian biochemist Ivor Asbjorn Folling (1888–1973) discovered, in research published in *Hoppe-Seyler's Zeitschrift für physiologische Chemie*, that a cause of **mental retardation**—one of the so-called "inborn errors of metabolism"—was a genetic inability to metabolize the amino acid L-phenylalanine. As a result, toxic amounts of a metabolite of phenylalanine accumulated in the brain, causing a disease known as phenylketonuria (PKU)—so-called because the ketone metabolite phenylpyruvic acid in the urine has a peculiar smell and turns green in the presence of ferric chloride (phenylpyruvic acid was known, somewhat cruelly, to insiders as "the idiot acid").

PKU turned out to have a significant genetic source. In 1935, Lionel S. Penrose (1898–1972), a physician on staff at the Royal Eastern Counties' Institution at Colchester—an asylum for mental retardation—studied the genetics of mental retardation (MR) by carefully interviewing the families of 1280 patients; in research published in the *Lancet* in 1935, he found that PKU was inherited as an autosomal recessive trait.

In 1953, Horst Bickel (1918–2000)* and co-workers at the Children's Hospital in Birmingham described in the *Lancet* the success of a diet low in phenylalanine in reducing PKU. In 1963, Robert Guthrie (1916–1995) at the Children's Hospital in Buffalo, New York, announced in *Pediatrics* a simple screeing test for PKU that entailed inhibiting the growth of bacteria. Then, Seymour Kaufman (1924–), chief of the Laboratory of Neurochemistry at the **National Institute of Mental Health**, wrapped up a virtual lifetime of doing basic research on the biochemistry of PKU by introducing folinic acid in 1987 in the treatment of one form of PKU that is caused by a lacking coenzyme; this research was published in the *Journal of Pediatrics*. This whole chain of research from Folling's discovery on has touched off a hunt for other biological causes of mental retardation. (Indeed, some observers consider PKU the only established abnormality in psychiatry.)

PHOBIA. *See* **ANXIETY AND PHOBIAS.**

PICHOT, PIERRE (1918–). Responsible for the introduction of quantitative techniques into French psychopharmacology, Pichot was born in the Vendée department, gaining his M.D. in Paris in 1948. He was a psychiatry intern and resident at the **Salpêtrière hospice** and **Ste.-Anne mental hospital** under **Jean Delay**, then from

* Bickel was later professor of pediatrics at **Heidelberg**.

1949 on Delay's assistant at Ste.-Anne. In 1964, he received a personal chair in medical psychology. As early as 1948, Pichot began publishing on psychological tests in psychiatry; this was a time, he, said, "when clinical psychiatrists in France scorned any appeal to quantification and statistics" (Shepherd, *Psychiatrists on Psychiatry*, p. 126). In 1955, his book on the **Rorschach** as a projective test appeared simultaneously with his work on *Clinical Psychometric Methods* (*Méthodes psychométriques en clinique*), a pioneering study of quantitative analysis. From 1972 to 1986, he was Delay's successor as head of the department of clinical psychiatry of the University of Paris. Just as **Pierre Deniker** was responsible for developing **chlorpromazine** at Ste.-Anne, a few years later Pichot undertook early trials of the antipsychotic drug haloperidol. In 1983, he wrote a major history of psychiatry, *A Century of Psychiatry*, demonstrating a better understanding than any previous historian that psychopharmacology is a method of discerning the nature of mental illness and not just a therapy.

PINEL, PHILIPPE (1745–1826). One of the founders of modern psychiatry, Pinel was born into a medical family in a village near Castres in southwest France, graduating as doctor of medicine from Toulouse in 1773. In 1778, he came up to Paris, making a meager living as a medical journalist. In 1786, he received a staff post at the "Maison Belhomme," a boarding house for psychiatric patients owned by a non-physician. Pinel greeted the French Revolution in 1789, and between 1793 and 1795 found himself chief physician of the Bicêtre hospice, a large institution for men in need of care that also included a psychiatric division. Here, he attempted to introduce psychological treatments of various kinds (called **moral treatment**, or le traitement moral). To generally make the care of patients more benevolent, Pinel gave the nonmedical supervisor Jean-Baptiste Pussin (1746–1811) latitude to remove the chains from the patients (for which Pinel himself, rather inexactly, has historically received the credit). In 1794, he became a professor at the newly founded École de santé (health school) of revolutionary Paris, and in 1795 became the chief physician of the **Salpêtrière hospice**, the equivalent of Bicêtre for women, where he remained until his death. In addition to his enlightened techniques for the management of psychiatric hospitals, Pinel is remembered for his 1785 translation of **William Cullen's** nosology (in French as *Institutions de médecine pratique*) and for a classification of mental illnesses in his big textbook, *Medical-Philosophical Treatise on Mental Illness* (*Traité médico-philosophique sur l'aliénation mentale*) (1801), one not based on Cullen.

By the second edition of his *Treatise* in 1809, Pinel's nosology had migrated from an emphasis on mania (which he understood as generalized insanity [délire général]) to include melancholia (or partial insanity [délire exclusif]); "dementia" (or "abolition of thought"), usually meaning in the writings of these older authors incoherent thought rather than loss of intelligence; and finally "idiotism" (or "obliteration of the intellectual and affective faculties"), either primary (from birth) or acquired. As French historian of psychiatry Jacques Postel points out, this second edition of Pinel's book, which now included his experiences at the Salpêtrière, "showed the importance of relations with the family, the community and other patients in the origins, the duration, and the exacerbation of mental illness. He emphasizes discipline, the regulation of the patients' daily lives, their rigorous classification, and the isolation of the most dangerous" (Postel, in Morel's *Dictionnaire biographique de la psychiatrie*, p. 196).

As for pharmacotherapy, Pinel held little of it: "Pinel was one of those physicians who reacted most strongly against the abuses of polypharmacy [multiple medications]," wrote René Semelaigne in 1888, a later-born psychiatrist whose family had memories of Pinel (Semelaigne, *Pinel*, p. 130). Of Pinel's many pupils, **Étienne Esquirol** later became most noted.

PMS. *See* **PREMENSTRUAL SYNDROME.**

POSITIVE VS. NEGATIVE SYMPTOMS (from 1887). "Positive" symptoms in the context of schizophrenia mean thought disorder, hallucinations and delusions, "negative" mean such symptoms as social withdrawal and flattening of affect. The use of the terms in psychiatry goes back to British neurologist John Hughlings Jackson (1835–1911), who applied "positive" and "negative" (already available in the medical literature) first to such neurological affections as epilepsy, then to mental illness. Jackson explained in the *Journal of Mental Science* in 1887 that, "The levels of evolution vary in the different kinds of insanity. . . . Disease, in the strict sense of pathological process, produces the negative physical change dissolution only, answering to negative affection of consciousness; disease is not the cause of positive mental symptoms. He who is studying the physical conditions of positive mental symptoms in any case of insanity is dealing with evolution" (*Selected Writings*, II, p. 78). Although Jackson expressed himself obscurely, this does mark the beginning of an important distinction.

At a meeting of the British Medical Association in Leeds in 1889, Jackson clarified this polarity: "All the positive mental symptoms in . . . insanities occur during activities of healthy nervous arrangements remaining in the maimed highest centres; they are . . . parts of the insane man's mentation . . . signs of his lowered consciousness; his illusions, as we call them, are his perceptions, and his mental symptoms altogether are lower homologues of his normal mentation." "Negative lesions," by contrast, involved paralysis and loss of consciousness. Jackson explained his theory more amply in an article in the *Medical Press and Circular* in 1894, accompanied by a diagram showing successive dissolution of function from highest levels of "cerebral centres" to lowest. This schema of successive downward dissolution in the central nervous system was later highly influential in French psychiatry.

"Basic vs. accessory" (1911). When Bleuler (*see* **SCHIZOPHRENIA: EMERGENCE: Bleuler** [1911]) distinguished between "basic" symptoms of schizophrenia such as thought disorder and "accessory" symptoms such as hallucinations and delusions, he had something different in mind from Jackson, and indeed Bleuler seemed unacquainted with Jackson's views. Bleuler did use the expressions positive and negative but only in the specific sense of "positive" and "negative" thoughts.* Yet, his "basic" symptoms of thought disorder might be considered negative symptoms and his accessory ones of hallucinations, et cetera, might be seen as positive.

Positive vs. negative revived (1974). Making specific reference to Jackson's earlier use, John S. Strauss (1932–) at the University of Rochester (and collaborators at the

---

* *See* Bleuler's article on "schizophrenic negativism" in the *Psychiatrisch-Neurologische Wochenschrift*, 1910, p. 184.

National Institute of Mental Health), in an article in *Schizophrenia Bulletin* in 1974, revived the concepts of "positive" and "negative" symptoms in schizophrenia. This use was reinforced by researcher **Nancy Andreasen** (1938–), who developed a scale for measuring negative symptoms in the disease. In 1982, Andreasen wrote in the *Archives of General Psychiatry*, "Although Hughlings Jackson's conceptual model of brain function may not apply precisely . . . his distinction between positive and negative symptoms is very useful for descriptive phenomenology" (p. 785).

Type I vs. Type II syndromes of schizophrenia (1980). **Timothy J. Crow** suggested in 1980 in the *British Medical Journal* that schizophrenia was really two different diseases. Type I schizophrenia, marked by so-called positive symptoms such as hallucinations, delusions, and thought disorder, was the acute form of the disease and was caused by abnormalities in the transmission of dopamine. Type II schizophrenia, characterized by such "negative" symptoms as flat affect, poverty of speech, and loss of drive, was the chronic form, or "defect" state, and was probably unrelated to dopamine. The hypothesis stimulated a good deal of research, although it was not ultimately accepted.

POSTTRAUMATIC STRESS DISORDER (PTSD). (*See also* **PSYCHOSIS: EMERGENCE: psychogenic [reactive] psychoses** [1916].) Interest in the psychiatric consequences of trauma initially arose following the enactment of health and accident insurance systems in the second half of the nineteenth century. The consequences of accidents became litigable in court. The initial trigger of litigation was "railway spine," supposed injuries to the spinal cord following a railway accident.

"Railway spine" (origin vague but in common use from the 1860s). In 1866, London surgery professor John Eric Erichsen (1818–1896), in six published lectures entitled *On Railway and Other Injuries of the Nervous System,* argued that physical symptoms following railway and other accidents that otherwise had left no evidence of a lesion were in fact organic in nature. ("No injury of the head is too trivial to be despised.") In his *On Concussion of the Spine: Nervous Shock, and Other Obscure Injuries of the Nervous System,* published in 1875, Erichsen spelled out his ideas more fully: "[I] direct your attention to a class of cases in which the injury inflicted upon the back is either very slight in degree, or in which the blow, if more severe, has fallen upon some other part of the body than the spine, and in which, consequently, its influence upon the cord has been of a less direct . . . character. Nothing is more common than that the symptoms of spinal mischief do not develop for several days after heavy falls on the back" (pp. 36–37). For a while, spinal concussion was referred to as "Erichsen's disease." This "organicity" argument became a target for more psychologically minded researchers to shoot at in coming decades. Erichsen abjured the "absurd appellation of the 'railway spine' " and did not use it.

In 1881, Carl Moeli (1849–1919), a staff psychiatrist at Berlin's Charité hospital, without mentioning Erichsen, discussed frank psychiatric changes following railroad accidents in four patients whose injuries were minor; it was, he said, clearly the traumatic psychological experience of the accident itself that had produced psychiatric changes. This is probably the first partial description of what was later known (in the ***DSM-III*** in 1980) as "posttraumatic stress disorder," or PTSD. Moeli's article "On Psychic Disturbances Following Railroad Accidents" ("Über psychische Störungen nach Eisenbahnunfällen") appeared in the *Berlin Clinical Weekly* (*Berliner Klinische Wochenschrift*).

In the English-speaking world, Herbert Page's (1845–1926) *Injuries of the Spine and Spinal Cord Without Apparent Mechanical Lesion and Nervous Shock in Their Surgical and Medico-Legal Aspects* (1883) undertook a specific refutation of Erichsen. Page, who graduated in medicine in 1870, had his practice in London's fashionable Harley Street and consulted to several railway companies as well as being surgeon to St. Mary's Hospital. "There is something so altogether indefinite in the expression 'concussion of the spine'—the 'spine' being so commonly used as a comprehensive term for muscles, ligaments, bones, joints, membranes, spinal fluid, spinal marrow and nerves going off from it—that when we speak of 'concussion of the spine' we must perforce use an expression scientifically inaccurate, and either more or less than adequate to describe a lesion affecting one only of the elements of which the 'spine' is composed" (p. 52). This kind of imprecision could only encourage litigation, he said. Nervous shock, for Page, was essentially psychological: "The collapse from severe bodily injury is coincident with the injury itself, or with the immediate results of it, but when the shock is produced by purely mental causes the manifestations thereof may be delayed" (p. 148).

The issues raised by Erichsen, Moeli, and Page continued to reverberate in medicolegal settings for decades thereafter, and even today it is litigable to what extent trauma from accidents has psychological as well as physical causes.

"Traumatic hysteria" (traumatic neurosis) (from 1877). In a lecture at the **Salpêtrière hospice** in December 1877, **Jean-Martin Charcot** described as "local hysteria" the disability of a body part arising from minor, local trauma. Charcot acknowledged that the English surgeon Benjamin Brodie (1783–1862) had floated the concept in 1837. Yet, Charcot's was a more comprehensive description. The lecture was summarized in *Progrès médical* on May 4, 1878.

In 1888, Hermann Oppenheim (1858–1919) in Berlin, the leading neurologist of his day, coined the phrase "traumatic neurosis" in the *Berlin Clinical Weekly* (*Berliner Klinische Wochenschrift*) in reference to railways accidents. There were, he said, psychiatric symptoms: "Most of the core symptoms concern the psyche and especially the affective domain. Mood changes and reactivity constitute the core of the mental side of the disorder" (p. 167). Yet, he considered the apparent neurological changes organically caused. Following the legislation on health-insurance in 1889 of the German chancellor Otto von Bismarck (1815–1898), the Imperial Insurance Office accepted "traumatic neuroses" (traumatische Neurosen) as an official diagnosis. As well, in 1889 Oppenheim published *Traumatic Neuroses* (*Die traumatischen Neurosen*), insisting that functional symptoms following accidents had in all likelihood an organic basis. He refused to believe such symptoms were an aspect of hysteria. This remained the single most influential work on the subject until the First World War, during which Oppenheim's beliefs about organicity became widely discredited.

From the fourth edition of his textbook *Psychiatry* (*Psychiatrie*) in 1893 onward, **Emil Kraepelin** incorporated Oppenheim's traumatic neurosis, or "fright neurosis" (Schreckneurose), the term Kraepelin preferred, in his nosology.

The war neuroses: "shell shock," et cetera (from 1915). (*See also* **ANXIETY AND PHOBIAS: "irritable heart" [soldiers' heart]** [1871].) In the tradition of

Oppenheim, previous posttraumatic diagnoses had focused more on pseudoneurological symptoms. With the rise of the war neuroses, psychiatric symptoms as such become attributable to trauma. Such terms as "soldiers' heart," "war neuroses" (Kriegsneurosen), and "general nervous shock" had been used to refer to the psychological casualties of combat even before the First World War. Yet, it was in 1915 that Charles S. Myers (1873–1946), a medically qualified psychologist with the British Expeditionary Force fighting in France, used, in an article in the *Lancet*, the new military term "shell shock" for the large numbers of psychological casualties who had started to be evacuated home as early as December 1914. (The war began in August 1914.) The term became enormously popular as way of explaining posttraumatic stress in soldiers without attributing it to "hysteria."

In the United States, it was Thomas W. Salmon (1876–1927), medical director of the National Committee for Mental Hygiene (*see* **Clifford Beers**), who helped create a psychiatric service for the United States Army. According to historian Ben Shepherd, author of *A War of Nerves*, Salmon advocated diminishing shell shock by keeping out of military service "all insane, feeble-minded, psychopathic and neuropathic individuals" (p. 125).

During the Second World War, the U.S. military used the term "operational fatigue" (or "combat fatigue") for what had previously been called shell shock. As Roy R. Grinker, Sr. (1900–1993) and John Paul Spiegel (1911–?), medical officers in the Army Air Forces, noted in their book *Men Under Stress* in 1945, "[Such] terms are temporary expedients to hide the neurotic nature of the illness to which they are usually applied. . . . Unlike the diagnosis of neurosis, which is prejudicial, this diagnosis permits the grounding of a man and his subsequent return to flying status" (p. 208). Yet, Grinker and Spiegel stipulated that the phrase "operational fatigue" was just a synonym for "war neuroses." (On Grinker and Spiegel, *see* **BARBITURATES: narcotherapy**.)

"Acute grief" (1944). Following a fire at the Coconut Grove night club in Boston on November 28, 1942, 491 people died and psychiatric symptoms set in among many of the survivors and relatives of the victims. Harvard psychiatrist Erich Lindemann (1900–1974), who was already interested in the consequences of grief for gastrointestinal disorders, was called in to counsel the afflicted, and in the *American Journal of Psychiatry* in 1944, he described preventive intervention—meaning counselling and "verbalizing his feelings of guilt"—in the management of "acute grief." "It is of the greatest importance," Lindemann said, "to notice that not only over-reaction but underreaction of the bereaved must be given attention, because delayed responses may occur at unpredictable moments and the dangerous distortions of the grief reaction, not conspicuous at first, be quite destructive later and these may be prevented" (p. 147). The article placed trauma on the map for American psychiatry as a source of psychiatric symptomatology. The techniques he described became part of the counseling of patients with posttraumatic stress disorder (*see below*).

"Posttraumatic stress disorder" (1980 and after). Following a persistent political campaign by the Vietnam War veterans, led in part by such figures as Yale psychiatry professor Robert Jay Lifton (1926–), in 1980 the American Psychiatric Association accepted in its new diagnostic manual, ***DSM-III***, the diagnosis posttraumatic stress disorder (PTSD), listing both acute and "chronic or delayed" versions. Classified under the anxiety section, PTSD was said to occur "following a psychologically traumatic event that is generally outside the range of usual human experience." The syndrome consisted of (1) "reexperiencing of the trauma," as evidenced by recurrent recollections of it, by dreams, and by the sudden feeling that it was reoccuring; (2) a psychological "numbing," characterized by diminished interest in normal events, feelings of detachment, and emotional narrowing; (3) two out of six such symptoms as "exaggerated startle response" or "trouble concentrating" (pp. 237–238).

DSM-III-R (1987) considerably increased the number of symptoms, any two of which would permit a patient to qualify for the diagnosis, adding, for example, "anniversaries of the trauma," and "persistent symptoms of increased arousal" such as irritability and reactivity to events somewhat resembling the circumstances of the trauma (p. 250).

DSM-IV (1994) added characteristic symptoms that might be expected in young children with PTSD, such as "repetitive play . . . in which themes or aspects of the trauma are expressed" (p. 428).

According to medical historians Mark Micale and Paul Lerner in their book, *Traumatic Pasts*, "At the beginning of the twenty-first century, PTSD is perhaps the fastest growing and most influential diagnosis in American psychiatry" (p. 3). PTSD clinics proliferate, and the U.S. Society for Traumatic Stress, founded in 1985, has given risen to a far-flung international network of traumatic-stress societies. The concept has not remained without sceptics, however, and readers may the consult *The Harmony of Illusions: Inventing Post-Traumatic Stress Disorder* (1995) by McGill University anthropologist Allan Young (1938–), on the conversion of what was formerly known as shell shock into a growth industry. In 2000, the Pfizer company began indicating its product Zoloft (sertraline), initially launched in 1992 as an antidepressant, for "posttraumatic stress disorder." (*See* **SELECTIVE SEROTONIN REUPTAKE INHIBITORS**.)

PREMENSTRUAL SYNDROME (PMS). Although some observers are troubled by the notion that a bodily function so universal as menstruation could have an intrinsic psychiatric pathology, menstruation is in fact disrupted in some psychiatric illnesses, such as in late schizophrenia. There are menstrual anomalies in about 40% of the cases of epilepsy. Yet, the extent to which menstruation produces psychiatric illness remains unclear. The whole subject of mind–body relations in gynecology is so drenched in prejudice that Helen Flanders Dunbar (1902–1959), a psychiatrist at Columbia University with a specialty in psychosomatic matters, wrote in 1935 in her magisterial overview *Emotions and Bodily Changes*, "Physicians since the time of Hippocrates and Galen have been dominated by the idea that diseased genital organs were the *sedes morbi* for the manifold hysterical disturbances of bodily function" (p. 330 of 2nd ed.). One must therefore be wary of identifying "landmark" scientific findings in this wasteland of bias.

What one can say is that physicians have long believed in the existence of a premenstrual syndrome, assigning to it such terms as "menstrual insanity." As **Emil Kraepelin** noted in the fifth edition of his textbook in 1896, "In women the physiological process of menstruation is regularly accompanied by a mild increase in nervous and psychic irritability that in certain individuals may reach an almost pathological level (depression, excited agitation)." "We even see cases of periodic mania [Tobsucht] that are so narrowly coupled to the menses that one is entitled to speak of 'menstrual insanity' " (p. 53).

In 1931, Robert T. Frank (1875–1949), a New York gynecologist with a Park Avenue practice (he had founded the endocrine research laboratory at Mt. Sinai Hospital in 1925), turned a page in the *Archives of Neurology and Psychiatry* by arguing that "premenstrual tension" was caused by hormonal changes, rather than by local changes in the uterus: "Continued circulation of an excessive amount of female sex hormone in the blood may in labile persons produce serious symptoms, some cardiovascular, but the most striking definitely psychic and nervous (autonomic). These periodic attacks are incapacitating and lead occasionally to extreme unhappiness and family discord. They can be directly ascribed to the excessive hormonal stimulus" (p. 1056).

The term "premenstrual syndrome" was coined in 1953 by (Charles) Raymond Greene (1901–1982), an endocrinologist at the Royal Northern Hospital in the London suburb of Hampstead (and brother of novelist Graham Greene), and Katharina Dorothea (Kuipers) Dalton (1916–2004), a London family doctor, in the *British Medical Journal*. They said, " 'Premenstrual tension,' as it has hitherto been called, is the commonest of the minor endocrine disorders." It was no longer necessary for women to "pass through one week of discomfort in every month, usually without complaining to their doctors but not necessarily without disturbing the tranquility of their homes" (p. 1007). The authors recommended treatment with the progestogen hormones. In 1953, Dalton established at University College Hospital the first "Premenstrual Syndrome Clinic" in the world. (She later wrote the bestselling *Premenstrual Syndrome* [1964]. In 1971 she became the first woman to serve as president of the general practice section of the Royal Society of Medicine.)

With the cornucopia of psychoactive medications hitting the market in the 1960s and after, "PMS" soared in popularity as an indication for drug therapy.

The whole concept of premenstrual complaints has undergone some bizarre contortions in the ***DSM*** series. ***DSM-III*** in 1980 contained nothing on it. ***DSM-III-R*** in 1987 proposed in an appendix the diagnosis "late luteal phase dysphoric disorder," a "pattern of clinically significant emotional and behavioral symptoms that occur during the last week of the luteal phase" (p. 367). Nothing was said about PMS. The clunky diagnosis did not catch on. Then, in ***DSM-IV*** in 1994, the disease designers tried again, with "premenstrual dysphoric disorder" (quickly abbreviated as PMDD). Although the diagnosis was intended for the mood disorders section of the *Manual*, the American Psychiatric Association once again consigned it to an appendix after a protest campaign by feminist organizations.

In 1993, in work published in the *International Journal of Psychiatry in Medicine*, psychiatrist Uriel Halbreich (1943–) at the State University of New York at Buffalo, discovered "altered serotonergic activity in women with dysphoric premenstrual syndromes." This suggested a possible role for **selective serotonin reuptake inhibitor** (SSRI) drugs. Thus, a seal of approval of a kind for PMDD came rather via the back channel, as in November 1999, the Psychopharmacologic Drugs Advisory Committee of the U.S. Food and Drug Administration accepted PMDD as a legitimate indication for Lilly's SSRI antidepressant drug fluoxetine (Prozac).

PRICHARD, JAMES COWLES (1786–1848). Best known for his concept "moral insanity," Prichard was born at Ross in Herefordshire, England, into a cultivated Quaker family but was raised in Bristol. He earned his M.D. from Edinburgh in 1808, and shortly thereafter began practicing medicine in Bristol. There, he began studies of an anthropological nature (e.g., why do Africans have black skin). In 1811, he was elected physician to St. Peter's Hospital, which had many psychiatric patients. Based on this experience, in 1822 he wrote his *Treatise on Diseases of the Nervous System . . . Comprising Convulsive and Maniacal Affections* (1822), which pioneered a number of concepts in epileptology, including that of "partial epilepsy," involving some particular part of the body. (*See* **EPILEPSY**.) In an article in *The Cyclopaedia of Practical Medicine* (1833–1835), Prichard first proposed the notion of moral insanity as a form of partial insanity involving mainly the passions and the will but not otherwise "madness," meaning no hallucinations or delusions. He enlarged his notions in 1835 in *Treatise on Insanity and Other Disorders Affecting the Mind*. Prichard said, "This form of mental derangement has been described as consisting in a morbid perversion of the feelings, affections, and active powers, without any illusion or erroneous conviction impressed upon the understanding." Intelligence was preserved in the disorder: "They often display great ingenuity in giving reasons for the eccentricities of their conduct . . . and justifying the state of moral feeling under which they appear to exist. In one sense, indeed, their intellectual faculties may be termed unsound; they think and act under the influence of strongly excited feelings, and persons accounted sane are, under such circumstances, proverbially liable to error both in judgment and conduct" (pp. 20–21).

Yet, Prichard did not otherwise well delineate the term, and it was quickly overtaken by the more careful definitions of the French and German nosologists. (The English have never been in the international forefront of disease-naming.) Nonetheless, in the judgment of psychiatry historians Richard Hunter and Ida Macalpine, "It was Prichard who first put at the centre of the psychiatric map the many mental disorders which reveal themselves only by disturbances of affect and behaviour and which had been largely neglected at the periphery" (*Three Hundred Years of Psychiatry*, p. 837). For later generations, "moral insanity" came to be synonymous with sociopathy and psychopathy, although that is not what Prichard understood by it.

PROZAC (fluoxetine). *See* **SELECTIVE SEROTONIN REUPTAKE INHIBITORS (SSRIs).**

PSYCHIATRIC GENETICS. Since the eighteenth century, psychiatrists have suspected that family genetic history played something of a role in their patients' illnesses. Articulated first as "inheritance," then "degeneration" and "eugenics," then finally after the Second World War as psychiatric genetics, patterns of inheritance represent the main physical evidence of the biological nature of major psychiatric illness. Yet the concept of patterns of inheritance spills easily into "race" and "degeneration," putting science at the service of its social masters.

Degeneration theory introduced to psychiatry (1857). In his *Treatise on Degeneration* (*Traité des dégénérescences physiques, intellectuelles et morales de l'éspece humaine*, 1857), French psychiatrist **Bénédict-Augustin Morel** ascribed major psychiatric illnesses to the process of degeneration, the corruption of the germ plasm from generation to generation. This popularized a concept already in use in scientific circles, and introduced a notion of inheritance comparable to that of an express train gathering speed across the generations, as ever more degenerate "seed" was transmitted from one generation to the next. The notion of degeneration is comparable to the modern doctrine of "genetic anticipation," as the penetrance of a disorder increases over successive generations, as for example in "fragile-X," a form of mental retardation, or Huntington's disease. As Morel wrote in 1857, "The degenerate human being, if he is abandoned to himself, falls into a progressive degradation. He becomes . . . not only incapable of forming part of the chain of transmission of progress in human society, he is the greatest obstacle to this progress through his contact with the healthy portion of the population." (On Morel, *see* **PSYCHOSIS: EMERGENCE: mania and melancholia as a result of degeneration** [1857].)

See **LOMBROSO** on the genetics of genius and criminality (from 1864).

Francis Galton on the inheritability of genius (1869). Galton (1822–1911), an independently wealthy Englishman involved in the administration of science, introduced in his 1869 book, *Hereditary Genius: An Inquiry into its Laws and Consequences,* the "pedigree," or family history, method into the study of inheritance. Yet, Galton himself did not use the diagrams showing how positive and negative traits migrated down the family tree that later became so popular. Galton concluded, "It follows that the human race has a large control over its future forms of activity—far more than any individual has over his own, since the freedom of individuals is narrowly restricted by the cost, in energy, of exercising their wills" (p. 375). This doctrine of control of the genetic pool became a basic tenet of eugenic theory. In 1905, Galton established the Eugenics Record Office at University College London (later baptized the Galton Laboratory), and in 1907 he became a cofounder of the Eugenics Education Society, an organization founded, as medical historian Pauline Mazumdar has put it in her book on the history of the Eugenic Society, "to press for legislative remedies for what it saw as the fundamental cause of pauperism," namely low physical fitness and high fertility (p. 2). Galton coined the term "eugenics," meaning positive heredity. Galton was responsible for the (in retrospect quite correct) idea that certain traits have a heavy genetic component, but he was not responsible for the notion that undesirable traits may be weeded out through such measures as sterilization—later a central eugenist tenet. (He was knighted, becoming "Sir Francis," in 1909.)

Emil Kraepelin declared that 70% of schizophrenia patients have a hereditary predisposition (1896). **Kraepelin** had always believed that "dementia praecox," as he called schizophrenia, was highly inheritable, as indeed were all psychiatric illnesses in his view. In the fifth edition of his textbook *Psychiatry* (*Psychiatrie*) in 1896, he wrote, "Hereditary predisposition [erbliche Veranlagung] was present in around 70 percent of the cases in which information was available; correspondingly, the so-called signs of degeneration were frequently observed" (p. 437). "It goes without saying," he said, "that hereditarily loaded individuals have a general tendency to be constitutionally ill, continually ill, or ill in frequently recurring episodes. The more that the actual cause of insanity has its locus in the overall predisposition of the person, the more trivial need be the external impetus that brings about a lasting and customarily incurable disorder of the entire personality" (p. 88).

The first large family study of psychiatric illness (1916). Although Swiss-born psychiatrist Ernst Rüdin (1874–1952) later made himself notorious as an apologist for Nazi sterilization practices, he was in fact the founder of psychiatric genetics on a demographic basis (following up systematically the patients' relatives at large in the population rather than haphazardly studying "interesting cases"). Rüdin spent most of his academic career in Munich, first at **Kraepelin's** psychiatric clinic, then after 1918 at the German Psychiatric Research Institute (Deutsche Forschungsanstalt für Psychiatrie) that Kraepelin had founded. Rüdin's 1916 monograph, *On the Inheritability and Causation of Dementia Praecox* (*Zur Vererbung und Neuentstehung der Dementia praecox*), was based on 701 families with 4823 children, the majority of probands coming from the Munich clinic and from a provincial Bavarian asylum. Rüdin obtained information on the first-degree relatives of schizophrenics in correspondence with the parish priests, among other sources. He found that 4.5% of the children with healthy parents had schizophrenia and 6.2% of the children with at least one ill parent. Commented psychiatry historian Matthias Weber, "Through Rüdin's work, the genetic viewpoint won a prominent position in scientific psychiatry and gained its own methodology" (*Ernst Rüdin, eine kritische Biographie* [1993], p. 113).

The twin-study technique of demographic research on psychiatric genetics (from 1928). The logic of a twin-study is that monozygotic twins (identical twins that developed from the same egg) have identical genes; if indeed schizophrenia has a genetic cause, both twins will often have the illness. Dizygotic twins, on the other hand (nonidentical twins), develop from different ova and would have no higher risk of schizophrenia than any two sibs. A measure, therefore, of genetic risk is the difference between the percent of monozygotic and dizygotic co-twins who have schizophrenia (or any other psychiatric illness). This approach was initiated by a junior member of Kraepelin's German Psychiatric Research Institute, Hans Luxenburger (1894–1976), in a 1928 article in the *Journal of Combined Neurology and Psychiatry* (*Zeitschrift für die gesamte Neurologie und Psychiatrie*). He collected from all Bavarian asylums lists of schizophrenic patients who were twins, then tracked the other co-twin down by writing to the parish priests and communal record offices, collecting in this manner 211 twin-sets in which one twin had been institutionalized for schizophrenia, manic-depressive illness, or epilepsy. Luxenburger found that among identical twins, 64% of the co-twins had schizophrenia; among nonidentical twins, none of the co-twins had become ill.

Following Luxenburger's work, other important twin studies included the following.

In 1932, Aaron J. Rosanoff (1878–1943), who then had a private psychiatric practice in Los Angeles, published in *California and Western Medicine* a study of 127 twin pairs in which one twin had been institutionalized. Of the 48 monozygotic pairs, both twins had been affected in 41 cases, or 85%; of the 79 dizygotic twin pairs, only 34% had a co-twin with a psychiatric illness. Rosanoff published his findings more fully in 1941 in *The Etiology of Child Behavior Difficulties, Juvenile Delinquency and Adult Criminality with Special Reference to Their Occurrence in Twins.* (Rosanoff is also remembered for having started the process of deinstitutionalization in California after he became director of the state department of institutions in 1939.)

The schizophrenia twin-study of Franz J. Kallmann (1897–1965), a German emigré psychiatrist who had landed at the New York State Psychiatric Institute, published in the *American Journal of Psychiatry* in 1946, found that, among 691 "twin index families," in 86% of the monozygotic twin pairs both twins had schizophrenia, but in only 15% of the dizygotic. (When Kallmann's results were presented at the first World Congress of Psychiatry in Paris in 1950, they caused consternation: the largely psychoanalytically oriented participants found such findings incredible and totally inconsistent with psychoanalytic theory.)

Finally, among these early twin-studies, the most ample of all was conducted by English psychiatrist and geneticist **Eliot Slater**, presented in his 1953 book, *Psychotic and Neurotic Illnesses in Twins*. In schizophrenia, Slater found a concordance for the monozygotic twin pairs of 75% and for the dizygotic of 11%. Slater concluded, "These facts suggest that genetical causes provide a potentiality for schizophrenia, perhaps an essential one, though environmental factors play a substantial role" (p. 88).

These and other twin studies provided a kind of statistical battering ram for forcing open the biological door in the study of schizophrenia and were for many years among the most powerful arguments for the organicity of the disease (today, evidence from **neuroimaging** is very compelling as well). Later twin-studies, using refined techniques, found the concordance for schizophrenia in identical twins somewhat lower than in the above studies. Yet, Irving Gottesman (1930–), a psychologist then at the University of Virginia, summarizing the literature in his 1991 book, *Schizophrenia Genesis*, nonetheless put the concordance in monozygotic twins at around 50%, in dyzygotic at only around 20%, in nephews and nieces of schizophrenic patients at 5%, and the risk in the general population at less than 1%. He concluded, "The facts about the risks of schizophrenia obtained from family studies of schizophrenics—their parents, siblings, children, and more distant relatives—all suggest that schizophrenia is familial. . . . Genetic factors are important, though not adequate to explain all the observations" (pp. 126–127).

Penrose studies family genetics through careful interviewing (1938 and after). Lionel S. Penrose (1898–1972), a physician on staff at the Royal Eastern Counties' Institution at Colchester—an asylum for mental retardation—studied the genetics of mental retardation (MR) by carefully interviewing the families of 1280 patients and securing other sources of information as well. In *A Clinical and Genetic Study of 1280 Cases of Mental Defect* (1938), he determined that 7% to 9% of the first-degree relatives of the patients had themselves some form of MR. (At Colchester, Penrose also discovered that one cause of MR, known as **phenylketonuria**, was inherited as an autosomal recessive trait. Identifying the genetics of this "error of metabolism" in an article in the *Lancet* in 1935—one of the few then known as causes of MR—represented a big advance for genetics.)

In 1945, Penrose took up the chair of Galton Professor of Eugenics at University College London, established in 1911 with a bequest from Francis Galton. In 1963, after a long struggle owing to the wording of Galton's will, he succeeded in changing the name of the chair to Galton Professorship of Human Genetics. (As editor, in 1954 he had similarly changed the title of the journal *Annals of Eugenics* to *Annals of Human Genetics*.)

Adoption studies using a follow-up method as a means of separating genetic from environmental factors (from 1966). The issue of a "distorted family environment" as a possible source of illness continued to bedevil schizophrenia researchers. In 1966, Leonard L. Heston (1930–), then a resident in psychiatry at the University of Oregon Medical School, published a paper in the *British Journal of Psychiatry* on children of schizophrenic mothers who had been adopted away compared to controls. Five of the 47 children of the schizophrenic mothers were themselves schizophrenic;

none of the control subjects, who were children selected at random from the same foundling home that cared for the children of the schizophrenic mothers, had become schizophrenic at follow-up. Heston concluded, "The results of this study support a genetic aetiology of schizophrenia" (p. 823). (For a psychiatry resident in Oregon, the choice of journal is an interesting one. Heston subsequently explained: "The article appeared in the *British Journal of Psychiatry* because I was doing a fellowship year in London at the time and my supervisor was **Eliot Slater**, the editor of the *British Journal*. It seemed the politic thing to do. However, I was pleased to have Dr. Slater on my side as I did not expect a friendly reception from American editors. I had submitted grants to **NIMH** and a few foundations. All were rejected, I thought quite disdainfully in some instances. So I knew that my findings would not be popular.")

A year later, at a conference in Dorado, Puerto Rico, Seymour S. Kety (1915–2000), David Rosenthal (ca. 1919–1996), Paul H. Wender (1934–)—all at the **National Institute of Mental Health**—and Fini Schulsinger (1923–), a Copenhagen psychiatrist, reported the first results of an adoption study they had undertaken based on the adoption registers of Copenhagen, Denmark, a country having a recordkeeping system that permits the lifetime follow-up of individuals. They found that, of the 5483 adoptions in Copenhagen to unrelated adoptive parents from 1924 through 1947, 33 of the children had developed schizophrenia. How common was schizophrenia in the biological families of these children as opposed to those of controls? Of the 150 biological relatives of the schizophrenic children, 13 had a history of the illness, whereas in the adopted families of the 33 children, and among the controls, there was very little schizophrenia. The evidence pointed overwhelmingly to a genetic contribution to the illness. The authors concluded "that the roughly 10 percent prevalence of schizophrenia found in the families of naturally reared schizophrenics is a manifestation of genetically transmitted factors" (p. 359). The work was published in 1968 in the *Journal of Psychiatric Research* and created something of a sensation within psychiatry.

First positive linkage to schizophrenia using DNA markers (1988). Was there a schizophrenia gene? The first link between forms of the illness and specific loci on the DNA was discovered on chromosome 5 by a team led by Robin Sherrington and reported in *Nature* in 1988. Yet, the finding of a specific gene was not confirmed. (*See* **SCHIZOPHRENIA: RECENT CONCEPTS** [1988].) As this field has evolved, it appears that there are probably several DNA markers for schizophrenia, as indeed "schizophrenia" is likely to be a final common pathway for a number of biological conditions, some of them genetic in nature and having quite diverse DNA sources of susceptibility. (At this writing, it seems that "schizophrenia genes" as such probably do not exist, and that genetic influences affect mainly information processing within the brain.)

"PSYCHIATRY"—origin of term (1808). Johann Christian Reil (1759–1813), a professor of medicine in Halle, Germany, coined the term "psychiatry" to mean the third arm of the art of medicine, next to physic (medication) and surgery. In a journal of brief duration that he and Johann Christoph Hoffbauer (1766–1827) had founded, called *Contributions to Encouraging a Method of Treatment Using Mental Approaches* (*Beyträge zur Beförderung einer Curmethode auf psychischem Wege*), in 1808 Reil wrote "On the Concept of Medicine and its Branches, Especially in Relation to the Justification of the Topic of Psychiatry" ("Über den Begriff der Medicin und ihre Verzweigungen, besonders in

Beziehung auf die Berechtigung der Topik der Psychiaterie [*sic*]"). In a contribution published posthumously in 1816 by his students, 3 years after his death (*Entwurf einer allgemeinen Therapie*), Reil began spelling it in German "Psychiatrie" rather than "Psychiaterie." These facts were ascertained by Achim Mechler, in a 1963 article in *Der Nervenarzt*. The use of the new term spread rather slowly, yet already in 1818 we find it in Johann Christian August Heinroth's (1773–1843) *Textbook of Disturbances of Mental Life* (*Lehrbuch der Störungen des Seelenlebens*), as he complained, "There is as yet no proper system of psychiatry, certainly none based on the principles stated in this book" (p. 37 of George Mora's translation into English). (*See* **GERMAN "ROMANTIC" PSYCHIATRY: Heinroth.**)

PSYCHOANALYSIS. "Psychoanalysis" was the word Freud coined in 1896, in an article written in French in the *Revue neurologique*, for the new kind of psychological investigation that he and his Viennese colleague Josef Breuer (1842–1925) were devising: "I owe my results to the use of a new method of psychoanalysis [psychoanalyse], a procedure explored by J. Breuer; it is rather subtle but will establish itself as irreplaceable because it has demonstrated itself to be so fertile in illuminating the dark paths of unconscious ideation" (*Gesammelte Werke*, I, p. 416). (For details, *see* **FREUD; FREUDIAN DOCTRINE OF HYSTERIA; FREUDIAN INTERPRETATIONS OF OBSESSION AND COMPULSION; FREUDIAN INTERPRETATIONS OF PSYCHOSIS AND SCHIZOPHRENIA; FREUDIAN PSYCHOTHERAPY: TECHNIQUE; ID; NARCISSISM; NEUROSIS; PERSONALITY DISORDERS.**)

PSYCHOPATHOLOGY (as a movement). Because the term "psychpathology" springs so readily to the lips, it is difficult to ascertain the priority for its first use. It is mentioned in passing in some of the psychiatric writing of the early nineteenth century. The Viennese psychiatrist Ernst von Feuchtersleben (1806–1849), in commenting on the somaticist views of his colleague at the University of Würzburg, Johann Baptist Friedreich (1796–1862), said about the supposed physical causation of mental illness: "Psychopathology has not yet been able to cast enough light on these critical processes" (*Textbook of Medical Psychology* [*Lehrbuch der ärztlichen Seelenkunde*], 1845, p. 69).

The importance of psychopathology lies in the belief of its proponents that a disease is constructed from symptoms (the proponents of nosology, on the other hand, claim that there is a prior disease, and the disease determines the symptoms). After the work of **Karl Jaspers**, it would be the abnormal forms of symptoms, rather than the abnormal symptoms themselves (for example that hallucinations are taking place rather than the content of the hallucinations), that are relevant to the disease.

Guislain introduced the term "phenomenology" into psychiatry (1852). Within psychiatry, phenomenology came to have a meaning equivalent to psychopathology. The German philosopher Georg Wilhelm Friedrich Hegel (1770–1831) first gave the term "phenomenology" its currency in the *Phenomenology of Spirit* (*Phaenomenologie des Geistes*) in 1807. Thus, the word was in the air when Belgian psychiatrist Joseph Guislain (1797–1860), offering the medical students at Ghent University detailed guidance on how to investigate a patient, coached them on how to pose questions: "When did you get married? When are you getting out of here?" Guislain told the students, "if you know how to formulate your questions along these lines, you will know how to address your patients in order to determine the phenomenology of the illness. . . . You will have taken a step ahead in the practical science of mental illness" (p. 45). Guislain published his lectures under the title, *Oral Lectures on the Phrenopathies, Or a Practical and Theoretical Treatise on the Mental Illnesses* (*Leçons orales sur les phrénopathies, ou traité théorique et pratique des maladies mentales*, 1852).

Concept of "general pathology" applied to the psyche (1859). Adolph Wachsmuth (1827–1865), having trained in medicine at Göttingen University, decided in the mid-1850s to go over to psychiatry. After a study trip to some of the larger asylums, he started to lecture on the subject in Göttingen (while remaining an assistant in the medical clinic), and in 1859 wrote *General Mental Pathology* (*Allgemeine Pathologie der Seele*), saying that psychiatry was now open to the same kind of progress that internal medicine had been making: "Our understanding of somatic physiology and pathology now permits no doubt that a scientific physiology and pathology of mind [Seele] are possible in exactly the same manner" (pp. 4–5). He broke down psychic illnesses into those affecting mood (Gemüt), hallucinatory illnesses (Sinnestäuschungen), thought disorder (Wahnsinn), and the "conditions of psychic weakness" (psychische Schwächezustände).

The launching manifesto of the psychopathology movement: Kahlbaum's *Catatonia* (1874). In his book on *Catatonia* (*die Katatonie*), **Karl Kahlbaum** said at the outset that all previous psychiatry textbooks, despite their stated intentions of moving beyond such fixed categories as "mania" and "melancholia," had nonetheless arrayed their case material upon this traditional disease scaffolding. For the sake of the "clinical method," it was time to "evaluate as many as possible of the individual patient's symptoms for the sake of the correct diagnosis and to ascertain the prognosis." Then, one might see which symptoms could empirically be grouped into psychiatric diseases, with the understanding that the symptom picture down the road might be very different from the picture at the beginning. Furthermore, previous efforts to link clinical pictures with brain lesions had largely failed, and now it was time to concentrate on careful clinical observation rather than on postmortem microscopy. "Only the comprehensive and intensive application of the clinical method can serve here and advance the science of psychiatry to ever deeper insights into psychopathic processes" (p. viii). Kahlbaum rejected the previous psychology of the Romantic psychiatrists (*see* **GERMAN "ROMANTIC" PSYCHIATRY**) as filled with useless moralizing. "But there exists a whole world of individual psychological phenomena that currently . . . remain terra incognita and that may only be discovered through meticulous investigation" (p. xi). Kahlbaum concluded: "The penetrating observation and frequent analysis of psychological phenomena of mentally-ill individuals—as well as the launching of a disease-specific psychological symptomatology—are the next urgent agenda of clinical psychopathology" (pp. xi–xii). Many younger psychiatrists now responded to this clarion call with the same enthusiasm that had once drawn earlier generations of physicians to identify the basic organic diseases of the human body using the same clinical method.

A psychologist lays the basis of psychopathology in France: Ribot (1875 onwards). Théodule Armand Ribot (1839–1916), whom **Pierre Pichot** calls the "father of French scientific psychology," was keen to break with past metaphysical traditions in psychology about whether the mind had knowledge of itself and put the discipline on a scientific basis in order to classify mental phenomena, normal and pathological. (He recommended that psychologists should begin as psychiatrists.) In 1875, he described in *Contemporary English Psychology* (*La psychologie anglaise contemporaine*) the recent empirical contributions of the English. His own principal contributions to psychopathology were *Disorders of Memory* (*Maladies de la mémoire*, 1881), *Disorders of Will* (*Maladies de la volonté*, 1883), and *Disorders of Personality* (*Maladies de la Personnalité*, 1885). In 1885, he began teaching a course in experimental psychology at the University of Paris and in 1888 was appointed professor of experimental and comparative psychology at the Collège de France.

The term "general psychopathology" becomes current (1878). In the same year that Hermann Emminghaus (1845–1904) became the professor of psychiatry in Dorpat (Tartu), 1878, he published his psychiatry textbook, *General Psychopathology: An Introduction to the Study of Mental Illness* (*Allgemeine Psychopathologie: Zur Einführung in das Studium der Geistesstörungen*). Yet, the work was more a general psychiatry textbook than a discussion of symptoms as such.

Kraepelin: psychopathology and psychiatric diseases (1909). The eighth edition of **Emil Kraepelin's** classic textbook represents the most elaborate classification in his work of diseases and symptoms. In the first volume of this edition, published in 1909, Kraepelin turned his hand—more so than in previous editions—to the fine description and differentiation of psychiatric symptoms, to objective psychopathology in other words, although Kraepelin did not use the term "psychopathology" and preferred to speak of "the manifestations of insanity" (die Erscheinungen des Irreseins). He divided symptoms into "disorders of perception," "disorders of mental activity," "disorders of emotional life," and "disorders of will and activity," for each domain describing how normal psychological function is distorted in illness. Indeed, Kraepelin made ample use of the kinds of psychometrics he had learned when studying with Wilhelm Wundt (1832–1920) in Leipzig. In the following volumes of this edition, published in 1910 and after, Kraepelin went on to a nosology of disease.

Reconciling psychopathology and psychoanalysis: an English attempt (1912). On the face of it, **Sigmund Freud's** psychoanalysis was more concerned with limning unconscious processes than with the fine description of symptoms as such. Yet in 1912, Bernard Hart (1879–1966), an English psychiatrist then at Long Grove Asylum in Epsom (who advanced to a consulting room on London's Harley Street), defined psychopathology in his little book, *The Psychology of Insanity*, as "the science which attempts to explain the problems of mental disorder by psychological principles" and suggested that psychoanalysis qualified under that rubric because "Freud slowly and tentatively built up his theoretical conceptions in accordance with the facts which were continuously elicited by investigation of his patients" (p. xxviii). Yet, most psychopathologists held psychoanalysis at arm's distance, and vice versa.

Jaspers's textbook *General Psychopathology* (*Allgemeine Psychopathologie*) (1913) as the most important milestone in the history of the psychopathology movement. **Karl Jaspers** was influenced by the German philosopher Georg W. F. Hegel's (1770–1831) concept of "phenomenology," by which Hegel meant the sum total of the productions of the mind. More specifically, Edmund Husserl's (1859–1938) "descriptive phenomenology," articulated in Husserl's 1890 book, *Logical Investigations* (*Logische Untersuchungen*), shaped Jaspers's thinking (*see* Husserl, I, p. 212). Jaspers later wrote in his autobiography (1977) of Husserl's impact: "Describing what patients innerly experienced as phenomena of consciousness turned out to be possible, and productive. Not only hallucinations, but delusions as well, the ways in which patients experienced their consciousness of themselves [Ichbewusstsein] and their feelings, could be described so clearly in the patients' self-reports as to make sure that the phenomena would be recognizable again in other cases. Phenomenology became a research method" (p. 23). Phenomenology for Jaspers and the **Heidelberg** school did not therefore mean the objective classification and description of symptoms, as others often understood the term, but the subjective phenomena of pathological mental experiences.

In his 1913 book, Jaspers was hostile to Kraepelin's big disease concepts (the task of nosology) and differentiated the various areas of psychopathology: phenomenology, objective performance, the psychology of expression, and so forth. He recognized the distinction between meaningful connections (verstehen) and causal explanation (begreifen); yet, psychopathology cannot be understood as the science of empathic understanding alone: some additional dimension of grasping the issues was involved. In particular, Jaspers distinguished between the form of psychosis and its content, saying the former was the more important. "The mode in which the experience appears is the form (whether as a perception, an image, or a thought.) Thus hypochondriacal ideas, for example, are contents of [such forms as] calling voices, compulsive ideas, or . . . delusions. The form of psychosis may be contrasted with its particular contents: for example, the periodic episodes of depression represented the form of the illness but its various contents may be suicide, alcoholism . . . and so forth" (p. 19). Jaspers-style psychopathology would thus lose interest in what the patients were actually saying, or hallucinating, in favor of studying the form of the psychosis—yet with the nuance that Jaspers and his school were highly interested in empathically placing themselves in the patients' shoes for the sake of determining whether the patients' psychology before the illness had been roughly congruent with the content of the illness—or whether the symptoms had come out of the blue. (*See* **PARANOIA: Jaspers's "pathological jealousy"** [1910].)

After Jaspers, phenomenology came to be used in two senses: (1) as by Jaspers, meaning the inner life of the patient, (2) as descriptions of clinical phenomena. Determing which phenomena are commonly held makes it possible to close in on causes of psychiatric diseases.

The first monograph of the Heidelberg phenomenology school (1924): **Willi Mayer-Gross** on *Self-Descriptions of Confusion: Oneiroid Experiences* (*Selbstschilderungen der Verwirrtheit: die oneiroide Erlebnisform*). He attempted to let the patients describe events occurring in their conscious processes. (*See* also **HEIDELBERG**.)

Ludwig Binswanger's study of "flight of ideas" (Ideenflucht), the beginning of existential psychiatry (1933). Binswanger (1881–1966), director of his family's private nervous clinic "Bellevue" in Kreuzlingen, Switzerland, had been interested in phenomenology since 1917, when he published an article in a Swiss medical weekly on that subject. In 1933, he took a careful look at mania from the manic patient's viewpoint, excerpting long passages of manic speech. The book is generally considered the beginning of a version of phenomenology, or of existential analysis, that Binswanger called in 1942 Daseinsanalyse (pronounced DA-zines-anah-loo-zuh), after the German philosopher Martin Heidegger's (1889–1976) concept of "Dasein," or being-in-the-world.

Freyhan's concept of "target symptoms" (1956). Fritz A. Freyhan (1912–1982), a young German-Jewish medical graduate who qualified in Berlin in 1937, then fled the Nazis and trained in psychiatry at the Delaware State Hospital in Farnhurst, remained imbued with German concepts of psychopathologic thinking. At Delaware, he presided over early trials of some of the new **antidepressants** and **antipsychotics**, realizing that for highly heterogeneous groups of "depressed" and "psychotic" patients the drugs were rather ineffective. In a paper given at a **National Institute of Mental Health** conference in 1956 that launched the Psychopharmacology Service Center, he spoke of his experiences with **chlorpromazine** and **reserpine**, arguing that research in psychopathology should be shifted from a Kraepelinian interest in outcome to responsiveness to drugs. "What we have to decide first and foremost is the effect of a pharmacological agent on behavior. This we can study clinically and measure in terms of the modifiability of specific psychopathological symptoms. To do so, we have to record all clinical observations in 'double-bookkeeping' fashion, listing target symptoms as well as clinical diagnoses" (in Cole, *Psychopharmacology*, p. 375).

Freyhan expanded his views in an article in *Neuropsychopharmacology* in 1961: "To think in terms of 'anti-schizophrenic' or even 'anti-psychotic' action impresses me as reckless. There is certainly no evidence of correlations between response to drugs and assumed entities labeled schizophrenia or psychosis" (p. 193). Psychopathologic thinking, he said, demanded that these patients be sorted into treatment-responsive syndromes on the basis of "target symptoms"; the syndromes would then be more responsive to the new drugs: "melancholic syndrome" in depression, consisting of the target symptoms of psychomotor retardation, apathy, sadness, somatic disturbances, and insomnia, was more responsive to the new antidepressant drugs than an "ideational" syndrome consisting of hypochondriasis, phobias, guilt, and delusions.

Phenomenology: current understanding in U.S. psychiatry (1998). In the second edition of their book *Perspectives of Psychiatry* (1998), Paul R. McHugh (1931–) and Phillip R. Slavney (1940–), both professors of psychiatry at Johns Hopkins University in Baltimore, explain that phenomenology represents the patient's answers to such queries as "What is your mood today?" "Are your thoughts clear?" Acknowledging **Karl Jaspers's** views of phenomenology as, in their words, "the results of eliciting and describing the personal mental experiences of patients," the authors continue, "We can learn how another person is thinking and feeling by talking to that person." Thus, the mental status examination is merely "a systematic way of talking to patients" (pp. 9–10). The phenomenological aspect of such an interview is not the content of the patient's answers but how the patient processes his thoughts.

PSYCHOPHARMACOLOGY. The study of the differential use of drugs to understand and modify neuochemistry and the psychiatric disorders to which anomalies in neurochemistry give rise.

The first researcher in the modern history of medicine to use a psychoactive drug in order to study differences in the form of illness was Jacques-Joseph Moreau (1804–1884, called "Moreau de Tours" because he had studied medicine in Tours). In a well-known monograph in 1845 on *Hashish and Mental Illness* (*Du hachisch et de l'aliénation mentale*), Moreau said that the effect of hashish, given in steadily increasing doses, in melancholic depression was quite different from that in retarded depression (un aliéné stupide) or in dementia. "In the demented patients the results . . . were virtually null, despite the high dose. It was the same for stupidity. Two melancholic patients, after five or six hours, experienced a quite lively arousal with all the characteristics of merriment and banter that are normal." "As soon as the arousal had passed, both patients relapsed to their former state" (pp. 402–403). This was the first modern demonstration of differential effectiveness in different illnesses and represents a distant anticipation of the birth of psychopharmacology 100 years later. (The next efforts to use drugs to study mental pathology would be the LSD research of the late 1940s and after. *See* **HALLUCINOGEN.**)

The term "psychopharmacology" was coined in 1920 by David Macht (1882–1961), a pharmacologist at Johns Hopkins University, in the *Johns Hopkins Hospital Bulletin*, to describe "the effect of drugs on psychological functions" (p. 167). In a wider sense, as Thomas Ban (1929–), at the time founding director of the division of psychopharmacology at **McGill University**, pointed out in his textbook *Psychopharmacology* in 1970, it is "a new scientific discipline which encompasses all the aspects and interactions between psychoactive drugs and biological systems" (p. vii). Contemporary use of the term dates from an article by **Jean Delay** and Jean Thuillier (1921–), who was Delay's assistant, on "Psychiatrie experimentelle et psychopharmacologie" in the *Hospital Gazette* (*Semaine des Hôpitaux*) in 1956. It came into general use after a conference in Milan in 1957.

Psychopharmacology as a field of study has conventionally been dated from the introduction of **chlorpromazine** in 1952. Yet, there were several striking earlier successes in the use of drugs to improve psychiatric conditions, notably William J. Bleckwenn's introduction of intravenous injections of amobarbital in 1930 to relieve catatonia. (*See* **BARBITURATES; CATATONIA.** For further details on the history of psychopharmacology, *see* the entries for **ANTIDEPRESSANT; ANTIPSYCHOTICS; BENZODIAZEPINES; DOPAMINE; EXTRAPYRAMIDAL SIDE EFFECTS; IPRONIAZID; LITHIUM; PARKINSONISM; RESERPINE; SELECTIVE SEROTONIN REUPTAKE INHIBITORS; TARDIVE DYSKINESIA.**)

PSYCHOSIS: EMERGENCE OF CONCEPTS. (*See* also **FOLIE À DEUX; FRENCH CHRONIC DELUSIONAL STATES** [from 1909]; **PARANOIA; PARAPHRENIA; POSITIVE VS. NEGATIVE; SCHIZOPHRENIA: EMERGENCE; UNITARY PSYCHOSIS.**) In medicine, psychosis can mean (1) loss of contact with reality, in the form of hallucinations, illusions, and delusions; (2) a synonym for schizophrenia (though one bears in mind there are many psychotic patients, such as those with mania, delirium, or dementia who are not schizophrenic); (3) severe mental illness of any kind; in other words, psychosis on a continuum from neurosis. In fact, for many years every mental illness was referred to as a "psychosis."

"The history of schizophrenia is actually the history of psychosis in general," wrote **Heidelberg** psychiatrist and schizophrenia expert Hans Gruhle (1880–1958) in 1932, because "from what was called at the beginning of the discipline of psychiatry . . . insanity, mental derangement, madness, derangement of mind, alienation, maladie mentale, folie . . . pazzia, the exogenous psychoses were increasingly split off, and schizophrenia remained the actual core of insanity." (Gruhle wrote these lines in Oswald Bumke's [1877–1950] great *Handbook of Mental Illnesses* [*Handbuch der Geisteskrankheiten*], vol 5, p. 1.) Although the histories of psychosis and of schizophrenia are highly intertwined, for conceptual simplicity this *Dictionary* discusses them separately. (*See* **SCHIZOPHRENIA: EMERGENCE** for Kraepelin's introduction of dementia praecox in 1893 and after.)

Views at the birth of psychiatry (late eighteenth century). When psychiatry as a discipline was born late in the eighteenth century, there were two schools of thought about the nature of insanity. One school maintained that it was a mental reflection of general body illness. **Philippe Pinel**, for example, one of the first originators of the concept of the therapeutic asylum, believed that mental illness could arise in such peripheral woes as a spasm of the stomach or a missed period. A second school believed madness to be a poorly understood affliction of the brain itself. Johann Christian Reil (1759–1813), a Leipzig psychiatrist, maintained in 1803 that the brain possessed its own energy—the torpid portions of it having too little, the exalted too much—and that these energy imbalances caused madness (*Meditations about the Application of the Psychic Method of Cure to Mental Disorders* [*Rhapsodien über die Anwendung der psychischen Curmethode auf Geisteszerrüttungen*], pp. 47, 49). As for the forms of insanity, most authors agreed there were two, mania and melancholia, the former meaning a general derangement of the mind, the latter a partial (also including the depression of the mood).

On the whole, these older authors put much greater emphasis on the content of insanity—on so-called associations—than on its form. A patient who had cut his penis off, for example, and had expressed confused religious ideas would be classified as suffering from "religious enthusiasm" rather than psychosis. Of the various components of psychosis, such as delusional thinking, hallucinations, and illusions—all being forms of insanity—differentiation would take place only in the course of the nineteenth century.

Pinel's "emotional insanity" (manie sans délire) (1801). In his textbook *Traité médico-philosophique sur l'aliénation mentale* (1801), **Philippe Pinel** made a fundamental division that was to run through French, German, and English psychiatry for the rest of the century: distinguishing between madness that does affect intelligence (called "mania with delirium," or manie avec délire), and madness that affects only emotions and drives but not intelligence (emotional insanity), or manie sans délire. In France, virtually every influential psychiatrist except the Falret family picked up this distinction, elaborating it in ever more refined subcategories. The opposing view would be articulated in Germany as "**unitary psychosis**" (Einheitspsychose), stipulating that it is not possible to have lesions that affect only the drives and emotions but not the intelligence. (In French psychiatry, the term "délire" can mean a number of conditions—especially delusions [*see* **PARANOIA**], but Pinel used it to mean a disorder of intelligence.) Pinel's manie sans délire was a condition that shaded lightly into **personality disorders** as well as madness.

Esquirol's monomania (1816, 1838). "The passions of the insane are impetuous," wrote **Étienne Esquirol** in 1816, "above all in mania and monomania; they are sad in lypemania, in dementia, and in imbecility" ("On Madness" ["De la folie"], p. 14). Esquirol reckoned lypemania to our modern concept of depression. With Esquirol's monomania, the second important differentiation in the larger notion of insanity takes place (after Pinel's emotional insanity, or manie sans délire). Esquirol defined monomania generally as the overvaluation of a single idea, as opposed to the excess of all brain functions of mania, with delusions or hallucinations but with intelligence preserved. "We have at Charenton [a Paris mental hospital] a monomaniac, age 30, who is convinced that every night he is led down into the galleries under the Opera" (*Maladies mentales*, I, p. 214).

In volume 2 of his *On Mental Illness* (*Des maladies mentales*), published in 1838, Esquirol subdivided monomania into three parts—affective, instinctual, and intellectual (p. 2) (on intellectual monomania, *see* **PARANOIA**). His "instinctual monomania" may be taken as an early description of **obsessive-compulsive disorder**, obsessive thoughts or compulsive actions. Yet, monomania as a whole represented for Esquirol a kind of partial insanity in which the personality is preserved and the patient's thinking is not "demented," or chaotic.

Hallucinations (1817). Esquirol revived the traditional term "hallucinations" in order to describe the symptoms of psychosis (délire); he did so in an essay "On Hallucinations" ("Des hallucinations"): "Someone who has the profound conviction of perceiving a current sensation, while no exterior object apt to excite this sensation is within range of his senses" (Maladies mentales, I, p. 159). He uses the term in its modern sense of perceptions without a real external stimulus. The phenomena of hallucinations as such, however, were long familiar in psychiatric writing (**William Cullen** had assigned them to the "Morbi Locales"; Sinnestäuschungen is the customary phrase in German; John Haslam of Bethlem Hospital talked in 1809 of "false perception" [*Observations on Madness*, second ed., p. 28]).

Differentiating illusions from hallucinations (1832). Esquirol described illusions as a symptom of psychosis: "Illusions, so frequent among the insane, deceive these patients about the qualities, the meaning and the causes of impressions currently being received, and give rise to false judgments about their internal and external sensations; reason does not rectify the error" ("On Illusions" ["Des illlusions"], p. 204). Esquirol employed here the modern sense of the term: distortion or misinterpretation of a real perception. Normal people can commit these misinterpretations as well, without a predisposition to illness, but they are more frequent in people with mental illness.

Madness is one disease, from 1822. *See* **UNITARY PSYCHOSIS.**

"Moral insanity" (insanity without hallucinations or delusions). *See* **PRICHARD, JAMES COWLES** (1835).

Distinction between momentary symptom picture and underlying disease process in psychiatry (1844). To some extent, physicians have always been aware that the symptoms at any moment are conceptually different from the underlying disease producing them (mumps in one moment can produce a swelling, in another, a fever). Yet, psychiatry has long had a tendency to make symptomatic diagnoses (e.g., kleptomania as a separate disease). In 1844, Carl Friedrich Flemming (1799–1880), chief physician of the newly opened asylum Sachsenberg, near Schwerin, made the explicit distinction: "With mental disorders we are not dealing directly with diseases but initially only with symptoms of diseases or with forms of unwellness." He told readers it was important to discern the actual diseases (Krankheiten) (*General Journal of Psychiatry* [*Allgemeine Zeitschrift für Psychiatrie*], 1844, p. 122).

"Psychosis" introduced (1845). After Vienna's Ernst von Feuchtersleben (1806–1849) had become secretary of the Medical Society, in 1844 he initiated a series of lectures on psychiatry. With **William Cullen's** class of "neuroses" in mind—meaning disease of the central nervous system—Feuchtersleben in his lectures coined the term "psychosis": "Where psychic phenomena present themselves abnormally, we speak of mental illness [Seelenkrankheit]; it is rooted in the mind [die Seele], and insofar as these phenomena are transmitted through the brain [das sinnliche Organ], they are rooted in the body, because the brain is the organ of the mind." "Every psychosis [disorder of the psyche] is at the same time a neurosis [disorder of the brain], because without the mediation of the nervous system no mental change is able to become manifest; but every neurosis is not simultaneously a psychosis" (p. 265). Psychosis and neurosis soon acquired directly opposite meanings from those intended by Feuchtersleben, who associated psychosis with mind, and neurosis with brain. His lectures were published in 1845 as *The Principles of Medical Psychology* (*Lehrbuch der ärztlichen Seelenheilkunde*). (Cullen had introduced "neurosis" in 1777.)

The concept of "psychosis" was then disseminated within medicine by Carl Friedrich Flemming's influential 1859 textbook, *Pathology and Treatment of the Psychoses* (*Pathologie und Therapie der Psychosen*).

Mania and melancholia as a result of degeneration (1857). In his *Treatise on Degeneration* (*Traité des dégénéréscences physiques, intellectuelles et morales de l'éspece humaine*), French psychiatrist **Bénédict-Augustin Morel** (1809–1873), medical supervisor of the St.-Yon asylum near Rouen, ascribed major psychiatric illnesses to the process of degeneration, an inherited tendency to disease as a result of poisoned ancestry. "Mental illness is degeneration," he wrote (p. 682). Across the generations, the signs of degeneration would, he said, become steadily more evident, resulting ultimately in sterility. There was evidence of a lesion of some kind in degeneration because asylum patients often have a "special cachet in their physiognomy" (p. 346). This was not the first doctrine of genetics in psychiatry, but it reverberated powerfully over the years and into the Nazi period. (*See also* **HYPOMANIA AND MANIA; PSYCHIATRIC GENETICS.**)

Dementia praecox (démence précoce) (1860). *See* **SCHIZOPHRENIA: EMERGENCE.**

Kahlbaum's Vesania typica (typical insanity) (1863). *See* **SCHIZOPHRENIA: EMERGENCE.**

Delusions and hallucinations as a separate illness (not a late stage of melancholy) (1865, 1867). Two German psychiatrists share the priority in seeing delusions and hallucinations as a separate illness ("primary"), not as a stage of mania or melancholia.

Snell: In 1865, Ludwig Daniel Christian Snell (1817–1892), superintendent of the asylum in Hildesheim, Germany, and pioneer of asylum farm-colonies, proposed that delusions and hallucinations (Wahnsinn) represented a "primary form of mental disturbance," distinct from melancholia (because of patients' elevated self-esteem) and from mania (because of the absence of flight of ideas and similar manic symptoms). He thought "monomania" an appropriate term. In his experience, mania and melancholia went downhill into various psychic endstages, but did not turn into monomania. Hence, monomania must be "primary" (*Allgemeine Zeitschrift für Psychiatrie*, 1865, quotes pp. 368–369).

Griesinger: Two years later, in his lecture in May 1867 on the occasion of the opening of the new psychiatric clinic at the Charité Hospital in Berlin, **Wilhelm Griesinger** said that delusions and hallucinations were "primary" forms of insanity (Primordialdelirien) that arose de novo without pathological emotions such as melancholy as precursors. Common forms were persecutory ideas involving suffering or expansive expressions of grandiosity. Griesinger cited Snell (as well as **Morel's** 1860 book that mentioned démence précoce) but went one step beyond them: inspired by the model of neurosyphilis, he hypothesized underlying brain disease as the cause of the delusions: "the ganglion cells of the cerebral gray matter." In the first edition of his textbook in 1845, Griesinger had denied the primordial nature of delusions and had considered mania and melancholia to be "primary disorders" (Elementarstörungen) (p. 49). Now he had turned a page. The lecture was published in 1868 in volume 1 of Griesinger's new journal, *The Archive of Psychiatry and Nervous Diseases* (*Archiv für Psychiatrie und Nervenkrankheiten*).

Hebephrenia (1871). *See* **SCHIZOPHRENIA: EMERGENCE.**

Catatonia (1874). *See* **SCHIZOPHRENIA: EMERGENCE.**

See **PARANOIA**, 1883.

Chronic systematized delusional disorder (délire chronique à évolution systématique) (1886, 1888, 1892). Beginning in 1886, Paris psychiatrist **Valentin Magnan**, in charge of the intake service at the **Ste.-Anne mental hospital**, introduced colleagues at the Medical-Psychological Society to his conception of a chronic kind of well-circumscribed delusional disorder that went through four stages after a period of incubation: inquietude-hallucinations, persecution, manic-grandeur, and dementia. The delusions were highly structured, hence the adjective "systematic," or "systematized." In 1888, Magnan published a series of articles on it in *Le Progrès médical*, then in 1892 together with his colleague Paul Sérieux (1864–1947), he described the disorder in a monograph entitled *Le délire chronique à évolution systématique*. Magnan attributed great importance to degeneration in other psychiatric illnesses and built considerably on the work of his teacher Prosper Lucas (1808–1885), who in 1850 had highlighted the importance of heredity in psychiatry (Lucas, *Philosophical Treatise on Natural Heredity* [*Traité philosophique de l'hérédité naturelle*]), as well as on **Ernest Lasègue's** "delusions of persecution" in 1852. (*See* **PARANOIA.**) Yet, Magnan's chronic systematized delusional disorder was found more in the "predisposed normal" than in the degenerate. In retrospect, it is difficult not to see Magnan's creation as an early description of dementia praecox, although Magnan, like many French psychiatrists, detested Kraepelin's term. (*See also* **FRENCH CHRONIC DELUSIONAL STATES.**)

La Bouffée délirante, or transitory delusional psychosis (1886, 1891). In 1886, **Valentin Magnan**'s students Honoré Saury (1854–?) and Paul-Maurice Legrain (1860–1939), in books of their own, each described the master's notions of la bouffée délirante, a concept so intensely French that even today in the international literature the French term is used. Then, in an 1891 monograph on chronic systematized delusional disorder (*see above*), Magnan himself mentioned these transitory (reactive) psychotic states, "bouffées délirantes," in contrast to the chronic downhill variety. Affecting mainly the degenerate, they might arrive out of the blue and then fade again as suddenly. Bouffées délirantes were widely diagnosed in French psychiatry and remain a nosological staple even today. After about 1910, the diagnosis lost the degenerative note.

Meynert's "amentia" (1890). **Theodor Meynert** described in his 1890 clinical lectures a form of sudden-onset confusion (Verwirrtheit), often with such psychotic symptoms as hallucinations, that he called "amentia," a term long in use in psychiatry for major illness (although following **William Cullen's** "amentia congenita" [1777], many authors used amentia to mean mental retardation.) Meynert distinguished this from dementia. (Amentia was a thinking disorder, whereas "dementia" was a personality deterioration.) Symptoms of amentia ran the gamut from excitement to stupor. Meynert saw amentia as relapsing but only occasionally ending in deterioration. He attributed it to disorders in the association fibers between the frontal lobe and other centers. "In almost every episode of confusion, remissions alternate with intensive symptoms, in the form of recovery and exhaustion. Sometimes the patients are confused in the morning . . . clearer towards evening. . . . Even in episodes of confusion they respond with rational declarations to external events. . . . In milder cases, the physician must not expect to find the patients continuously confused, but always prone, indeed prepared, to relapse into deep exhaustion and confusion" (p. 107).

Meynert's diagnosis met a rather ignominious end as **Emil Kraepelin** took it up, then in the eighth edition of his textbook (1910) assimilated "acute confusion (amentia)" to the forms of febrile delirium. Yet, the memory of "amentia" lingered on in Vienna among such Meynert students as Josef Berze (1866–1958) as yet another Viennese equivalent of Kraepelin's all-conquering "dementia praecox." (*See* **SCHIZOPHRENIA: EMERGENCE: Stransky's intrapsychic ataxia** [1903].) In 1936, Berze wrote in his memoir, "Meynert and Schizophrenia," in the *Journal of Combined Neurology and Psychiatry* (*Zeitschrift für die gesamte Neurologie und Psychiatrie*), "Meynert . . . with his amentia had essentially the same kind of cases as Kraepelin and **Bleuler.**" Between Meynert's "deficit in association" and Bleuler's "loosening of association" there was not such a big difference, Berze said (p. 273). Berze believed that if Meynert had lived, he rather than Kraepelin would have had the priority.

Emil Kraepelin's dementia praecox (after 1893). *See* **SCHIZOPHRENIA: EMERGENCE.**

Bleuler's schizophrenia (1908, 1911). *See* **SCHIZOPHRENIA: EMERGENCE.**

See **FRENCH CHRONIC DELUSIONAL STATES** (from 1909).

Karl Jaspers's "pathological jealousy" (meaning a delusion with jealousy as its content; Eifersuchtswahn) (1910). (*See* **PARANOIA.**) **Jaspers** did not believe in Kraepelin's dementia praecox as a single large disease. But, he did recognize that some psychoses probably had an underlying organic basis. In order to distinguish between psychotic patients whose prognosis was good from those whose was not, Jaspers differentiated between patients whose delusional jealousy was simply an extension of their lifelong suspiciousness ("personality development" patients [Entwicklung einer Persönlichkeit]) and "process" patients, whose symptoms came out of the blue on top of a basically normal premorbid personality. The "developmental" patients had good prospects for recovery; the "process" patients, whose normal mental life had been interrupted by a somatic disease, did not. Jaspers was not the first to use the term "process" as implying an organic illness with inexorable change. (The concept goes back to Heinrich Neumann's *Textbook of Psychiatry* in 1859.) Yet, the distinction between development and process became fundamental for several generations of psychiatrists, and as late as 1998 Paul McHugh (1931–), chair of psychiatry at Johns

Hopkins University, and his colleague Phillip Slavney (1940–) mused about it in their book, *Perspectives of Psychiatry* (second edition). Jaspers' 1910 paper appeared in the premier volume of the *Journal of Combined Neurology and Psychiatry* (*Zeitschrift für die gesamte Neurologie und Psychiatrie*).

See **FREUDIAN INTERPRETATIONS OF PSYCHOSIS AND SCHIZOPHRENIA** (1907).

Psychogenic (reactive) psychoses (1916). August Wimmer (1872–1937), then director of St. Hans Psychiatric Hospital near Roskilde, Denmark, and chair of psychiatry at the University of Copenhagen from 1921 to 1937, published in 1916 the first comprehensive account of the reactive psychoses, *Psykogene Sindssygdomsformer* (*Psychogenic Forms of Mental Diseases*). "[Their] distinctive feature is that they most often occur on a predisposed terrain that is exposed to psychological traumata," in the words of biographer Johan Schioldann-Nielsen (*History of Psychiatry*, 1993, p. 414). Wimmer did not actually discover the concept of reactive psychoses, which had been widely discussed in psychiatry at the turn of the century. He had been influenced by **Magnan's** 1893 concept of bouffées délirantes and by his 1895 book, *Les Dégénérés* (although Wimmer's key concept was reaction, whereas Magnan's was degeneration). Unlike the chronic conditions described by the French and Germans, these psychotic episodes remitted quickly. Wimmer's work was never translated into English but became a building block of Scandinavian psychiatry.*

In 1968, **Erik Strömgren** revived Wimmer's concept in an influential paper on "reactive psychoses," a term that he changed in 1974 to "psychogenic psychoses." (This appeared in a volume of classic papers in European psychiatry edited by Steven R. Hirsch [1937–] and **Michael Shepherd**.) "It must be stressed that these psychoses are regarded as being psychogenic in a restricted sense," he wrote. "The mental trauma must be of such a nature that the psychosis would not have arisen in its absence." He divided them into three groups: emotional reactions, disorders of consciousness, and paranoid states" (pp. 100–101). Strömgren later expressed bafflement that the concept of psychogenic psychosis, which represented around 10% of all admissions to Danish psychiatric hospitals, was viewed by the World Health Organization in its *International Classification of Diseases* as "rare" (Shepherd, *Psychiatrists*, p. 166).

Sensitive delusions of reference (sensitiver Beziehungswahn) (1918). This was the first important concept of Tübingen psychiatrist **Ernst Kretschmer**. His chief, Robert Gaupp, was intent upon demonstrating the existence of delusional disorders in patients who did not have schizophrenia (but rather reactive **paranoia**) and doubtless steered Kretschmer in this direction. Kretschmer postulated delusions as an independent illness in patients who did not have the underlying brain disease schizophrenia but rather were vulnerable because of specially "sensitive" premorbid personalities. The distinction that **Karl Jaspers** had made in 1910 between developmental illnesses in individuals with healthy personalities (in whom the illness was "understandable") and "process" illnesses in individuals with underlying brain disease

---

*Johan Schioldann-Nielsen, an Adelaide psychiatrist of Danish origin, currently has an English translation forthcoming from Adelaide Academic Press, with forewords by German Berrios and Nils Retterstol.

(in whom the illness was not "understandable") was quite influential in German psychiatry in those years, and Kretschmer identified here a series of transitions involving delusions and hallucinations between developmental forms and process forms. Kretschmer's book *Sensitive Delusions of Reference: A Contribution to the Question of Paranoia and to the Doctrine of Character in Psychiatry* (*Der sensitive Beziehungswahn: ein Beitrag zur Panaroiafrage und zur psychiatrischen Charakterlehre*) was published in 1918 and translated into several languages, being reissued as late as 1966. The diagnosis did not really catch on until after the Second World War. Some observers believe, however, that many patients with this diagnosis in fact have schizophrenia (Gruhle in Wilmanns, *Schizophrenie*, p. 30).

Kretschmer's constitutional psychoses (1921). Trying to make a link between physical type, personality, and illness, **Kretschmer** postulated in his book *Body Type and Character* (*Körperbau und Charakter*) the existence of three basic body types: athletic, meaning robustly developed skeleton, muscles, and skin, slightly prone to schizophrenia; asthenic, meaning thin bodies and limbs, prone to schizophrenia; and pyknic, large body-cavities (abdomen, thorax, cranium), tendency to fat, plus rather delicate limbs, prone to manic-depressive illness. "The manner in which these three types are distributed within schizophrenic and manic-depressive illness (circular) is very diverse and quite remarkable. Among healthy people as well, we find these types recurring everywhere, so they do not entail anything pathological in themselves. . . ." (seventh ed., 1929, p. 17). These associations between body type and psychiatric illness had a large impact on research in the next decades. In 1932, **Kurt Schneider** judged Kretschmer's body-type classification "the only really big contribution to clinical psychiatry since Kraepelin" (Schneider, *Problems of Clinical Psychiatry* [*Probleme der klinischen Psychiatrie*], 1932, p. 12).

Periodic catatonia (1932 and after). In 1932, Rolf Gjessing (1889–1959) of the Dikemark Psychiatric Hospital in Oslo, Norway, began the first of his lifelong investigations of the periodic forms of psychosis that Kraepelin (*see* **SCHIZOPHRENIA: EMERGENCE**) in 1913 had assigned to dementia praecox. By the time of Gjessing's 1938 article in the *Journal of Mental Science*, he linked the attacks to sharp periodic shifts in the body's nitrogen balance. The abnormal levels of nitrogen were treatable with the thyroid hormone thyroxin. This represents the first successful attempt to connect a schizophrenic syndrome with a biochemical body change. (Such conditions are rarely seen today because antipsychotic drugs have obliterated their periodicity.)

For further developments, *see* **SCHIZOPHRENIA: CURRENT CONCEPTS.**

PSYCHOSOMATIC. *See* **HYSTERIA-PSYCHOSOMATIC-SOMATIZATION.**

PSYCHOSURGERY. The modern history of operating on the brain to relieve mental illness begins with Swiss psychiatrist Gottlieb Burckhardt (1836–1907), who in 1882 became director of the private Préfargier Clinic in Marin, near Neuchâtel. Starting in December 1888, he operated on the brains of six patients to relieve the symptoms of schizophrenia. These largely unsuccessful operations, when reported at a medical congress in Berlin in 1890—and then in the *Allgemeine Zeitschrift für Psychiatrie* in 1891—caused disquiet in German medical circles; no further psychosurgery was done in Central Europe until leukotomy in the late 1930s. (*See* **LOBOTOMY.**)

Almost simultaneously, as historian German Berrios tells the story in *150 Years of British Psychiatry*, in 1889 Thomas Claye Shaw (1841–1927), a psychiatrist in a London asylum and lecturer in psychological medicine at St. Bartholomew's Hospital, asked surgeon Harrison Cripps (Fellow of the Royal College of Surgeons [FRCS], Eng. 1875) to open the cranium and resect the dura of a patient suffering from neurosyphilis, in order to drain off fluid that was increasing intracranial pressure. Reported in the *British Medical Journal* in the same year, this operation stimulated a wave of similar procedures in neuosyphilis as well as in other mental diseases—on the grounds that "relieving intracranial pressure" was therapeutic—in Britain, France, and the United States; this boom in psychosurgery continued until about the mid-1890s. Thereafter, little more psychosurgery was performed until the first leukotomy in late 1935 in Lisbon, Portugal. (*See* **LOBOTOMY**.)

PSYCHOTHERAPY. The last half of the eighteenth century saw a big upsurge of interest in using the doctor–patient relationship therapeutically, which is the essence of medical psychotherapy. In France after 1750, there had been much writing on "la médecine de l'esprit," or psychological medicine, and a number of English physicians had discoursed on the subject as well. The first systematic psychotherapies do not, however, appear until the 1880s.

On "moral treatment," in the sense of psychological treatment, ca. 1800, *see* **MORAL TREATMENT**.

Bernheim introduces the first systematic psychotherapy of "suggestion" (1883). Hippolyte Bernheim (1840–1919), professor of medicine at the University of Nancy in France, had learned from a general practitioner in Nancy (Ambroise-Auguste Liébeault [1823–1904]) how to reproduce "hysterical" phenomena with hypnotism, or "suggestion." Yet, Bernheim discovered as well that nonhypnotic suggestion, simply giving the patients instructions in a normal voice, could also produce and abolish hysterical phenomena. In an eight-part series of articles in the *Eastern Medical Review* (*Revue Médicale de l'Est*) in 1883, Bernheim explained that nonhypnotic suggestion had applications going beyond the treatment of hysteria. He asked rhetorically, "To what point are passions, instincts, tastes, and psychic faculties capable of being modified by prolonged and skilfully conducted suggestive therapy, either in the waking state or under hypnosis?" (p. 93 from his 1884 book, *On Suggestive Therapy under Hypnosis or in the Waking State* [*De la suggestion dans l'état hypnotique et dans l'état de veille*]).

First modern use of term "psychotherapy" (1887). Under the influence of Bernheim and the "Nancy school," two Dutch physicians, Frederik Willem van Eeden (1860–1932) and Albert Willem van Renterghem (1845–1939), opened in 1887 a "clinic for suggestive psychotherapy" in Amsterdam. The clinic was devoted entirely to hypnotherapy, and the two doctors reported their first results in 1889 in the book *Clinic in Suggestive Psychotherapy* (*Clinique de psycho-thérapie suggestive*), published in Brussels.

See **FREUDIAN PSYCHOTHERAPY: TECHNIQUE** (from 1893).

Dubois' "rational psychotherapy" (1904). Paul Dubois (1848–1918), a family doctor in Berne, Switzerland, who drifted into psychotherapeutics via electrotherapy, was the wellspring of the most important international psychotherapy movement before Freud: Dubois's rational psychotherapy, sometimes called "the persuasion method." Dubois, who shared the confidence of the liberal middle classes of the late-nineteenth century in reason, believed that psychoneurosis could be overcome in rational discussions with patients about their personal histories and the origin of their symptoms. He became the professor of neuropathology in Berne in 1902, and in his influential book *The Psychoneuroses and their Psychological Treatment* (*Les Psychonévroses et leur traitement moral*) that he published 2 years later (1904), he wrote that "for neurasthenia there is another psychotherapy altogether [than Bernheim's suggestion], a kind of psychological training that does not try to conjure away fatigue but to make it disappear by slowly suppressing its principal cause: emotivity" (p. xxiii). Dubois's rational psychotherapy may be seen as an ancestor of today's "**cognitive-behavioral therapy.**"

Jungian psychotherapy (from 1911). *See* **JUNG, CARL GUSTAV.**

"Milieu therapy": beginning of (1925). In 1918, August Aichhorn (1878–1949), a child-welfare specialist working for the city of Vienna in charge of organizing pediatric emergency services during the First World War, was asked to oversee a residential center for delinquent youth on the site of a former refugee camp in the Viennese suburb of Oberhollabrunn. Shortly thereafter, Aichhorn began his own training in psychoanalysis and attempted to model the education of these youngsters along psychoanalytic principles.

His book about these experiences, *Wayward Youth* (published in 1925 in German as *Verwahrloste Jugend* and translated into English in 1935), represented the first attempt to implement the principles of milieu therapy, recognizing the therapeutic nature of interactions within the setting itself. (*See* **CONDUCT DISORDER.**) Aichhorn and the school's pediatric-psychiatrist consultant Erwin Lazar (1877–1932) first allocated the pupils [Zöglinge] into psychologically more or less homogeneous groups, then resolved to let the groups themselves undertake the work of reform: "The more that the collective life of the pupils in the group alone—without further pedagogic measures—therapeutically improves dissocialization, the better is the allocation to the groups. So the question is: which delinquents have to be sorted with which, in order to achieve from the simple act of living together the best preconditions for re-socialization?" (p. 187 of the German ed.).

Aichhorn contrasted his own residential school with the typical Austrian reform schools for bad adolescents: "It was clear to us from the very beginning at the simple emotional level that we had to bring some fun [Freude] into the lives of boys and girls and young people from the ages of fourteen to eighteen. It had never occurred to any of us to see them as delinquents or even criminals from whom society had to be protected; for us they were people on whom life had imposed too great a burden, whose negative attitudes and hate of society was justified; a milieu therefore had to be created for them in which they could feel at ease. And in fact that just sort of happened automatically" (p. 192).

Narcotherapy. *See* **BARBITURATES: narcotherapy** (1930).

Group psychotherapy. Since the nineteenth century, psychiatrists have realized that therapeutic benefits occur when patients work, play, and collaborate together. In 1842, William Alexander Francis Browne (1805–1885), who had just become medical officer of the newly established Crichton Royal Hospital in Dumfries, Scotland, began to encourage patients to stage amateur theatricals involving "farces, vaudevilles [and] comedies by members of their own community, by those participating in their own infirmities." He saw these efforts as an aspect of "mental therapeutics," "a means of calling forth neglected energies, of diffusing bustle, and expectation, and enjoyment where all is generally dead and dull and dark, of creating sources of happiness on the very limits . . . of surveillance" (*Journal of Mental Science*, 1864, p. 333).

Beginning in 1911, Jakob Moreno-Lewy (1892–1974), at the time a medical student in Vienna, began organizing for young people, in entirely nonmedical settings such as taverns, a kind of impromptu theater, or "immediate" theater, that he called Stegreiftheater. He went on to train briefly in psychiatry under **Wagner-Jauregg**; in 1922, while serving as a factory doctor in the Viennese suburb of Bad Vöslau, Moreno established in the city center a permanent impromptu theater; he described his dramaturgical techniques the following year in the small book *Impromptu Theater* (*Stegreiftheater*). In passing he noted that impromptu techniques could have medical applications as well (later called "psychodrama"): "Life is the inhaling of the soul, impromptu the exhaling. Through inhaling, poisons (conflicts) arise; through impromptu they are once again discharged. On this basis rests its therapeutic significance" (p. 71). Yet, at this point he did not use the term "group therapy," however implicit it may have been in his approach.

Moreno emigrated to the United States in 1925. At a luncheon for the National Committee on Prisons and Prison Labor in 1931, Moreno had suggested the introduction of group psychotherapy at Sing Sing Prison in New York State. This proposal received written form in the National Committee's *Application of the Group Method to Classification* ("second edition") in 1932, and Moreno reprinted parts of it in 1971 under the title *The First Book on Group Psychotherapy*, "third edition."

It must be pointed out, however, that group psychotherapy was already a reality at several U.S. institutions as early as 1930, although these innovations were not widely reported. In 1930, Louis Wender (1890–1966), chief psychiatrist at Hillside Hospital, then at Hastings-on-Hudson, introduced for economic reasons what he called "group psychotherapy": Sitting about and talking with the patients was cheaper than individual psychotherapy.

In an article in *Mental Hygiene* in 1939, **Paul Schilder** explained that classical psychoanalysis was too long and expensive to be practical for most patients. "A year and a half ago," he said, "I began an experiment in group psychotherapy in the Out-Patient Department of the Psychiatric Division of Bellevue Hospital [in New York]." Groups of two to seven patients under the leadership of a physician would meet several times a week. The patients were encouraged to gain psychoanalytic insights, and they would have to file a written report after they had achieved them. Schilder also handed out "elaborate" questionnaires. Subsequent techniques of group therapy differed so radically from Schilder's that it is difficult to see him as having priority with the concept of "group." Yet he appears to have popularized the phrase.

Apparently ignorant of Schilder's usage, in 1943 in the *Lancet*, two British military psychiatrists, Wilfred R. Bion (1897–1979) and John Rickman (1891–1951), seconded from the **Tavistock Clinic** and who had been at Northfield Military Hospital near Birmingham, described the analysis of "intra-group tensions" as the task of "group therapy." They wrote as though the term were already quite familiar. Bion drafted the part of the report dealing with rehabilitation ("therapeutic cooperation" at group meetings discussing the program) (p. 678) and Rickman the part on "group therapy in a small ward": He dilated upon patients' "personal difficulties in putting the welfare of the group in the first place during their membership of group" (p. 680).

"Therapeutic community" (from 1939). Also known as "milieu therapy" (*see above*). In 1938, Joshua Bierer (1901–1984), a Viennese psychologist who had trained with Alfred Adler (1870–1937) and had acquired experience doing group psychotherapy in Palestine in the 1920s and Vienna in the 1930s, fled to England. In 1939, he was taken on as a psychotherapist at Runwell Hospital, an asylum in Essex, where he proceeded to help the patients organize a self-governing social club, the first therapeutic community in a psychiatric setting. (He described this work in the *Journal of Mental Science* in 1941, then again in an article on "Group Psychotherapy" in the *British Medical Journal* in 1942.) Bierer referred to the technique as "'community' treatment."

Shortly thereafter, at Mill Hill Emergency Hospital, where part of the **Maudsley Hospital** had removed during the Second World War, Maxwell Jones (1907–1990), a young Scottish staff psychiatrist, noted that a self-help group the patients themselves had organized was having an energizing effect. He encouraged them to begin doing some psychodrama and, by 1944, it was clear to Jones that group interactions in and of themselves were therapeutically beneficial. Beginning in 1945, Jones and co-workers organized these ideas on a larger scale at the Southern Hospital at Dartford in Kent, where interest in "therapeutic communities" was now considerable. Jones described this work in 1952 in his book *Social Psychiatry: A Study of Therapeutic Communities*.

The phrase "therapeutic community" itself was coined by English psychiatrist Thomas ("Tom") Main (1911–1990) in an article in the *Menninger Clinic Bulletin* in 1946 on a therapeutic "setting" he had encouraged at Northfield Military Hospital, as toward the end of the war he was appointed there. (*See* **TAVISTOCK CLINIC**.) Main's concept emphasized close emotional contacts among staff themselves and between staff and patients. Under the subheading "a therapeutic community," he explained that "The Northfield Experiment is an attempt to use a hospital not as an organization run by doctors in the interests of their own greater technical efficiency, but as a community with the immediate aim of full participation of all its members in its daily life and the eventual aim of the resocialization of the neurotic individual for life in ordinary society" (p. 67).

Bion and John Rickman helped import the notion of group therapy to the Tavistock Clinic once they resumed work as staff members.

The American story (after 1945). After the Second World War, the United States came to dominate the international psychotherapy story. Ironically, it was in psychotherapy systems practiced more by psychologists than psychiatrists that American psychiatry first started to make its world impact. After the Second World War, virtually no more novel psychotherapy systems originated in Europe: all were American. Owing little to Freud, Jung, or any of the other classic writers, the American psychotherapies disclaimed the doctor–patient hierarchy and could also be administered by psychologists and social workers to "clients." In international persective, they proved to be world-beaters.

"Therapeutic community" in the United States (from the late 1940s.) Anglo-Saxon notions of therapeutic community crossed the Atlantic quickly. Beginning in the late 1940s, patient self-government in the United States blossomed at the Boston Psychopathic Hospital—in 1956 renamed the Massachusetts Mental Health Center ("Mass Mental")—under the leadership of assistant superintendent Robert W. Hyde (1910–?), who is also remembered for having brought research on LSD (*see* **HALLUCINOGEN**) to the United States. In the mid-1950s, Milton Greenblatt (1914–1994), who had been on staff during this reform period and who became director of clinical psychiatry at Mass Mental, headed a team sponsored by the Russell Sage Foundation that aimed at implementing such reforms at other Massachusetts mental hospitals. Greenblatt's 1955 report, *From Custodial to Therapeutic Patient Care in Mental Hospitals*, concluded that various new somatic therapies together with "the therapeutic use of the social environment" could return a large number of patients to the community.

In 1961, these concepts received a powerful push in the United States with the report of the Joint Commission on Mental Illness and Health, *Action for Mental Health*. The commission had been struck in 1955 as a joint project of the American Medical Association and the American Psychiatric Association and was supported by Congress. Headed by Jack R. Ewalt (1910–), the Massachusetts commissioner of mental health, it was ultimately joined by 36 other organizations. Among the reports subcontracted by the joint commission, there was one on patient care by Brandeis University sociologist Morris S. Schwartz (1916–), who had been co-author with psychiatrist Alfred H. Stanton (1912–1983) in 1954 of an influential study of the hospital as social setting (*The Mental Hospital*). Their basic recommendation of the principles of the therapeutic milieu made it into the main 1961 report ("the new mental hospital: a therapeutic community," p. 46), although Schwartz's book, cowritten with Charlotte Green Schwartz, *Social Approaches in Mental Patient Care*, was not published until 1964. The authors argued that creating a "therapeutic milieu" in a psychiatric hospital involved (1) making the institution as a whole "democratic, treatment-oriented [and] flexible"; (2) encouraging the staff to be "sympathetic, friendly, and respectful to patients"; and (3) using the milieu to achieve specific effects with patients, such as "accept[ing] the idea that he is ill, develop[ing] insight into the reasons for his illness," among other objectives (pp. 164–165).

Carl Rogers's "client-centered therapy" (from 1946). With Rogers, the transition of psychotherapy begins from the hands of physicians and psychoanalysts to those of clinical psychologists and psychiatric social workers. Rogers's client-centered therapy was "humanistically" oriented, unlike theory-based Freudian, biological, and behavioral therapies, and opened a new chapter in the history of psychotherapy. As Harry Specht (1929–1995), Dean of the School of Social Welfare at the University of California at Berkeley, noted in the *Social Service Review* in 1991, "The journey of the [social work] profession over this century appears to end here [with Rogers] as social workers become part of the institution of popular psychotherapy, one of the major battalions in the armies of the secular priesthood to carry forth the tenets of the church of individual repair" (p. 353).

Carl Rogers (1902–1987) graduated with a Ph.D. in clinical psychology at Columbia University in 1931 and taught at Ohio State University until 1945, when he went to the University of Chicago to start a counseling center. In 1940, in the *Journal of Consulting Psychology*, Rogers outlined some of his ideas without using the term "client-centered therapy." His landmark article, "Significant Aspects of Client-Centered Therapy," appeared in *American Psychologist* in 1946, describing a therapeutic procedure with a "predictable" outcome in which the therapist played only a "cathartic role." The article seized what was to be the core of Rogers's approach and that of the human potential movement: "Within the client reside constructive forces whose strength and uniformity have been either entirely unrecognized or grossly underestimated." The therapy was orderly and predictable because the therapist simply relied upon those forces. Catharsis and insight in therapies were not new, he said. "But we have not known or recognized that in most if not all individuals there exist growth forces, tendencies toward self-actualization, which may act as the sole motivation for therapy." "All of these capacities I have described are released in the individual if a suitable psychological atmosphere is provided."

After a brief stint at the University of Wisconsin, Rogers took a research position at an institute in La Jolla, California, remaining there until his death. Rogers's first book on the subject was his *Client-Centered Therapy* (1951).

As Rogers's approach developed, it came to have the following features (as he explained in Silvano Arieti's psychiatry textbook [1966]): (1) a therapeutic climate in which the therapist conveys to the patient his "congruence," or genuineness, his "unconditional positive regard" for the patient (meaning complete acceptance of the patient as he or she is); and a "sensitively accurate empathic understanding." (2) "Client-centered" meant the therapy's focus on the patient's "phenomenal world," the patient's immediate thoughts and experiences rather than offering advice or interpretations from outside. (3) The central objective of therapy was change and growth in the human personality, feeding into the "human potential movement," with which Rogers's name was closely associated alongside Friedrich ("Fritz") Perls (1893–1970) (*see* **GESTALT THERAPY**) and others.* By the early 1960s, it was clear to Rogers and his circle that this kind of growth could be stimulated in intensive group experiences, sometimes called "T-Groups," "Sensitivity Training Groups," "Basic Encounter Groups," and the like.

Rogers thought of his client-centered approach as a kind of "third force" in American psychology, alongside Freudian psychoanalysis and behaviorism. Rogers played "a major role," as Peter Steinglass puts it, "in wresting the practice of psychotherapy from psychiatry alone and distributing it into the hands of psychology and other disciplines" (Steinglass in Kaplan, *Comprehensive Textbook of Psychiatry*, sixth ed., p. 1866).

The term "milieu therapy" becomes popularized by Bruno Bettelheim (1948). Bettelheim (1903–1990), another Viennese, had studied psychology at the University of Vienna (he had a year of psychoanalysis with Richard Sterba [1898–1989]), then emigrated to the United States in 1939 where he began an academic career in the Chicago area teaching psychoanalytically oriented psychology, mainly at the University of Chicago. In 1944, he became director of the Sonia Shankman Orthogenic School, a residential treatment center for disturbed children at the university. Many of the children were autistic, and it was in this context that, in an article in the

---

* Fritz Perls's **Gestalt therapy** is the one exception to the claim that the postwar psychotherapy systems in the United States were homegrown.

American Journal of Orthopsychiatry in 1948 on "A therapeutic milieu," he and collaborator Emmy Sylvester (1910–), a child psychiatrist and psychoanalyst, elaborated the term "milieu therapy": "A therapeutic milieu is characterized by its inner cohesiveness which alone permits the child to develop a consistent frame of reference. . . . Emphasis on spontaneity and flexibility . . . makes questions of schedule or routine subservient to the relevance of highly individualized and spontaneous interpersonal relationships" (p. 192). As the authors observed in the *Psychoanalytic Review* in 1949, "Milieu therapy is not new as a psychotherapeutic technique. It is no more than the application of psychoanalytical concepts to the specific task of creating a setting for emotionally disturbed children who are in need of residential treatment."

Among Bettelheim's many publications arising from the Orthogenic School, perhaps his best known is *The Empty Fortress* (1967). (*See* **AUTISM**.) The book had virtually nothing to say about therapeutic community and analogized at length between the situation of autistic children and concentration camp inmates: "Infantile autism is a state of mind that develops in reaction to feeling oneself in an extreme situation, entirely without hope," comparable to those death-camp prisoners, called by the prisoners "moslems," who too had abandoned hope (p. 68). The nature of the therapies Bettelheim actually practiced at his school has subsequently become enveloped in controversy (*see* Nina Sutton, *Bruno Bettelheim: the Other Side of Madness*, translated from French in 1995), but the principles that he enunciated in his publications have been highly influential.

Family therapy (from 1956). Although mental-health professionals have always considered the patient's relationship to other family members, "family therapy" as a field implies counseling various family members together in the same room, usually with schizophrenia as the focus. Nathan Ackerman (1908–1971) is generally considered the founder of the field. While a staff psychiatrist at the **Menninger** Clinic (where he had trained), in 1937 Ackerman wrote an article in the *Bulletin of the Kansas Mental Hygiene Society* on the centrality of the family in mental illness. The landmark event in the history of family therapy is his cofounding in 1956 of the "family mental health clinic" (of which he was director) at the Jewish Family Service in New York; he was also an associate clinical professor at Columbia University. In 1958, Ackerman wrote in his book *The Psychodynamics of Family Life: Diagnosis and Treatment of Family Relationships*, "Over a span of time the critical focus of conflict and anxiety may move from one family member to another or gravitate first to one family pair and then to another. . . . The patterns of interpersonal conflict within the family affect the vicissitudes of control of internalized conflict" (p. 11). In other words, it was the family as a whole, not the identified patient, that was ill.

Simultaneously, a group was forming in Palo Alto, California, to examine the psychotherapy of schizophrenia. In 1952, Gregory Bateson (1904–1980), an anthropologist at the Palo Alto Veterans Administration hospital, had received a Rockefeller grant to study communication, and in 1954 he launched a research project on "schizophrenic communication." In 1956, Bateson, Donald D. Jackson (1920–1968), who was a psychiatrist and psychoanalyst, Jay Haley (1923–), a psychotherapist whom Bateson recruited for the schizophrenia project, and psychotherapist John H. Weakland (ca. 1919–1995) contributed an article to the first volume of the journal *Behavioral Science*, in which they described a family communications theory of schizophrenia. They maintained that within the family the patient is in a "'double bind'—a situation in which no matter what a person does, he 'can't win.'" As part of this project, in 1959 Jackson founded the Mental Research Institute in Palo Alto, the focus of which was schizophrenia.

Even though the leaders of family therapy declared their debt to the European psychoanalytic tradition, family therapy and Rogers's client-centered therapy count as the first genuinely American contributions to the international science of psychiatry in the twentieth century. They owed little to psychoanalysis and instead, as "popular psychotherapies," had their roots in American "mind cure" traditions of the nineteenth century.

Cognitive-behavioral therapy (CBT) (from 1963). (*See* **COGNITIVE-BEHAVIORAL THERAPY.**) CBT in the United States is heavily associated with the work of psychiatrist Aaron Beck (1921–). Its roots go back to the work of **Pierre Janet** and Paul Dubois (1848–1918) at the turn of the century.

"Interpersonal psychotherapy of depression" (from 1967). Inspired by the approach of **Harry Stack Sullivan** to interpersonal relations in illness, beginning in 1967 the members of the New Haven-Boston Collaborative Depression Research Project, led by **Gerald Klerman**, set out to develop a brief, focused form of psychotherapy for the ambulatory depressed patients in the project. They first field-tested the procedure on 150 "neurotic depressed female patients," finding no significant difference between those on the antidepressant amitriptyline (*see* **IMIPRAMINE AND TRICYCLIC ANTIDEPRESSANTS**) and those on psychotherapy (announcing their findings in 1974 in the *American Journal of Psychiatry*). After extensive field testing, there followed in 1984 a definitive manual of IPT: *Interpersonal Psychotherapy of Depression: A Brief, Focused, Specific Strategy*. The authors were Klerman, who died just before the book was published; his wife **Myrna Weissman** (1935–), a professor of psychiatric epidemiology at Yale University; and Bruce J. Rounsaville (1949–), a professor of psychiatry at Yale. As they explained, "We are convinced . . . that clinical depression occurs in an interpersonal context and that psychotherapeutic interventions directed at this . . . context will facilitate the patients' recovery from the acute episode and possibly have preventive effects against relapse" (pp. 5–6). Although the authors acknowledged the influence of several psychoanalytic thinkers, they emphasized that IPT was not intended to work upon the unconscious, but rather upon "current disputes, frustrations, anxieties, and wishes" arising from the patient's current social relations: "The work focuses on the 'here-and-now'" (p. 7).

The discovery that psychotherapy produces brain changes (1996). A team of researchers at the University of California at Los Angeles led by Jeffrey M. Schwartz (1951–) of the department of psychiatry discovered that successful treatment of obsessive-compulsive disorder (OCD) with psychotherapy—**cognitive-behavioral therapy**—produced actual physiological changes (changed glucose metabolism) in those parts of the brain thought to be responsible for producing the symptoms of OCD; namely, the caudate nucleus and adjacent circuits. The research, published in the *Archives of General Psychiatry* in 1996, involved **neuroimaging** with positron emission tomography (PET) and a radiolabeled form of glucose. The discovery is of interest because it suggests the effectiveness of psychological treatments at the biological level.

PTSD. *See* **POSTTRAUMATIC STRESS DISORDER.**

Q–R

RADÓ, SÁNDOR (1890–1972). Born in Kisvarda, Hungary, Radó first earned a Ph.D. in political science before graduating with an M.D. from the University of Budapest in 1915. After a residency in psychiatry and some psychoanalytic training (in 1913 he was a founding member of the Hungarian Psychoanalytic Society), in 1923 he left Hungary for Berlin and taught at the Berlin Psychoanalytic Institute. From this base he became a movement insider. In 1926, Freud appointed him editor of two psychoanalytic journals, *Zeitschrift für Psychoanalyse* and *Imago*. In 1931, Abraham Brill (1874–1948) asked him to come to New York and organize training at the just-founded New York Psychoanalytic Institute. Radó left the psychoanalytic institute in 1941 after some disagreements with the more orthodox members, part of the tumult known as the "New York psychoanalytic civil wars." In 1944, he was appointed professor of psychiatry at Columbia University, and early in 1945 he became head of the newly opened Columbia University Psychoanalytic and Psychosomatic Clinic for Training and Research, the first such training institute within a university (and for that reason much opposed by the analytic community, who disliked the idea of university control of psychoanalytic training). In 1957, he retired from Columbia and became professor of psychiatry and dean of the New York School of Psychiatry, from which he retired as dean emeritus in 1967. Radó's name is associated with a number of concepts in psychiatry, including depression (*see* **DEPRESSION: EMERGENCE: depressive neurosis** [1927]); schizotypal personality (*see* **SCHIZOID PERSONALITY** [1953]); and "adaptational psychodynamics," a term he coined in 1956. He explained it as follows in 1959 in Silvano Arieti's (1914–1981) psychiatry textbook: "Freud attributed irrational thought to the influence of instincts, with emotions implied; we attribute irrational thought to the influence of emotions, with nothing implied but the organism which has them. We place emotions in the forefront of investigative interest" (Arieti, *Handbook*, I, pp. 327–328).

RAPID EYE MOVEMENT SLEEP. *See* **REM SLEEP.**

REACTIVE DEPRESSION. *See* **DEPRESSION: EMERGENCE: vital vs. reactive depression** (1920).

REES, WILLIAM LINFORD LLEWELYN (1914–). Pioneer of controlled drug trials in psychiatry, Rees was born in rural Wales, the son of a family of teachers (he said that he entered medicine "to avoid becoming a teacher"), and received his medical degree from the Welsh National School of Medicine in 1938. After serving as a house officer at the Worcester asylum in Powick, he came down to London in 1940 to do a Diploma in Psychological Medicine at the **Maudsley Hospital** (which had already moved to its wartime location at Mill Hill). In 1947, he left the Maudsley, where he had become a staff psychiatrist, for several mental-hospital posts in Wales, returning to London in 1954 as a consultant physician to the now combined Bethlem Royal Hospital and

Maudsley Hospital. In 1966, he became professor of psychiatry at St. Bartholomew's Hospital ("Barts").

It was, however, when Rees was in South Wales running outpatient clinics that he and Carl Lambert carried out several important trials. In 1950, Rees reported at the First World Congress on Psychiatry in Paris a study of **insulin coma therapy**, **electroconvulsive therapy**, and leukotomy (**lobotomy**) in the treatment of schizophrenia, compared to a randomized group of historic controls (patients admitted to hospital before these treatments were available). He found insulin coma therapy most effective of all.

Then, Rees and Carl Lambert carried out a controlled trial of **chlorpromazine** in anxiety states. Designed as a crossover study (one half of the patients took chlorpromazine, another half took the dummy tablets, then unknowingly switched halfway through), it did not employ the standard later technique of randomized parallel groups. "It didn't take me long to get a hundred anxiety states," Rees later said. "Colleagues in London were flabbergasted but it was different there because I had an unlimited supply of patients." He presented the findings in 1955 at a conference in Paris that **Jean Delay**, **Pierre Deniker**, and **Pierre Pichot** had organized on chlorpromazine, then published them the same year in the *Journal of Mental Science*. He found that the drug was only of marginal utility in anxiety "because people with executive or responsible positions had their anxiety relieved but it also eroded their enthusiasm and motivation," Rees said in a later interview (with David Healy). Rees and collaborators went on to do a long series of controlled trials on various psychiatric drugs, with the further refinement that the patients were usually randomized to the treatment group or the control group. This technique of randomized control trials (RCTs) became the gold standard for clinical trials in psychopharmacology.*

REM (RAPID EYE MOVEMENT) SLEEP. REM sleep is the lightest of the various sleep stages and is characterized by rapid movement of the eyeballs back and forth. Its existence was discovered by Eugene Aserinsky (1921–1998), a graduate student in the physiology laboratory of Nathaniel Kleitman (1895–1999), professor of physiology at the University of Chicago, who established the world's first sleep laboratory after joining the faculty in 1925 and who is generally considered "the first scholar of sleep." Working on the physiology of sleep, Aserinsky established with the electrooculogram that children's eyelids move frequently at certain times of night. Then, he and Kleitman studied brain activity in adults with an electroencephalograph (EEG). By waking subjects up during REM and non-REM sleep, they determined that dreams often occur in the REM phase, reporting their findings in 1953 in *Science*. The authors referred to "rapid, jerky eye movements" or "eye motility periods" rather than to "REM" as such. It was said of Aserinsky's first findings that Kleitman thought either he had made a remarkable discovery or that the old EEG machine that Aserinsky found in a university basement was

---

* With the exception of Myron Prinzmetal's trial of amphetamine in 1935 (*see* **narcolepsy**), the first controlled trial in American psychopharmacology was conducted by pharmacologist Louis Lasagna (1923–2003) at Johns Hopkins University, comparing some of the new hypnotic drugs to the barbiturates (the latter won); it was published in the *Journal of Chronic Diseases* in 1956.

broken. (It was also said that Aserinsky left Chicago because he was miffed at having to include Kleitman as co-author.)

William Charles Dement (1928–), another student of Kleitman who worked as Aserinsky's research assistant, began monitoring subjects' sleep continuously all night rather than just over short periods. In 1955, he published in the *Journal of Nervous and Mental Disease* on the difference in "rapid eye movement" and dream recall between schizophrenics and controls. In 1957, the year he received his Ph.D. (he had earned an M.D. in 1955), he and Kleitman defined the normal human sleep cycle in *Electroencephalography and Clinical Neurophysiology*, dividing sleep into four stages, rapid eye movement sleep occuring predominantly in stage one, the lightest stage.

The question of REM sleep was of enormous interest in neurophysiology, of course, because it opened new ways of understanding the brain. Clinical psychiatry in the 1950s was mainly interested in sleep and dreams as a hoped-for avenue to the unconscious. Sleep REM became of renewed curiosity later because psychoactive medications often diminish REM sleep as well as the deep stages of sleep. In 1969, Allan Rechtschaffen (1927–), professor of psychology at the University of Chicago, together with Dement who by now was professor of psychiatry at Stanford University and director of its Sleep Research Laboratory, proposed in an article in A. Kales's *Sleep: Physiology and Pathology* that in certain kinds of **narcolepsy**, the sleep episodes are attacks of REM sleep.

RESERPINE, AN EARLY PSYCHIATRY DRUG (from 1954). Although Ayurvedic practitioners in India had used the roots of the Rauwolfia plant for centuries in the treatment of mental illness, it was only in the early 1950s that the drug became part of the revolution in psychopharmacology then underway. In 1952, three scientists of the Ciba company in Basel—J. M. Müller, E. Schlittler, and H. J. Bein—in an article in *Experientia,* isolated the alkaloid reserpine as the sedative principle of *Rauwolfia serpentina* Benth. Clinical use began, as Albert Kurland (1914–), director of research at Spring Grove State Hospital in Catonsville, Maryland, tells the story, on a spring Sunday in May 1953, as **Nathan Kline** was reading an article in the *New York Times* about R. A. Hakim, an Indian psychiatrist "of the Western school" at the Hospital for Mental Health of Ahmedabad, who had received a medal for his work on the cure of schizophrenia with a preparation from the Rauwolfia plant. Two U.S. pharmaceutical companies were already making Rauwolfia and its alkaloids available for the treatment of hypertension; from Squibb and Sons, Kline got a preparation of the whole root marketed as Raudixin, and from Ciba he obtained the alkaloid reserpine, which had been marketed under the trade name of Serpasil. Kline and co-workers gave them both to psychotic inpatients at the Rockland State Hospital in Orangeburg, New York. In April 1954, Kline reported in the *Annals of the New York Academy of Sciences* on the effectiveness of both the extract (reserpine) and the root; this was almost exactly at the time that **chlorpromazine** was being launched in the United States. In July 1954, **Jean Delay** and **Pierre Deniker** gave a similar account of reserpine in the *Congrès des aliénistes et neurologues de langue française*.

These findings were confirmed in 1955, in a randomized controlled trial, as David Lewis Davies (1911–1983) and **Michael Shepherd** of the **Maudsley Hospital** established that reserpine had some effectiveness in the treatment of anxious and depressed patients.* This important research, published in 1955 in the *Lancet,* was widely ignored.

On August 26, 1955, at the Laboratory of Chemical Pathology of the National Heart Institute, Alfred Pletscher (1917–), who was a guest scientist from Roche in Basel, Parkhurst A. Shore (1924–), and Bernard B. Brodie (1909–1989), the head of the laboratory, announced in *Science* that administering reserpine to rabbits seemed to drive down the levels of serotonin in the cells of their intestines (the drug caused release of serotonin, in other words).† Because there was already evidence that reserpine affected behavior, the authors speculated that, "some of the central [brain] effects of reserpine are mediated through the release of serotonin. It is conceivable that the beneficial effects of reserpine in mental disturbances result from the liberation of serotonin" (p. 375). This was one of the earliest empirical findings pointing to the psychiatric role of the **neurotransmitter** serotonin and really represents the birth of biochemical psychiatry (although later psychopharmacologists sought to keep the level of serotonin up rather than to drive it down, or "liberate" it). (*See* **SELECTIVE SEROTONIN REUPTAKE INHIBITORS.)**

Using Brodie's reserpine model, Swedish pharmacologist Arvid Carlsson (1923–), then at Lund University, and his colleague Bertil Waldeck discovered in 1958 that **dopamine** ("3-hydroxytryptamine") was a neurotransmitter (*see* his article in *Science,* February 28; he actually submitted the article in 1957); in 1959 in *Pharmacological Reviews,* Carlsson speculated that it might be deficient in Parkinson's disease.

In 1961, reserpine ceased being marketed for psychiatric indications because of side effects. Yet, interest in reserpine as a potentially useful psychiatric drug has continued, and in 1998, in an article entitled "Reserpine exhumed" in the *British Journal of Psychiatry,* Irish psychiatrist David Healy (1954–) suggested that reserpine should be reexamined for its potential as an antidepressant.

ROBINS, ELI (1921–1994). A pioneer in the United States of rigorous diagnostic thinking, Robins was born in Rosenberg, Texas, into an immigrant family from Russia. He earned his M.D. at Harvard in 1943, then trained in psychiatry and neurology at **McLean Hospital** and the Massachusetts General Hospital, coming under the influence of the intensely anti-psychoanalytic Harvard psychiatrist-turned-neurologist Mandel Cohen (1907–2000). Robins initially considered Washington University in St. Louis because he wanted to work there with pharmacologist Oliver Lowry (1910–1996).

---

* Davies succeeded **Aubrey Lewis** as Dean of the Institute of Psychiatry at the Maudsley, holding office from 1950 to 1966.

† To clarify priorities, in *Science* on August 12, 1955, Parkhurst Shore, Stanley L. Silver, and Bernard Brodie suggested that "certain actions of reserpine may be mediated through the liberation of serotonin" (p. 285). Yet, the thrust of that article was about the "interaction of reserpine, serotonin and lysergic acid diethylamide in brain." The article on August 26, with Pletscher the chief author, established "by direct analysis that reserpine effects the release of serotonin" (p. 374).

Robins' main interest was in establishing psychiatry as a rigorously scientific discipline, supported by work in the basic sciences from genetics to pharmacology. As his obituarist Philip Majerus, a medical student at Washington University in the late 1950s, said, "I didn't really appreciate, at the time, how revolutionary Eli's ideas about psychiatry were. His contention that psychiatric illness had an organic basis that was discoverable, and that diagnoses could be made by classical clinical methods, seemed to me . . . obvious and logical" (*Annals of Clinical Psychiatry*, 1995, p. 6). In 1972, Robins was co-author of what turned out to be one of the most cited papers in the field of psychiatry: "Diagnostic Criteria for Use in Psychiatric Research" in the *American Journal of Psychiatry*; the main author was John Feighner (1937–), at the time a resident in the department—this was in keeping with a generous policy of giving first-author credit to junior clinicians—and the criteria became known as "the **St. Louis** criteria," or "the Feighner criteria." In establishing objective guidelines for psychiatric diagnoses, the 1972 paper helped pave the way for ***DSM-III***.

Robins wrote one of the classics in suicide studies, *The Final Months* (1981), and was editor of the English translation of the fifth edition of Karl Leonhard's *The Classification of Endogenous Psychoses* (1979). (*See* **WERNICKE–KLEIST–LEONHARD PATHWAY.**)

RORSCHACH TEST. Hermann Rorschach (1884–1922) grew up in Schaffhausen, Switzerland, and studied medicine in Zurich under **Eugen Bleuler**; as a student he was befriended by the artist Konrad Gehring and conceived the idea of determining whether successful students had a richer fantasy life than less successful. To this end, he prepared a number of ambiguous inkblots and quizzed his fellow students about them. After graduating in 1909, he became a staff physician at various Swiss asylums, ending finally at Herisau asylum in Appenzell Canton. After 14 years of experimentation at these institutions, with 300 psychiatry patients and 100 normal controls, in 1921 he published his famous projective test, limited by the publisher to 10 inkblots: *Psychodiagnosis: Methods and Results of Diagnostic Experiments in Perception* (*Interpretation of Random Forms*) (*Psychodiagnostik. Methodik und Ergebnisse eines wahrnehmungsdiagnostischen Experiments* [*Deutenlassen von Zufallsformen*]). Rorschach was also a psychoanalyst, in these years of febrile interest in psychoanalysis under Bleuler at the **Burghölzli**, and later became founding vice-president of the Swiss Psychoanalytic Society.

Rorschach's inkblot test (Formdeutversuch) became the most frequently used individual test in American psychiatry and psychology. Five of the blots were in black and white, five included color. The test was believed to be of use in the diagnosis of mental illness on the basis of psychoanalytic criteria: patients project their needs onto the blots, revealing their internal psychodynamics. (Patients who saw "a bat" in form I, for example—and who identified the bat's "anus" on the blot—were often thought "paranoid.") The test could be scored, the number of "P" responses, for example, showing the extent to which the patient was still in contact with reality. With the arrival of more objective tests for measuring personality such as the Minnesota Multiphasic Personality Inventory (MMPI) (first published in 1940 but popular only with the second edition in 1951), the Rorschach test went somewhat out of fashion. It was also shaded by the advent in 1980 of ***DSM-III***, with its "operational criteria" for making such diagnoses as schizophrenia.

RUSH, BENJAMIN (1746–1813). Called "the father of American psychiatry," Rush was born in Byberry, Pennsylvania, the son of a gunsmith. He began the study of medicine, as was common in those days, as an apprentice, then in 1768 graduated with an M.D. from Edinburgh University. (It is therefore unsurprising that he was influenced by the ideas of **William Cullen**.) From 1769 until his death he served as physician to the medical faculty of the College of Philadelphia, and after 1787 was occupied with the care of the mentally ill in Pennsylvania Hospital in Philadelphia. In 1791, he initiated the first course of psychiatry lectures in the United States. His 1812 book, *Medical Inquiries and Observations upon Diseases of the Mind*, is said to be the first psychiatry text by an American born in the United States. Notably, in 1776 he was one of the signatories of the Declaration of Independence. He was a strong advocate of bleeding in the relief of psychiatric illness and also recommended an early form of psychological therapy, namely, the "eye": "The first object of a physician, when he enters the cell or chamber of his deranged patient, should be to catch his EYE, and look him out of countenance. The dread of the eye was early imposed upon every beast of the field. The tiger, the mad bull, and the enraged dog, all fly from it; now a man deprived of his reason partakes so much of the nature of those animals, that he is for the most part easily terrified, or composed, by the eye of a man who possesses his reason" (*Medical Inquiries*, 3rd ed., 1827, p. 173).

RUTTER, MICHAEL. (*See also* **MAUDSLEY HOSPITAL**.) The founder of non-psychoanalytic child psychiatry in England, Rutter was born in 1933 to English parents who were living at the time in Lebanon. After spending the war years in the United States, he read medicine at Birmingham, graduating in 1955. He trained in psychiatry at the Maudsley Hospital, then spend a postgraduate year at the Albert Einstein College of Medicine in New York, joining the Medical Research Council social psychiatry unit at the Maudsley in 1962. Four years later, in 1966, he became senior lecturer, remaining there for the rest of his career. In 1973, he was appointed professor of child psychiatry and head of the department; in 1984, he set up the child psychiatry research unit at the Maudsley and in 1994 the research center for social, genetic, and developmental psychiatry, from which he retired as director in 1998, acquiring the post of professor of developmental psychophathology. (He was knighted in 1992.)

After 1979, Rutter became known in particular for his work on protective factors and vulnerability in children. Writing in 1987 in the *American Journal of Orthopsychiatry*, he said, "We need to ask why and how some individuals manage to maintain high self-esteem and self-efficacy in spite of facing the same adversities that lead other people to give up and lose hope. . . . The search is not for broadly defined protective factors but, rather, for the developmental and situational mechanisms involved in protective processes" (p. 317). Rutter and co-workers at the department of child and adolescent psychiatry at the Maudsley also pioneered the epidemiology of psychiatric disorder in children, finding, in an article published in the *British Journal of Psychiatry* in 1975, twice as much deviance and psychiatric disorder among 10-year-old children in an inner London borough as on the Isle of Wight.

S

SADISM. Just as with its mirror image **masochism**, sadism has come to have three meanings: (1) the voluntary infliction of suffering; (2) in psychoanalysis, a compulsive kind of personality characterized by regression to the anal-sadistic phase of infant development; (3) a kind of sex play among consenting adults called "SM" for "sadomasochism" but involving more the transfer of control in erotic situations than the administration of pain.

The referent for the term "sadism" is the French nobleman Donatien Alphonse François, Count de Sade (1740–1814), known as "the Marquis de Sade" (pronounced Sahd), who in two famous novels, *Justine* (1791) and *Juliette* (1798)—in addition to a host of other writings—portrayed fantastical orgies in which most of the participants end up dead and in which both male and female figures inflict much stylized violence upon the other players. (The scenes were intended to be allegorical, not masturbatory.) **Richard von Krafft-Ebing**, a somewhat prudish individual who was deaf-eared to allegory, missed Sade's intent and in 1890 in *New Research in the Area of Psychopathia Sexualis* (*Neue Forschungen auf dem Gebiete der Psychopathia sexualis*) proposed the term "sadism," already current in France, to mean voluntary cruelty to others. In the sixth edition of his *Psychopathia sexualis* in 1891, Krafft defined sadism as "the association of active cruelty and violence with sexual passion" and gave such examples as "sex murders."

Sigmund Freud first used the term "sadism" in 1905 in his *Three Essays on Sexual Theory* (*Drei Abhandlungen zur Sexualtheorie*), calling "the tendency to cause pain to the sexual object . . . the commonest and most significant of all perversions." He adopted Krafft-Ebing's term "sadism." "The sexuality of most men shows an adjuvant of aggression, a tendency to rape, the biological significance of which must be based on the necessity of overcoming the resistance of the sex object through other techniques than the act of courtship" (*Gesammelte Werke*, V, p. 57). Later in the essay, he outlined the stages of infantile libidinal development: first came the "oral" phase," then the phase of "sadistic-anal organization." "The dominance of sadism and the cloaca-role of the anal zone give [to this phase] an exquisitely archaic stamp." Freud emphasized that sadism and masochism were often to be found together (*Gesammelte Werke*, V, p. 99).

In his 1920 book *Beyond the Pleasure Principle* (*Jenseits des Lustprinzips*), Freud made sadism a more or less normal component of the human psyche, which is to say, part of the "death instinct" (der Todestrieb), the existence of which he announced in this work: "How can one possibly derive the sadistic drive, which is directed towards damaging the [love] object, from the life-giving notion of eros? Are we not actually close to the assumption that this sadism really is the death instinct, which under the influence of the narcissistic libido is flung away from the ego, so that it makes its first appearance on the object" (*Gesammelte Werke*, XIII, p. 58).

In his book *Escape from Freedom* (1941), psychoanalyst Erich Fromm (1900–1980), a German-born sociologist who had been a member of the Institute for Social Research in Frankfurt (the "Frankfurt School") and had emigrated to the United States in

1934, announced the existence of a "sado-masochistic character." Writing under the influence of contemporary events, he said, "For great parts of the lower middle class in Germany and other European countries, the sado-masochistic character is typical, and . . . it is this kind of character structure to which Nazi ideology had its strongest appeal." In neurotics, Fromm thought the term "sado-masochistic character" appropriate. When this character type was found in non-neurotic individuals, Fromm preferred the phrase "authoritarian character." To wit: "He admires authority and tends to submit to it, but at the same time he wants to be an authority himself and have others submit to him." The term "authoritarian character" thus represented for Rank "the personality structure which is the human basis of Fascism" (pp. 185–186).

In the ***DSM*** series, "sadism" first appeared in the second edition of the *Manual* in 1968 as one of several "sexual deviations." ***DSM-III*** (1980) included a full discussion of "sexual sadism": (a) on a nonconsenting partner; (b) on a consenting partner who is not seriously injured; (c) on a consenting partner who is seriously injured. Sexual sadism vanished from the official diagnoses in ***DSM-III-R*** in 1987, although "sadistic personality disorder" was proposed in an appendix as a possible diagnosis ("a pervasive pattern of cruel, demeaning, and aggressive behavior directed toward other people"). ***DSM-IV*** in 1994 gave up on the whole issue, as indeed it had given up on masochism, in possible recognition of the fact that sadomasochism for the most part belonged to a subculture of sex play among consenting adults.

According to sexuality historian Robert Bienvenu, in his Indiana University sociology dissertation (1998), sexual subcultures of "SM" begin to emerge in Europe in the late 1920s, in the United States in the early 1930s, and among "gay leather" circles in the early 1950s. It is interesting that, just as much sexual behavior became "psychiatrized" with the generation of sexologists of Richard von Krafft-Ebing's day—the 1880s—it became "de-psychiatrized" with the later editions of *DSM* a century later.

ST. ELIZABETHS HOSPITAL, Washington, D.C. Owing to the efforts of American psychiatry reformer Dorothea Dix (1802–1887), in 1852 Congress passed an act founding the Government Hospital for the Insane under the Department of the Interior. Intended to serve as a receptacle for members of the armed services with psychiatric illnesses, as well as for citizens of Washington, D.C.—at the time little numerous—the hospital opened its doors in 1855. (The capital later acquired a separate asylum, and thereafter the Government Hospital took only the spillover from it.) During the Civil War, the St. Elizabeth building of the hospital served as a general hospital for wounded soldiers, and because the troops were reluctant to have their address characterized as a hospital for the insane, the use gradually began of calling the entire institution St. Elizabeth Hospital. In 1916, it was renamed St. Elizabeths Hospital (the "s" officially lacking an apostrophe). Of its superintendents, Charles H. Nichols was the first, who came in 1852 just after Congress had appropriated funds and left in 1877 to take charge of the Bloomingdale Hospital for the Insane then in New York City (after 1894 in White Plains, NY). The best known superintendent was doubtless the psychoanalyst William Alanson White (1870–1937), who arrived in 1903 and on whose watch the hospital expanded greatly its scientific work. In 1907, White added a psychological laboratory, and in 1914 he appointed a full-time psychoanalyst. In

1924, under White's direction, hospital psychiatrist Nolan D. C. Lewis (1889–1979)* and co-investigators introduced to the United States **Julius Wagner von Jauregg's** malarial-fever cure for **neurosyphilis**. When White died in office in 1937, the hospital had over 5000 beds.

In 1957, English psychiatrist **Joel Elkes** moved to the United States at the invitation of Seymour Kety (1915–2000) and Robert A. Cohen (1909–?) of the **National Institute of Mental Health** to set up a clinical neuropharmacological research center (CNRC) at the hospital. Remaining until 1963, Elkes furthered some pathbreaking work in the neurosciences at the hospital, and such clinical investigators as German emigré psychiatrist Fritz Freyhan (1912–1982), previously at a mental hospital in Delaware, and British psychiatrist Anthony Hordern (1925–), who had just finished training in London, undertook clinial trials.

In a series of reorganizations, the hospital came under the Federal Security Agency in 1940, then under the Department of Health, Education and Welfare in 1953, then ultimately under the National Institute of Mental Health (NIMH) in 1967; finally, after further churning, it devolved in 1987 to the District of Columbia.

Erving Goffman's *Asylums: Essays on the Social Situation of Mental Patients and Other Inmates* (1961), one of the cornerstone documents of the antipsychiatry movement, was based on St. Elizabeths. (*See* **ANTIPSYCHIATRY MOVEMENT: Goffman.**)

"ST. LOUIS SCHOOL OF PSYCHIATRY" (at Washington University in St. Louis) (from 1942). The St. Louis school of psychiatry is significant because it introduced biological thinking into American psychiatry at a time when the prestigious teaching institutions were all dominated by psychoanalysis.

Founded by psychiatrist David Rioch (1900–1985) in 1938, the department of psychiatry at "Wash U" started to resound as the main voice for biological psychiatry in the United States in 1942 when Edwin Gildea (pronounced GIL-day) (1898–1977) became head of the department. (Rioch was a psychoanalyst.) The university was already a national center of innovative medical research, and it is said to have been the Washington University biochemist Carl Cori (1896–1984) who plumped for the appointment of Gildea. Gildea, born in Colorado Springs, had received his M.D. from Harvard in 1924, trained in psychiatry at the Boston Psychopathic Hospital between 1926 and 1928, and taught neuropathology at Harvard before going to Yale in 1929 as a member of the department of psychiatry. In 1942, he was called to Wash U as professor of psychiatry and head of neuropsychiatry. His wife, Margaret Crane-Lillie Gildea (1903–?), was also a psychiatrist. Gildea set out to give the department, at that point full of psychoanalysts, a biological spin.

In 1949, Gildea brought **Eli Robins** (1921–1994) to Washington University as an instructor in neuropsychiatry. Robins became head of the department of psychiatry in 1963 when Gildea retired, retiring in 1975 himself as a result of his advancing illness. (Robins's wife, Lee Nelken Robins [1922–] was a distinguished medical sociologist

---

* Lewis, a noted child psychiatrist, later became head of the New York State Psychiatric Institute, which is affiliated with the department of psychiatry of Columbia University's College of Physicians and Surgeons.

who, together with Darrel A. Regier (1944–), led the first major epidemiological study in U.S. psychiatry, the Epidemiological Catchment Area Study, funded by the **National Institute of Mental Health** and published in 1991 as *Psychiatric Disorders in America.*)

Between 1975 and 1989, **Samuel Guze** succeeded Robins as chair of psychiatry.

A third member of the triumvirate was **George Winokur**, who came to Wash U in 1951 as an instructor in the psychiatry department and remained there until becoming chair of psychiatry at the University of Iowa in 1971.

The "St. Louis school," under Robins, Guze, and Winokur, began to take on a collective existence as the three of them presented a plan for future resident training to a somewhat taken aback Gildea. During the years, they established their distinctive imprint of conducting long-term follow-up studies and doing genetic research. They trained many influential American figures in biological psychiatry after the Second World War, including C. Robert Cloninger (1944–), Paula J. Clayton (*see* **WOMEN IN PSYCHIATRY**), Robert A. Woodruff, Jr. (1934–), and Rodrigo Muñoz (1939–). Known as the "neo-Kraepelinians," they replaced the previous insider group in American psychiatry, the Group for the Advancement of Psychiatry based at the **Menninger** Clinic, as the intellectual leadership in American psychiatry.

Much later, American psychiatrist David Sheehan (1947–), at the Institute for Research in Psychiatry of the University of South Florida in Tampa, Florida, reflected about the significance of the St. Louis school: "It's an invisible network. Those involved know it. They never comment on it. It is understood, like they are all wearing the same college tie. . . . It's the equivalent of the **Maudsley** or the **Salpêtrière** in Paris or **Kraepelin**'s group in Munich" (Healy *Psychopharmacologists*, III, p. 503).

STE.-ANNE MENTAL HOSPITAL (1867), Paris. Given that at mid-nineteenth century, the Seine department (Paris) disposed of only two mental hospitals, Bicêtre and the **Salpêtrière**, in 1860 Baron Georges Haussmann (1809–1891), the prefect of the Seine, ordered a commission to consider the reform of institutional care. Two years later, the administration of the department decided to build a central asylum in Paris at the Ste.-Anne "farm" where clinical teaching would take place and where a separate building would house the admissions service. (The Ste.-Anne farm had previously been an annex of Bicêtre hospital for agricultural work for the mentally ill.) In 1867, the new Ste.-Anne mental hospital was opened, and **Valentin Magnan** and his medical-school friend Louis-*Gustave* Bouchereau (1835–1900) were placed in charge of the emergency department, which turned out to be an immense fountain of psychiatric pathology given that many of the desperately ill patients in the city of Paris, referred from the emergency department of the prefecture of police (called L'infirmerie spéciale), passed through it. The admissions service also received patients from the Paris general hospitals (l'Assistance publique) and direct admissions via the patients' families. From the admissions department of Ste.-Anne, the patients would be redistributed to the other psychiatric hospitals in the Seine department, including the Ste.-Anne teaching service.

Among the professors of psychiatry in the teaching service until the Second World War were Benjamin Ball (1833–1893), who initiated instruction in 1879 in the newly founded (1877) "chair of mental and brain diseases" ("maladies mentales et de l'encéphale"); Alix Joffroy (1844–1908), who held the chair until his death; *Gilbert*-Louis-Siméon Ballet (1853–1916), who is remembered for precise descriptions of chronic hallucinatory psychosis (1911) (*see* **FRENCH CHRONIC DELUSIONAL STATES**) and other nervous disorders, in office until his death; *Ernest*-Ferdinand-Pierre-Louis Dupré (1862–1921), whose major contribution is the délire d'imagination (1910) (*see* **FRENCH CHRONIC DELUSIONAL STATES**), also died in office; **Henri Claude**, who retired from the chair in 1939 and the following year brought out, with Pierre Rubenovitch, a major guide to the physical therapies, *Thérapeutiques biologiques des affections mentales* (*Biological Treatments of Mental Illness*); Paul-Marie-*Maxime* Laignel-Lavastine (1875–1953), who coined the term "endocrine psychiatry" (1908), retired at reaching the age limit in 1942; Joseph Levy-Valensi (1879–1943), elected Laignel's replacement by the Faculty in 1942 despite his Jewish origins—Levy-Valensi was never permitted to begin teaching and died in Auschwitz in 1943; thereafter **Jean Delay** offered interim instruction in psychiatry until his own ascension to the chair in 1946; the chair was modified at Delay's retirement in 1970 (*see* **Pierre Deniker**), and **Pierre Pichot** continued on as head.

SALPÊTRIÈRE HOSPICE (Hospital), Paris. Founded in the seventeenth century by a 1656 decree of Louis XIV as one of four great hospices in Paris, the former "little arsensal" (or Salpetery—la Salpêtrière) was dedicated to receiving sick, destitute, and aged women of all descriptions. Several wings were subsequently added, such as one for criminal women in 1684 where prostitutes were incarcerated in the eighteenth century. Late in the eighteenth century, a medical division (infirmary) was authorized and the psychiatric wards renovated. **Pinel** famously installed gentler methods of treatment during the French Revolution, and in 1882 a chair for **Jean-Martin Charcot** in nervous diseases was created at the Salpêtrière, after which it became a noted center for neuropsychiatric training. Charcot's successors in the chair after 1893 were Fulgence Raymond (1844–1910) and, after Raymond's death, Jules-Joseph Dejerine (1849–1917). (In 1900, Dejerine wrote an important two-volume work on the *Symptomatology of Neurological Illness* [*Sémiologie des affections du système nerveux*], in which was added a fair amount of psychiatry as well.)

SARGANT, WILLIAM (1907–1988). A pioneer of physical and pharmacological treatments in British psychiatry, Sargant was the son of a devout Methodist businessman; it was said of Sargant himself that even though his religiousness lapsed, he applied the same enthusiasm to the treatment of his patients. After reading medicine at Cambridge, Sargant qualified in 1929 and served as a house officer at St. Mary's Hospital in London. After experiencing a bout of depression, he turned from internal medicine to psychiatry, and entered the **Maudsley Hospital** in 1935 under Edward Mapother (1881–1940). As the Maudsley was split in two during the war, Sargant and **Eliot Slater** ended up together at the branch at Sutton Emergency Hospital, where Slater was clinical director and Sargant his deputy. At Sutton, they put into practice many of the new somatic therapies that were just becoming available: **insulin coma**, metrazol convulsion (*see* **CONVULSIVE THERAPIES: CHEMICAL**), **electroconvulsive therapy**, **deep-sleep therapy**, and **leukotomy**.

In 1941, Sargant and Nellie Craske (née Wilson, M.B. 1929) described in the *Lancet* "modified insulin therapy," or insulin subcoma therapy, for high-grade anxiety in the war neuroses. Sargant was keen to try everything, and in 1944 he was senior author together with Slater of *An Introduction to Physical Methods of Treatment in Psychiatry*, one of the first such manuals. (This interest in physcial treatments and psychopharmacology harvested the active dislike of **Aubrey Lewis**, an advocate of social and community psychiatry and uneasy about treating the brain itself.) In 1948, he became head of psychiatry at St. Thomas's Hospital in London, where he helped introduce into Britain the first drug set of the psychopharmacological revolution, particularly the antidepressant monoamine oxidase inhibitors (*see* **iproniazid**), such tricyclic antidepressants as amitriptyline (*see* **imipramine** for details), and the diagnosis of "atypical depression." (*See* **DEPRESSION: RECENT CONCEPTS: atypical depression** [1959].) In the United Kingdom, Sargant is perhaps best known for his book *Battle for the Mind* (1957), written at the height of Cold War scares about "brain-washing." His bluff enthusiasm always made him a bit of a figure of fun in the eyes of the psychotherapeutically and social-psychiatrically oriented British establishment, but he lived to have the satisfaction of seeing many of the physcial therapies and the new drugs vindicated.

SCHILDER, PAUL FERDINAND (1886–1940). Highly influential in bringing European approaches to the United States, Schilder was born in Vienna, his father a silk merchant. In 1909, he graduated with an M.D. from the University of **Vienna**, then trained in psychiatry first with Gabriel Anton (1858–1933) at the university psychiatric clinic in Halle on the Saale, then in 1912–1914 with Paul Flechsig (1847–1929) at the university psychiatric clinic in Leipzig. In 1917, he earned a Ph.D. in philosophy in Vienna, then served from 1918 to 1928 as an assistant to **Julius Wagner von Jauregg** at the university psychiatric clinic in Vienna. He received his Habilitation in psychiatry and neurology from Vienna in 1920 (1925 associate professor, or ausserordentlicher professor). It was said that he left Vienna for Johns Hopkins University in 1928 because Wagner, on the verge of retirement, had pushed him out, fearful that the gifted young Schilder would become the next professor of psychiatry. (Wagner-Jauregg tended to be anti-Semitic and Schilder was Jewish; yet, Schilder had renounced the Jewish religion in 1918, and there were other Jews such as Emil Redlich (1866–1930) of whom Wagner was fond; the story seems more a personality clash; also, Schilder spoke in a high voice that many found distracting.) After a year at Hopkins, Schilder moved to New York in 1929 to start lecturing in psychiatry at New York University Medical School, and in 1930 became clinical director of psychiatry at Bellevue Hospital. He died in a traffic accident in 1940.

Schilder was adept in reaching across disciplines, sometimes focusing primarily on neurology—producing an enormous body of writing on neurological syndromes including Encephalitis periaxalis diffusa, "Schilder's disease" (1913)—sometimes interested in psychoanalytic formulations (he was prominent in Europe, yet was rejected for membership in the New York Psychoanalytic Society), and sometimes interested principally in the exact description of symptoms in the European tradition of psychopathology. In Vienna he often collaborated with such emerging stars as Hans Hoff (*see* **VIENNA**), Josef Gerstmann (1887–1969), and psychoanalyst Heinz Hartmann (1894–1970); in Baltimore, he collaborated with child psychiatrist Leo Kanner (1894–1981; author in 1935 of the first American textbook with the title *Child Psychiatry*; *see* **AUTISM**), and also with child psychiatrist Lauretta Bender (1897–1987) (*see* **WOMEN IN**

PSYCHIATRY: Bender), whom Schilder married as his second wife in 1936; at Bellevue he worked with Walter Bromberg (1900–2000). In 1939, in an article in *Mental Hygiene*, he described how at Bellevue Hospital he had initiated the practice of group psychotherapy, an early attempt at group therapy by a psychiatrist. (*See* **PSYCHOTHERAPY: group psychotherapy.**) Some of the books for which he is best known in the United States were published after his death: *Psychoanalysis, Man and Society* (1951), which is a collection of his articles edited by his widow Lauretta Bender; and *Medical Psychology* (the English translation in 1953 of his *Medizinische Psychologie* (German orig. 1924). In Europe, his German-language books, such as *Thoughts on Natural Philosophy* (*Gedanken zur Naturphilosophie*, 1928) made him a leading figure (also a heretical one, because he said the causes of melancholia were unplumbed). Schilder's interest in breakdowns of the mind–body relationship gave a lifelong focus to his work, and his *Image and Appearance of the Human Body* (1935) set the stage for much psychosomatic investigation. (*See* **BODY IMAGE: DISTURBANCES OF** [1935].)

SCHIZOID PERSONALITY, a personality disorder, in *DSM* (from 1952). When the patient is not psychotic or manifestly thought-disordered, yet withdrawn, unable to express hostility, and "**autistic**," ***DSM-I*** and ***DSM-II*** employed the concept "schizoid personality."

Interest in the schizoid personality goes back to the turn-of-the century view that psychotic symptoms might represent accentuations of preexisting personality states. In 1908, as **Eugen Bleuler** was still calling schizophrenia "dementia praecox," he distinguished in the *Zentralblatt für Nervenheilkunde* between a latent form and an active. "Thus the arrival of a stressful event [ein Affekt] can convert a latent dementia praecox to a manifest form. The disease had previously existed but was just not visible" (p. 225). **Ernst Kretschmer's** 1921 book put schizoid personality as such firmly on the map. (*See also* **PSYCHOSIS: EMERGENCE: Kretschmer's constitutional psychoses.**) In 1922, Bleuler had written about "Schizoidie" in the *Zeitschrift für die gesamte Neurologie und Psychiatrie*. But the train that leads to *DSM*'s version of schizoid personality begins with the German-Jewish geneticist Franz Kallmann (1897–1965), who in 1936, following his opposition to the Nazi laws on forced sterilization, emigrated to the United States, landing at the New York State Psychiatric Institute. On the basis of his research on twins, Kallmann said in 1953 that genetics predisposed to a schizoid personality, which in itself might lead to "involutional psychosis" (*Heredity in Health and Mental Disorders*, pp. 181, 183).

In New York, Kallmann was a close friend of psychoanalyst **Sándor Radó**, and despite their obvious theoretical differences, Kallmann sparked Radó's interest in what Radó called in the *American Journal of Psychiatry* in 1953 "schizotypal disorders." By schizotype, Radó meant the "underlying ensemble of psychodynamic traits which . . . is demonstrable in the patient during his whole life. This finding will identify him as a schizotype from birth to death. The ensemble of psychodynamic traits peculiar to the schizotypes may be called schizotypal organization." Radó thought that many genetic schizotypes never developed schizophrenia and that the stage of open psychosis itself was merely the third and final stage of the schizotype. (The second stage corresponded to Hoch and Polatin's "pseudo-neurotic schizophrenia.") (*See* **SCHIZOPHRENIA: RECENT CONCEPTS** [1949].) (Radó, "Disordered Behavior," in his collected works, *The Psychoanalysis of Behavior*, I, 274, 283–284.)

In 1962, psychologist Paul E. Meehl (1920–2003) at the University of Minnesota introduced the concept of "schizotaxia." Writing in *American Psychologist,* he said, "I believe we should take seriously the old European notion of an 'integrative neural defect' . . . which I shall christen schizotaxia." He said this represented the only aspect of schizophrenia that could be inherited. The schizotaxic individual would carry the schizotypic personality around with him, without ever necessarily becoming schizophrenic. "He will be like the gout-prone male whose genes determine him to have an elevated blood uric acid titer, but who never develops clinical gout" (pp. 829–830).

In this context in 1963, physiologist Seymour Kety (1915–2000) (who later became professor of psychiatry at Harvard) began his research in Copenhagen on children who had been adopted away and later developed schizophrenia, as opposed to adopted-away controls who remained normal; Kety and co-workers found that in some of the schizophrenics' biological families there were individuals who were bizarre and eccentric, part of the "schizophrenia spectrum" as they put it, without having formal schizophrenia; in such persons, whom **Robert Spitzer** defined in ***DSM-III*** in 1980 as "schizotypal," there did seem to be a familial loading, suggesting a genetic basis. ***DSM-III*** therefore included two new personality diagnoses: "schizoid personality disorder," meaning roughly what *DSM-I* and *-II* had had in mind, and "schizotypal personality disorder," for subthreshold schizophrenia, or individuals who had sufficient "oddities of thought, perception, speech, and behavior" that there seemed to be a problem, yet who were not formally schizophrenic. These categories were not essentially changed in subsequent editions of *DSM.*

SCHIZOPHRENIA/DEMENTIA PRAECOX: EMERGENCE OF THE CONCEPT. (*See also* **PSYCHOSIS: EMERGENCE; SCHIZOPHRENIA: RECENT CONCEPTS; UNITARY PSYCHOSIS; WERNICKE–KLEIST–LEONHARD PATHWAY.**) Schizophrenia remains among the most puzzling of all diseases in psychiatry because there is no single symptom characteristic of it. Nor is there a common course for all patients, for some do well, although the majority do not. Nor is there a common outcome of treatment, for some patients respond nicely to antipsychotic drugs, others not at all. (Nor a characteristic family history, for some have family trees laden with illness; for others, the illness comes, sometimes as late as mid-life, as a complete surprise.) It is tempting, of course, to see in "schizophrenia" a collecting basin for a number of different illnesses. Yet to date, despite decades of intense research, distinctive subtypes have not been teased out.

The concept of schizophrenia emerged as an amalgam of earlier diagnoses. It became conceived as an outcome rather than a typical symptom picture at any moment in time. Many diverse clinical presentations could end up having the same outcome, namely, in the language of the day, "dementia."

Dementia praecox (démence précoce) (1860). In his *Textbook of Mental Illnesses* (*Traité des maladies mentales*), **Bénédict-Augustin Morel** characterized a distinctive kind of adolescent insanity (folie) that he considered hereditary and degenerative in the sense of worsening from one generation to the next. Striking in the teenage years, dementia praecox ultimately eventuated in premature "dementia" (in the nineteenth-century meaning of incoherence rather than low intelligence). Although Morel had used the term in passing in 1853, only here did he characterize it more fully, describing for example a youth of 14 years of age who "progressively forgot all he had learned at school; his brilliant intellectual faculties underwent a very disquieting interruption. A kind of torpor close to hebetude took over from his earlier activities and when I saw him again [later in adolescence], I felt that the fatal transition to the state of premature dementia [démence précoce] was underway. This desperate prognosis is ordinarily far from the minds of parents and even of the physicians who care for these children" (p. 566).

Morel was the first psychiatric writer to use the label "premature dementia" for what was later called schizophrenia. But, he also was the first psychiatrist to classify psychotic illnesses on the basis of outcome rather than clinical presentation at a given moment in time. He drew up an entire class of insanity, of varying causes and symptoms, that had in common the termination in dementia: "The special state designated by the term dementia will be the terminal form of various mental afflictions, and will represent the most numerous class of patients accommodated in our asylums" (p. vi.)

Kahlbaum's Vesania typica (typical insanity) (1863). Part of the nosology of the Prussian psychiatrist **Karl Ludwig Kahlbaum** was based on outcome rather than momentary clinical picture. In his *Classification of Mental Disorders* (*Die Gruppirung der psychischen Krankheiten*, 1863), Kahlbaum was struck that there seemed to be two classes of illness than ran downhill irreversibly ("progressively") into dementia. One was what Bayle described (understood only in hindsight) as the syphilitic infiltration of the central nervous system, later called neurosyphilis (at the time progressive paralysis). The other Kahlbaum simply labeled Vesania typica, "typical insanity of the brain that includes all functions . . . until finally the onset of dementia occurs and mental life sinks away" (pp. 84–85). There is no doubt that many cases of what later was called schizophrenia were included in this set of outcomes.

Hebephrenia (1871). After **Kahlbaum** left the Allenberg asylum in 1867, he acquired a post at a private nervous clinic in the East Prussian town of Görlitz, and took his assistant Ewald Hecker (1843–1909) with him. At Görlitz, in the youth division of the clinic, the two men saw a number of young male patients with premature dementia. In 1871, in an article in the *Archive of Pathological Anatomy and Physiology for Clinical Medicine* (*Archiv für pathologische Anatomie und Physiologie für klinische Medizin*), Hecker offered a portrait of these patients, who presented a constantly changing series of clinical pictures before ending in dementia, suffering from what Kahlbaum had called in his lectures "hebephrenia."

Of the perhaps 500 adolescent patients whom Kahlbaum and Hecker had seen in Allenberg and Görlitz, 14 had the characteristic course of "hebephrenic dementia": Hecker emphasized the disorganized nature of their late-adolescent behavior (hence the Greek "hebe" for youth plus "phrenia" for mind): "First of all they show a distinctive deviation from logical sentence building . . . a characteristic indifference in the stringing together of sentences and the inability to conclude a thought in a precise way" (p. 404). Hecker continued, "There is also a very pronounced tendency . . . to mix up the language and to speak and write in a strange jargon." The young patients then progress, via mixed episodes of mania and melancholia, to a dulled form of dementia, interrupted by momentary bursts of agitation and periodic bouts of hallucinations, especially of the auditory variety. The dementia is terminal. No other psychiatric illnesses are characterized by onset at the time of puberty and an inevitable progression to early dementia. This description served **Emil Kraepelin** as a model for dementia praecox (*see* below).

Catatonia (1874). Catatonia means motor (muscle or movement) abnormalities—in the context of psychiatric illness—and today one distinguishes conventionally between catatonic excitement (an increase in spontaneous and purposeless movements) and catatonic stupor (the opposite); motor stereotypies, waxy flexibility, proskinesis, parakinesis and numerous mannerisms constitute additional motor symptoms. Yet catatonia figures in the schizophrenia narrative mainly because **Kraepelin** considered certain aspects of it as hallmarks of dementia praecox. (Catatonia may be found as well in delirium, depression, and in manic-depressive illness, but certain symptoms such as posturing [remaining in a fixed position], echolalia [repeating a doctor's question], and echopraxia [doing as the examiner is doing] are virtually pathognomic for schizophrenia.)

The term "catatonia" was coined by **Karl Ludwig Kahlbaum** in an 1874 monograph (*Die Katatonie, oder das Spannungsirresein*), but he had used it in public lectures since 1868. The phenomenon had, however, been long familiar in psychiatry and was recognized as part of the immobile apathy traditionally called melancholia attonita (attonita = thunderstruck). Schizophrenic symptoms were part of the clinical course that Kahlbaum depicted: "Catatonia is a brain disease with a cyclically variable course, in which melancholia, mania, stupor, confusion and finally dementia succeed one another" (p. 87). As for a cause, Kahlbaum attributed it to some kind of neurological convulsion. In fact, as German Berrios has shown in a reanalysis of Kahlbaum's 31 cases, most of Kahlbaum's patients probably had some kind of organic delirium or psychotic depression rather than schizophrenia (*History of Mental Symptoms*, pp. 382–383).

Schizophrenia and Emil Kraepelin's dementia praecox (from 1893). **Emil Kraepelin**, who characterized the illness dementia praecox, emerges as arguably the central figure in the history of modern psychiatry. His achievements were (1) to differentiate schizophrenia as an independent illness and not just a late-stage consequence of some other primary disorder; (2) to establish diseases on the basis of outcome (course) rather than clinical picture at a given moment; and (3) to erect "dementia praecox" (later called schizophrenia) and manic-depressive illness as the chief disease entities of psychiatry. Even today these traditions, for better or worse, are much alive in psychiatry.

It was only in the fourth edition of his textbook, in 1893, a year after arriving in Heidelberg, that **Kraepelin** used the term "dementia praecox." Kraepelin cited **Karl Kahlbaum** and Hecker as intellectual forbears rather than **Bénédict-Augustin Morel**. In the time since Morel had written, numerous European psychiatrists had described the same clinical picture of premature "dementia." It was Kraepelin's accomplishment to bring together under a single roof these various partial descriptions of démence précoce, Vesania typica, hebephrenia, catatonia, and the like: making of them a single well-defined disease—distinct from depression and manic-depressive illness—having a familiar set of symptoms and a predictable, indeed, inevitable course, the convergent path of deterioration. In this fourth edition, he assigned dementia praecox (DP) to the "psychic degenerative processes," alongside catatonia and "dementia paranoides" (a form of illness that Kraepelin had separated from Kahlbaum's "paranoia," by which Kraepelin meant sudden-onset psychosis that progresses to "feeble-minded confusion"

(p. 456). The prognosis of DP was gloomy: "The further course of these cases diverges to the extent that sometimes dementia sets in quickly, sometimes more slowly, and may cease to advance at often highly variable stages" (p. 438).

In this and several subsequent editions, Kraepelin left psychoses that were confined mainly to delusional disorders without deterioration as a separate category: "Madness (paranoia)" (die Verrücktheit [Paranoia]); they were not part of any larger disease class. (*See* **PARANOIA.**)

In the fifth edition of his text in 1896, Kraepelin made DP part of the "metabolic disorders leading to dementia," again alongside catatonia and dementia paranoides.

In the sixth edition in 1899, Kraepelin distinguished between the two great psychiatric diseases that would imprint psychiatry for the next 100 years: dementia praecox and manic-depressive illness, today called "bipolar disorder." (*See* **MANIC-DEPRESSIVE ILLNESS** [1899].) DP now included dementia paranoides and catatonia, expressing itself in three forms: the hebephrenic, the catatonic, and the paranoid. These subdivisions as well would survive for decades.

In the seventh edition in 1904, Kraepelin changed little, merely adding a tiny ray of hope in the discussion of outcomes: "In a small number of cases of dementia praecox, a complete recovery does seem to take place." The point was grudgingly made. Yet, he added a second category that, in view of discussions of outcome in previous editions, also sounded rather optimistic: "In any event, much more frequent is recovery with a deficit" (Heilung mit Defekt). After all symptoms had fled, the patient remained rather enfeebled (*Psychiatrie*, 7th ed., II, pp. 261–262).

In the eighth edition, which started appearing in 1909, the last he was to complete himself, in volume III(2) (1913), Kraepelin took DP from the independent causal status it had occupied in the several previous editions (meaning not part of any larger illness) and attached it to "the endogenous dementias" (die endogenen Verblödungen). In the discussion of prognosis he now admitted that 26% of these patients experienced some form of remission, if even only of a few months (vol. III[2], pp. 862–863).

In this volume, Kraepelin shifted some periodic forms of psychosis from the manic-depressive group to dementia praecox. (*See* **PSYCHOSIS: EMERGENCE: periodic catatonia** [1932 and after].) The periodically repeating episodes appear to come out of the blue, with recovery just as quickly. Many patients, after a series of attacks stay well; others deteriorate.

Kraepelin had hoped that the resemblance of dementia praecox to **neurosyphilis** ("progressive paralysis") would ultimately vindicate his assertion that DP was a unitary disease with a common clinical course and outcome. The clinical picture of neurosyphilis at any given moment was quite varied, just as that of DP: "What turns out in the end to be Paralysis," he wrote in 1909, "is a disease process with a unitary cause, a definite clinical course and a clear anatomical basis. On the other hand, the momentary clinical pictures show such a confusing variegation that on the basis of symptom picture alone it never would have been possible to recognize their common identity. . . . It is to be expected that the clarification of our other tentative large clinical entities [such as DP] will be achieved in a similar manner" (eighth edition, 1909, pp. 526–527).

On balance, some contemporaries were enthusiastic about Kraepelin's great concept of the two different diseases because they thought it made possible the prediction of prognosis. As Tübingen psychiatry professor Robert Gaupp (1870–1953) pointed out in 1926, "Every clinical concept is obliged to demonstrate its merit in its ability to tell, for an individual patient, what happens next. The prognosis is the measure of all of our scientific accomplishment" (*Archiv für Psychiatrie und Nervenkrankheiten*, pp. 77–78). One notes that predicting treatment response was still far from anyone's mind in the uses of diagnosis, because there were no treatments.

Stransky's intrapsychic ataxia (1903). Vienna psychiatrist Erwin Stransky (1877–1962) was uneasy about Kraepelin's notion of "dementia," because in fact the patients seemed more to suffer from a loosening of associations than from dementia as such. He referred to this "functional disharmony" among various parts of the psyche as "intrapsychic ataxia," and emphasized such symptoms as language confusion, paralogia (perverted logic), and the "derailment of volition" (or Entgleisung). In brief, a dementia-psychosis had turned into a derailment-psychosis. Stransky's first contribution appeared in 1903 in the *Yearbook of Psychiatry and Neurology* (*Jahrbuch für Psychiatrie und Neurologie*). Stransky had formulated the concept of intrapsychic "schism" and was disappointed when in 1908 Bleuler coined it as schizophrenia. Stransky later said that his idea had been overwhelmed by the psychoanalytic express train coming out of Vienna and running through Bleuler's Zurich (*Swiss Archive of Neurology and Psychiatry* [*Schweizer Archiv für Neurologie und Psychiatrie*], 1954, p. 323). Kraepelin acknowledged Stransky's work in the eighth edition (1913) of his textbook (p. 747).

Bleuler's schizophrenia (1908, 1911). Bleuler rebaptized **Kraepelin's** dementia praecox as "schizophrenia" at the annual meeting of the German Psychiatric Association in Berlin in 1908, saying he preferred "schizophrenia" because dementia praecox lent itself so poorly to use as an adjective and because he considered that there was some kind of "split" in psychic function. Up to that point, 647 patients with the diagnosis schizophrenia had been admitted to the **Burghölzli** in Zurich, and Bleuler had a good overview. The disease Bleuler described was much milder and broader than Kraepelin's, fully 73% of the acute cases going on to have relatively normal lives (though none fully recovered). The paranoid variety had a better prognosis than the catatonic, although Bleuler despaired at isolating truly distinctive subgroups within the illness. So upbeat was Bleuler about the general course of the illness (in contrast to the substantial gloom of Kraepelin) that Bleuler preferred to speak of illness episodes (Schübe) from a presumably normal state rather than of relapses (Rezidiven) from an abnormal underlying state.

Most at variance from Kraepelin were Bleuler's notions of the "primary," or core, symptoms—meaning part of the basic illness process—and "secondary" reactions of the patient to the environment or to the illness. By secondary, Bleuler understood virtually all the symptoms that Kraepelin had considered usually present in dementia praecox: hallucinations, delusions, social isolation, even deterioration ("dementia"). Bleuler considered even such symptoms as negativism and mutism secondary because they were subject to "psychic influences." To the ranks of primary symptoms, Bleuler assigned the neurological changes, such as differences in the pupils of the eye, a certain intellectual slowing and dazedness, and most importantly, "changes in associations" (meaning logical thought): "In schizophrenia, it is as though the physiological controls and channels [of thought] go amiss; the familiar normal pathways are not so sought out and the train of thought is easily lost in unfamiliar, false pathways. Thus the train of associations is given over to incidental influences, above all, emotional in nature, which leads to a partial or a complete loss of logical function." It was this loss of logic in schizophrenia, rather than "dementia" (which Bleuler considered easily reversible) that characterized the illness (*General Journal of Psychiatry* [*Allgemeine Zeitschrift für Psychiatrie*], 1908, p. 457). (Kraepelin found distinctions between primary and secondary symptoms "artificial.")

By the time of his 1911 book, *Dementia Praecox, or The Group of Schizophrenias* (*Dementia Praecox oder Gruppe der Schizophrenien*), Bleuler was calling primary symptoms "basic symptoms" (Grundsymptome) and secondary symptoms "accessory." Later usage would deem the basic symptoms to be "negative," meaning social withdrawal and the blocking of affect, the accessory symptoms "positive," meaning hallucinations and delusions. (*See* **POSITIVE VS. NEGATIVE SYMPTOMS.**) By 1911, Bleuler had provisionally settled on four subtypes of the disease: paranoid, catatonic, hebephrenic and "simple" (only a few specific basic symptoms) (p. 7). Among the basic symptoms he had added "relationship to reality: **autism.**"* "The sickest patients . . . live in a world of their own; they have cocooned into themselves [verpuppen] with their wishes, which they see as fulfilled, or with the misery of their persecution, and they restrict contact with the outside world as much as possible. This dereism [Loslösung von der Wirklichkeit] together with the relative and absolute predominance of their interior life we refer to as autism" (p. 52).

The passage from dementia praecox to schizophrenia was a transition from clinical course to the structure of thought. The difference between Kraepelinian and Bleulerian concepts of schizophrenia would continue to resonate. Said Hans Walther Gruhle (1880–1958) at Heidelberg in 1931: "Physicians who see every eccentric personality, every lonely person, as an undiagnosed schizophrenic, will naturally have different views about the arrest of the illness, or its practical cure, than those who make a demonstrable acute psychotic phase a precondition of the diagnosis" (p. 25). Bleuler's schizophrenia greatly expanded the circumference of the diagnosis, as opposed to Kraepelin's more austere version. With Bleuler's definition, a number of rather vague symptoms could qualify as evidence of the disease. As psychopharmacologist Paul Janssen (1926–2003) observed later, "The etiology of schizophrenia is Dr. Bleuler" (Healy, *Psychopharmacologists*, II, p. 60).

First finding of large anatomical changes in brains of patients with schizophrenia (1914). In 1910, Elmer Ernest Southard (1876–1920), director of the psychopathic department of the Boston State Hospital and professor of neuropathology at Harvard, began the systematic microscopic and macroscopic examination of randomly selected brains of deceased schizophrenic patients, concentrating especially on structural abnormalities visible to the naked eye. Of the 50 brains he examined, he noted, in an article in the *American Journal of Insanity* in October 1914, that 45 showed "gross anomalies or other lesions" (p. 387). In particular, in the original group of 28 brains he had studied in 1910, nine had what he called "internal hydrocephalus," or dilatation of the ventricles (noted in the January 1915 issue, p. 639). This finding,

* In fact, Bleuler first describes "autism" ("der Autismus") in his 1910 article on "Schizophrenic Negativism" in the *Psychiatrisch-Neurologische Wochenschrift* (p. 185f).

which went widely unheralded, represents the first linking of schizophrenia to gross (meaning macroscopically visible) anatomical brain changes. Southard did not have a control group of brains of non-ill persons.

Kraepelin backpedals on the "disease" concept (1920). In 1920, toward the end of his life, **Kraepelin** grew increasingly pessimistic about the possibility of separating dementia praecox from manic-depressive illness on the basis of symptoms alone, so much did the symptoms overlap. Kraepelin now reflected upon Berlin psychiatrist Karl Birnbaum's (1878–1950) distinction in 1919, in the *General Journal of Psychiatry* (*Allgemeine Zeitschrift für Psychiatrie*), between the "pathogenetic" contributions to the clinical illness (meaning the underlying brain forms) and the "pathoplastic" contributions (meaning how the patient responded to illness and environment). Kraepelin thought that many symptoms belonged more in the pathoplastic than the pathogenetic group, and were not specifically distinctive, or pathognomonic, in revealing the underlying disease. He thus stepped back somewhat from the "nosological" concept that psychiatry consisted of disease entities and edged toward the notion of illness as nonspecific symptom groups generated by endogenous underlying patterns of brain activity, a viewpoint for which **Alfred Hoche** had argued. "Every day it becomes clearer that it is impossible to demarcate satisfactorily both illnesses [schizophrenia and MDI]. . . . Yet I believe it remains clear that the notion of basically different illness processes must be retained." His article on "The Manifestations of Insanity" appeared in the *Journal of Combined Neurology and Psychiatry* (*Zeitschrift für die gesamte Neurologie und Psychiatrie*) (p. 27).

Kurt Schneider said later of this important article, "In this contribution Kraepelin did nothing more and nothing less that give up the basic idea of his life's work" (*Problems of Clinical Psychiatry* [*Probleme der klinischen Psychiatrie*], 1932, p. 21).

"Athymhormie" (lack of vital impulse) (1922). Maurice Dide (1873–1944), chief of the Braqueville mental hospital, and Paul Guiraud (1882–1974), one of his staff psychiatrists, proposed in their 1922 textbook, *Psychiatry for the Medical Practitioner* (*La psychiatrie du médecin practicien*) a pathogenic mechanism for dementia praecox: disregulation of the suboptic centers of the midbrain—especially the locus niger—as a key factor in the lack of vital force in the illness (dementia praecox they called "a hereditary illness characterized by the fragility and elective involution of groups of neurons that regulate the cenesthetic synthesis and instinctive vital activity" [p. 209]). They proposed rebaptizing dementia praecox as "juvenile athymhormie," suggesting as its central quality "the loss of the élan of the cenesthetic [sense of the body] and affective capacity" (p. 178).

The choice of this neologism Guiraud explained in his *General Psychiatry* (*Psychiatrie générale*) in 1950 as follows: "We wanted to suggest that the essential element in hebephrenia is . . . a lack of vital dynamism . . . From athymhormie all the essential symptoms are derived: uninterest, inertia, lack of affectivity . . . A lack of physiological dynamism could thus be the result of a lack of cellular dynamism" (pp. 493–494). **Henri Ey** defined the condition in his 1960 textbook as "a change in affective life: the patient becomes withdrawn into himself, seems indifferent and inattentive to the pleasures and pains of life. This behavior ends up in sulkiness, moroseness, frequently interrupted with paradoxal acts, ideas or sentiments, such as a sudden interest in philosophy or the theater" (*Manuel de psychiatrie*, p. 479). Today in France, "athymhormie" counts as a deficit or autistic symptom in schizophrenia. Dide, who was active in the Resistance during the war, was arrested by the Gestapo and died in Buchenwald. (The notion of Hormé, or Greek for "I put into motion," enjoyed a certain psychiatric currency in the interwar years, and Zurich neurologist Constantin von Monakow [1853–1930] and psychiatrist Raoul Mourgue in their 1928 book, *Biological Introduction to the Study of Neurology and Psychopathology* [*Introduction biologique à l'étude de la neurologie et de la psychopathologie*], speak of the "vital activity" of the brain as part of the "matrix of instincts or Hormé" that differentiate the body and its capacity of self-regeneration from a machine that has been damaged [p. x].)

Schizoaffective psychosis (1933). The question of "combined psychoses"—meaning generally a combination of schizophrenia and manic-depressive illness—had long been discussed in clinical circles. In 1903 Tübingen psychiatry professor Robert Gaupp (1870–1953) had examined the "combined psychoses" in the *Zentralblatt für Nervenheilkunde,* and the phrase "mixed psychoses" (Mischpsychosen) was familiar to German psychopathologists. Identifying such combinations as a homogeneous clinical subgroup was the work of Jacob S. Kasanin (1897–1946), research director of the state hospital in Howard, Rhode Island, who proposed as a separate category of "the acute schizoaffective psychoses" a group of young men and women, "quite well integrated socially, who suddenly blow up in a dramatic psychosis and present a clinical picture which may be called either schizophrenic or affective." There was, Kasanin pointed out, a research tradition of finding so-called schizophrenic features such as catatonia in manic-depressive illness. Yet unlike the cases in the literature, the nine patients whom Kasanin presented did not deteriorate. "Stress" had typically precipitated the illness, which might then recurr over time. Premorbidly, they had healthy personalities. "The fact that there is comparatively little of the extremely bizarre, unusual and mysterious, is what perhaps gives these cases a fairly good chance of recovery" (p. 101).

In the discussion following Kasanin's paper at the American Psychiatric Association's annual meeting in 1932, one participant said, "We have been in the habit of labeling these cases as psychopathic personalities with schizoid make-up or personalities with schizoid substrata. I think the name of schizoaffective is more appropriate" (I. L. Polozker of Detroit, *American Journal of Psychiatry*, pp. 123).

Kurt Schneider's first-rank and second-rank symptoms of schizophrenia (1939). Although **Schneider** did not believe in the existence of schizophrenia as a separate disease, he nonetheless accepted it as a type of illness. In this type, he distinguished between symptoms that were distinctive to schizophrenia but not seen in normal people or in other types of psychiatric illnesses ("qualitatively abnormal"), and symptoms that represented an exaggeration of otherwise normal types of experiences ("quantitatively [gradmässig] abnormal"). The former he called "first-rank symptoms," the latter "second-rank." Among the first-rank symptoms were delusions (Wahnwahrnehmungen), audible thoughts (Gedankenlautwerden), voices arguing (Stimmen in der Form von Rede und Gegenrede), voices commenting on one's actions (Begleitung des eigenen Tuns mit halluzinierten Bemerkungen), the belief that one's bodily organs, especially the sexual organs, are driving one's behavior (körperliche, insbesondere sexuelle Beeinflussungen), thought withdrawal and influencing by others (Gedankenentzug und Gedankenbeeinflussung), everything "made" by others (alles "Gemachte") in the area of feelings, drives, and the will. (In the 1946 edition of his classification, *Contributions to Psychiatry* [*Beiträge zur Psychiatrie*], Schneider added thought-broadcasting (Gedankenausbreitung) to the list of first-rank symptoms [p. 54].)

Among the "second-rank symptoms" were hallucinations (Sinnestäuschungen), the experience of thought-slowing (Denkhemmung), the flight of ideas (Ideenflucht), distractedness and perplexity (Zerfahrenheit und Ratlosigkeit), compulsive behavior (der Zwang), sudden delusional notions (der Wahneinfall), out-of-body experiences (die Entfremdungserlebnisse), "most disgruntlements" (die meisten Verstimmungen), and emotional blunting (die erlebte Gefühlsverarmung) (*Psychiatric Findings and Psychiatric Diagnosis* [*Psychischer Befund und Psychiatrische Diagnose*], 1939, p. 25). Schneider prided himself on having derived these characteristic features from a careful study of psychopathology based on the work of **Karl Jaspers**. Schneider later said, "When first-rank symptoms are present, that always means schizophrenia to us, but first-rank symptoms are not always present" (in the journal *Progress in Neurology, Psychiatry* [*Fortschritte der Neurologie, Psychiatrie*], 1957, p. 490).

(Clive Sidney Mellor [1932–], a psychiatrist at Manchester University, later found that each of the first-rank symptoms occurs in only a minority of schizophrenic patients, the commonest being thought-broadcasting [in 21.4% of a sample of 173 schizophrenics], the least common, impulses "made" by others [2.9%]. *See* his article in the *British Journal of Psychiatry*, 1970.)

Yet Schneider's most reliable guide to the diagnosis of schizophrenia did not make it into the "first-rank" symptoms but was articulated, almost in passing, in his psychiatric lectures to family doctors (*Psychiatrische Vorlesungen für Ärzte*) in 1933: "Making the diagnosis from the doctor—patient relationship. [Erfassung aus der Beziehung]: This is in workaday psychiatry usually the method of diagnosis. It concerns what is referred to as rapport or contact. Here the relevant fact is that most schizophrenics simply seem to occupy another, alien space, that one cannot simply relate to them as to a healthy individual or to a psychopath or to a cyclothymic depressive. It is difficult to express it other than in images [elsewhere Schneider spoke of a "glass wall" between the doctor and patient], and it is impossible to articulate this method as a concept " (p. 182 from the second edition in 1936).

Schizophreniform psychosis (1939). In contrast to the deteriorating form of schizophrenia, there were patients with previously more or less normal personalities who became acutely ill, often in response to stress. It was this kind of reactive schizophrenia that Gabriel Langfeldt (1895–1983), a staff psychiatrist at the university psychiatric clinic in Vinderen, near Oslo, called "schizophreniform." "Schizophrenia-like cases and particularly those revealing manic-depressive features, a strong hereditary taint and reactive . . . precipitation . . . give the best results [with **insulin** or **cardiazol** shock treatment], while the typical endogenic process psychoses characterized by depersonalization do not react to the treatment" (pp. 10–11). Langfeldt singled out the "schizophreniform psychoses" as a distinct group after the "typical schizophrenias" have been removed. The former had high rates of spontaneous remission and did well on shock therapy. The diagnosis of "schizophreniform psychosis" became popular because it suggested the existence of a treatment-responsive subpopulation and because clinicians liked its milder prognosis. Langfeldt's book *The Schizophreniform States* appeared in 1939 (in Copenhagen, in English). (*See also* **CONVULSIVE THERAPY: CHEMICAL**.)

SCHIZOPHRENIA: RECENT CONCEPTS. (*See also* **SCHIZOPHRENIA: EMERGENCE.**) After the Second World War, two contradictory tendencies hallmarked the approach to the psychoses and schizophrenia. One was the growing predominance of psychoanalysis, with its tendency to use the term "schizophrenia" to mean any psychiatric illness not amenable to office-based psychotherapy. The second was the growing thrust of biological research in schizophrenia.

Pseudoneurotic schizophrenia (1949). Uneasy about the tendency among psychoanalytically oriented psychiatrists to make a diagnosis of neurosis rather than schizophrenia, in an article in the *Psychiatric Quarterly* in 1949, Paul Hoch (1902–1964) and Phillip Polatin (1905–1980) of the New York State Psychiatric Institute called attention to a form of schizophrenia without delusions or hallucinations but characterized by what **Bleuler** had called dereistic (**autistic**) thinking and by disturbances of personality sufficiently severe to be called "pan-neurosis." This was a bridge between psychodynamic and classical formulations. They considered it possible that these "borderline" patients would evolve into full schizophrenia with deterioration. Hoch, who was born in Budapest and had studied in Göttingen and in Zurich with Manfred Bleuler, was oriented toward **Eugen Bleuler's** concepts of schizophrenia.

Schizophrenia and psychosis in *DSM-"One"* (1952). This first volume in the series of diagnostic and statistical manuals of the American Psychiatric Association (APA) accepted the distinction between organic brain disorders ("impairment of brain tissue function") and "psychogenic" disorders. Among the psychogenic variety were involutional psychotic reaction ("involutional" being a Kraepelinian inheritance; *see* **DEPRESSION: EMERGENCE: involutional melancholia** [1896]), schizophrenic "reactions" (the notion of reaction borrowed from Adolf Meyer rather than Karl Jaspers), and paranoid reactions. In line with the psychoanalytic thinking that dominated American psychiatry in those years, "manic depressive reaction" and "psychotic depressive reaction" were also considered to be "psychogenic."

The actual psychopathological symptoms that the APA accepted for schizophrenia reflected the influence of **Eugen Bleuler's** definition (*see* **SCHIZOPHRENIA: EMERGENCE**): "The disorders are marked by a strong tendency to retreat from reality, by emotional disharmony, unpredictable disturbances in stream of thought. . . ." Only some deteriorated (p. 26).

Schizophrenia and psychosis in *DSM-II* (1968). The second edition of the *DSM* series tried to bring American nosology more into line with the European; namely, the World Health Organization's *International Classification of Diseases* (*ICD*, eighth edition), adopted in 1966. "Psychogenic" schizophrenia thus went out the window, and the American Psychiatric Association's *Manual* simply distinguished between Organic Brain Syndromes (whether psychotic or not) and "Psychoses not attributed to physical conditions listed previously." Otherwise, there were no big changes from *DSM-I*, except perhaps to stipulate the psychoanalytic conviction—a movement that by this time predominated in American academic psychiatry—that the delusions and hallucinations "frequently appear psychologically self-protective" (p. 33). In general, both *DSM-I* and *DSM-II* used the term "psychosis" as a synonym for "severe" rather than in some specific psychopathological sense.

The "St. Louis criteria" of schizophrenia (1972). As part of the diagnostic rethinking leading up to ***DSM-III***, John Feighner and the other members of the

St. Louis school published in 1972 in the *Archives of General Psychiatry* an article on "Diagnostic Criteria for Use in Psychiatric Research." For schizophrenia, they offered a revised set of criteria, including mainly delusions and hallucinations plus some evidence of thought disorder. (There were also several social criteria such as being single and having a poor work history.)

Three years later, in 1975, Michael Alan Taylor (1940–) and Richard Abrams (1937–) at the State University of New York at Stony Brook argued in the *American Journal of Psychiatry* that the St. Louis criteria set the bar too low, proposing more rigorous criteria of their own, including a "formal thought disorder" (not just difficulty in communicating), the presence of "emotional blunting," auditory hallucinations, or sudden, fully formed delusions. In a sample of 89 patients recently hospitalized for "schizophrenia," only 12% satisfied the St. Louis criteria, 11% satisfied the Taylor and Abrams research criteria, and only 5 patients were considered schizophrenic by both criteria.

Finding metabolic abnormalities in schizophrenia: frontal lobes (1974). Although previous researchers had discovered numerous scattered brain abnormalities in schizophrenia, none had been reliably reproducible. In 1974, *David* Henschen Ingvar (1924–2000), professor of clinical neurophysiology at Lund University in Sweden, and *Göran* Anders Franzén (1929–), on-staff in the psychiatry department, discovered with the aid of radiolabeled xenon gas that blood flow was reduced in the frontal lobes of schizophrenia patients, especially older ones, compared to controls. This pointed to lower metabolic activity in the frontal lobes, meaning less activity in the neurons. In their article in *Acta Psychiatrica Scandinavica* they commented, "The finding of a significantly low resting blood flow in the frontal lobes (the 'hypofrontal' rCBF [regional cerebral blood flow] pattern) . . . warrants discussion of similarities between the symptoms in frontal lobe lesions and in chronic schizophrenia" (p. 457). They went on to point out numerous similarities between schizophrenia and organic frontal lobe lesions and helped direct attention of psychosis researchers to this area of the brain.

First computerized tomography finding of brain abnormalities in schizophrenia (1976). A group of researchers led by Eve C. Johnstone (1944–), who had just received her M.D. from the University of Glasgow (*see* **WOMEN IN PSYCHIATRY**), and **Timothy J. Crow** in the Divisions of Psychiatry and Radiology of the Clinical Research Centre in Harrow, Middlesex, England, found that, compared to controls, 17 institutionalized patients with schizophrenia had larger cerebral ventricles, and that increased ventricular size was "associated with poor performance on cognitive testing." This was the first finding of structural change in schizophrenia involving controls. It was published in the *Lancet*. (Gerd Huber's [1921–] earlier finding in 1964 at Heidelberg University of organic defects in schizophrenia employed pneumoencephalography (*see* his article in Gruhle, ed., *Psychiatrie der Gegenwart*, vol. 1). (*See* **NEUROIMAGING**.)

Much "schizophrenia" turns out to be manic-depressive illness (1978). In the *Archives of General Psychiatry*, Harrison G. Pope, Jr. (1947–) and Joseph F. Lipinski, Jr. (1940–), both of the Harvard University department of psychiatry, found in a review of studies that "schizophrenia" had been greatly overdiagnosed in United States psychiatry; manic-depressive illness (MDI) was similarly underdiagnosed. They also concluded that "'Schizophrenic' symptoms [as then understood] have virtually no demonstrated value in predicting outcome in psychoses" (p. 826). Furthermore: "Given that a patient, once misdiagnosed, is often misdiagnosed again and again, it is possible that there are upwards of 100,000 patients in this country carrying a diagnosis of schizophrenia who in fact suffer from MDI" (p. 825). This article helped shift the emphasis in psychosis from schizophrenia to affective disorder.

Type I vs. Type II syndromes of schizophrenia (1980). *See* **POSITIVE VS. NEGATIVE SYMPTOMS.**

Schizophrenia and psychosis in *DSM-III* (1980). Based on preliminary work by the **St. Louis school**, Taylor and Abrams, and the "RDC" criteria (*see above*), in ***DSM-III*** the psychoanalytic and **Meyerian** traditions were cast aside, and the classical German interpretations of psychopathology were given a new lease on life. The *DSM* drafters drew upon **Emil Kraepelin** in insisting that "deterioration from a previous level of functioning" be present before the diagnosis was granted. They drew upon **Kurt Schneider's** first-rank symptoms in asserting that a certain "content of thought" was often present, involving such symptoms as thought insertion, thought withdrawal, and the delusion of thoughts being controlled by some outside power. And they drew upon **Bleuler's** "basic symptoms" in saying that schizophrenics often had a certain "form of thought" involving the loosening of associations: "When loosening of associations is severe, incoherence may occur, that is, speech may become incomprehensible" (p. 182). (The points in this section are referenced at **SCHIZOPHRENIA: EMERGENCE.**)

One can see virtually the entire European tradition of psychopathology culminating in the symptoms that the *DSM* drafters were willing to accept: disorders of perception involving, in particular, auditory hallucinations, the blunting of affect, the diminution of drive. Dereism, catatonia, and other symptoms from the classic tradition also received their toll.

Yet, the actual checklist of symptoms for which—in the familiar *DSM-III* style—the patient would have to qualify in order to receive the diagnosis was heavily weighted toward Kraepelinian "positive" symptoms (Kraepelin did not use the phrase "positive"). Of the six "class A" diagnostic criteria, five involved hallucinations and delusions. (Class B involved deterioration; class C stipulated a minimum 6 months' duration.) Thus, the American *DSM-III* shifted the balance away from the generous Bleulerian view with its optimistic prognoses and back to the restrictive Kraepelinian with its florid psychoses and dim prognosis. It was partly for this reason (and partly because *DSM-III* represented a revival of "disease-thinking" in general) that **Gerald Klerman** referred to it in 1990 as "neo-Kraepelinian."

DSM-III granted independent status to **schizoid personality**. As well, in *DSM-III* several other diagnoses once grouped under the schizophrenia umbrella became independent. "Paranoia," "schizophreniform disorder," and "brief reactive psychosis" all acquired statuses of their own. Psychotic depression became firmly arrayed under affective disorders, and "schizoaffective disorder" and "atypical psychosis" also struggled free.

When the definitions conventionally used in U.S. psychiatry in the 1960s were applied to a group of patients, 163 qualified for the diagnosis of schizophrenia. When the *DSM-III* criteria were applied to the same group, only 19 did so. As English psychiatrist Ian Brockington noted in *European Psychiatry* in 1992, "There must be something profoundly wrong with a concept which has proved so unstable in its usage" (p. 203). (*See also* **WERNICKE–KLEIST–LEONHARD PATHWAY**.)

First quantitative magnetic-resonance study of schizophrenia (1986). **Nancy Andreasen** at the University of Iowa led a team using the **neuroimaging** technique of magnetic resonance imaging (MRI) to establish that schizophrenic patients had smaller frontal lobe size and also smaller intracranial and cerebral volume. This led the group, publishing in the *Archives of General Psychiatry* in 1986, to reinforce the hypothesis that schizophrenia was a "neurodevelopmental" disorder. In this work, they also pioneered a technique for making quantitative measurements of MRI images that eventuated in "voxel-based morphimetry."

Weinberger launches the "DLPFC" hypothesis (1986). Although researchers had long known there was some kind of frontal lobe problem in schizophrenia, in 1986 Daniel Weinberger (1947–), of the Section on Clinical Neuropsychiatry of the **National Institute of Mental Health** at **St. Elizabeths Hospital** in Washington, D.C., suggested that some of the symptoms of schizophrenia—both positive and negative—were owing to a lesion in the dorsolateral prefrontal cortex (DLPFC). The researchers had looked at regional blood flood in schizophrenics as compared to controls as they inhaled radiolabeled xenon gas (Xe 133): While doing a card-sorting test, the controls experienced a clear rise in blood flow in that area, whereas that of the schizophrenics underwent no change, suggesting lowered responsiveness (lesion) in that area of the brain. "The changes were regionally specific, involving only DLPFC" (p. 114). This research in the *Archives of General Psychiatry* promised to "shed light on one of the most physiologically mysterious aspects of schizophrenia—its tendency to appear in late adolescence." Weinberger analogized to other kinds of central nervous system lesions "the clinical manifestations of which appear or change with maturation as the affected neural system comes 'on line' " (p. 123).

Location of a possible single-gene locus for schizophrenia (1988). In work led by Robin Sherrington in the psychiatry department of the former Middlesex School of Medicine of the University of London, a group of nine co-authors reported in an article in *Nature* that two DNA "polymorphisms" (variant forms) on the long arm of Chromosome 5 were reliably linked to seven families in Britain and Iceland with histories of schizophrenia. The finding remained tentative because other groups at the time were not able to reproduce it. (*See also* **PSYCHIATRIC GENETICS** [1988].)

Late onset schizophrenia (1997). In 1997 in the *American Journal of Geriatric Psychiatry*, Dilip V. Jeste (1944–) and co-workers at the University of California at San Diego proposed the concept of "late onset schizophrenia" (LOS). Three years later, in 2000, at a consensus conference led by Robert Howard (1961–) of the Institute of Psychiatry in London, late onset schizophrenia replaced such older concepts as "paraphrenia in the elderly." (*See* **PARAPHRENIA**).

SCHNEIDER, KURT (1887–1967). The leading psychopathologist after **Karl Jaspers**, Schneider was born in Crailsheim, a small town in southwest Germany, into the family of a jurist. He studied medicine in Berlin and Tübingen (graduated in 1912). Enthralled by Robert Gaupp's lectures in psychiatry at Tübingen, he trained in psychiatry at the Lindenburg clinic in Cologne, served as an army psychiatrist in the period 1914–1918, then returned for his Habilitation to Cologne, earning simultaneously a Ph.D. in philosophy under Max Scheler (1874–1928), an influential phenomenologist. In 1931, he became director of the clinical service of the German Psychiatric Research Institute (Deutsche Forschungsanstalt für Psychiatrie) in Munich and chief psychiatrist of the adjacent Munich-Schwabing Hospital. During the Second World War, he again served as an army psychiatrist in the campaigns in Russia and France, and at war's end, in late 1945 he became professor of psychiatry in Heidelberg, stepping down in 1955. Schneider is best known to international audiences for his distinction between vital and reactive depression in 1920 (*See* **DEPRESSION: EMERGENCE: vital depression**) and for devising in 1939 the first-rank criteria, thought to be almost pathognomonic for diagnosing schizophrenia. (*See* **SCHIZOPHRENIA: EMERGENCE: Kurt Schneider's first rank . . .**) He is not to be confused with Carl Schneider (1891–1946), professor of psychiatry in Heidelberg in the period 1933–1945, who committed suicide in an American military prison.

SEASONAL AFFECTIVE DISORDER (SAD). *See* **DEPRESSION: seasonal affective disorder** (1984).

SEDATIVES/HYPNOTICS. *See* **BARBITURATES; BENZODIAZEPINES.**

SELECTIVE SEROTONIN REUPTAKE INHIBITORS (SSRIs). SSRIs represent a class of drugs based on the concept that inhibiting the "reuptake" of the neurotransmitter serotonin in the brain, at the synaptic junction between neurons, could bring relief in depression and other illnesses. (*See* **NEUROTRANSMITTER; SYNAPSE.**) Reuptake means reabsorbing into the upstream (presynaptic) neuron the quantity of neurotransmitter that has just been discharged into the synaptic cleft in order to make the downstream (postsynaptic) neuron fire. Inhibiting reuptake would, in theory, increase the quantity of serotonin available at the synapse and thus relieve psychiatric symptoms. Inhibiting reuptake does relieve symptoms. What has never been confirmed scientifically, however, is that there was anything wrong with the serotonin system.

Zimeldine. The story: The study of serotonin uptake and its modification by drugs was initiated by Julius Axelrod (1912–) and a co-worker at the **National Institute of Mental Health** in 1963; the researchers used a radiolabeled form, reporting their first results in the *Journal of Pharmacology and Experimental Therapeutics*. Then in 1968, Swedish pharmacologist Arvid Carlsson (1923–) of Gothenborg University discovered that the tricyclic antidepressant **imipramine** blocked the reuptake of serotonin in serotonin-type neurons (work co-authored by Kjell Fuxe [1938–] and Urban Ungerstedt [1942–], published in the *Journal of Pharmacy and Pharmacology*). "This action may be of importance for its antidepressant properties," the authors said.* (In 2000, Carlsson won a Nobel Prize for Physiology or Medicine for his research on dopamine.) This work excited interest at a number of pharmaceutical houses in the

* This hypothesis was spelled out in greater detail in an article co-authored by Carlsson, Corrodi, Fuxe, and Tomas Hökfelt in the *European Journal of Pharmacology* in 1969.

development of SSRIs (although that acronym did not come into use until the early 1990s).

Yet, it turned out that another tricyclic antidepressant drug, clomipramine, had an even more powerful effect on serotonin than did imipramine. Around 1970, therefore, Carlsson and an organic chemist named Hans Corrodi (1929–1974) at the Hässle Company in Mölndal, Sweden (which shortly thereafter became part of the Astra company), set out to design a molecule that would have an elective effect on serotonin reuptake (and that could be patented). Using an antihistamine called chlorpheniramine as a base, they came up with a strong selective serotonin reuptake inhibitor that Astra called zimeldine (after the drug was patented in 1972) and that was marketed in Europe in 1982 under the brand name Zelmid. This was the first SSRI in psychiatry. (The antihistamines had always been SSRIs.) Unfortunately, Zelmid was withdrawn in 1983 because it caused isolated cases of Guillain–Barré syndrome, a polyneuritis that affects neuromuscular function. This was one of the first occasions in which rational principles of drug design had actually been used to sculpt a pharmaceutical.

Six further SSRIs followed and are listed below in the order in which they were patented.

Paroxetine (1974). Patented by the Ferrosan company, which in 1980 sold the license to the company then known as SmithKline Beecham (folded into Glaxo SmithKline after 2000), the drug was launched as "Paxil" in the United States in 1993 and was advertised under the catchy acronym "SSRI," which the company coined. (Ferrosan had also made in 1974 the SSRI femoxetine, which died in development.)

Fluvoxamine (1975). The Philips-Duphar Company patented the molecule in 1975; it was launched by Duphar as "Floxyfral" in Switzerland in 1983 for depression (in the United Kingdom as "Faverin") and in the United States by the Solvay Company as "Luvox" in 1995 for obsessive-compulsive disorder.

Fluoxetine (1975). Patented by Lilly in 1975, the company apparently considered bringing it out initially as a weight-loss drug, then launched it as Prozac in the United States in 1988 for depression. (It was approved by the Food and Drug Administration in December 1987.) Prozac was one of the most successful products in the history of pharmaceuticals and virtually gave its name to an era.

Indalpine (1977). Patented by the French firm Mar-Pha Société, Fournier Frères acquired the license and marketed it in 1983 as an antidepressant, "Upstène," "the first specific inhibitor of the reuptake of serotonin," the company claimed. The drug was later withdrawn because of liver toxicity.

Citalopram (1977). Patented by Kefalas A/S, a subsidiary of the Lundbeck Company of Denmark, Lundbeck brought out citalopram in Denmark in 1989 as "Cipramil"; Lundbeck sold U.S. rights to Forest Pharmaceuticals, which marketed it in the United States in 1998 as "Celexa," an antidepressant.

Sertraline (1981). Patented by Pfizer, the company launched sertraline in 1992 as "Zoloft": "Gets depressed patients back into the mainsteam." As with the other "American" SSRIs, Pfizer subsequently extracted a number of other indications for the compound in the anxiety area from the Food and Drug Administration, in this case, for panic disorder, obsessive-compulsive disorder, posttraumatic stress disorder, and social anxiety disorder, as well as for "major depression."

Sertraline was the last "SSRI."* The Achilles' heel of this particular drug class, as Anita H. Clayton (1956–) of the University of Virginia and collaborators pointed out in an article in the *Journal of Clinical Psychiatry* in 2002, was the 30% to 40% rate of sexual dysfunction the various SSRIs produce.

It is an ironical consequence of the long delays required for licensing a drug, and of the interplay between science and marketing, that a drug class conceived in the 1960s, with numerous "me-toos" in the 1970s, became the latest new thing in psychopharmaceuticals in the 1990s.

SEROTONIN. *See* **SELECTIVE SEROTONIN REUPTAKE INHIBITORS (SSRIs).**

SHELL SHOCK. *See* **POSTTRAUMATIC STRESS DISORDER (PTSD).**

SHEPHERD, MICHAEL (1923–1995). The founder of psychiatric epidemiology—and a major figure in social psychiatry—in Britain, Shepherd was born in Bournemouth, England. After reading medicine at Oxford, he qualified in psychological medicine at the **Maudsley Hospital** in 1949 under **Aubrey Lewis**. Becoming a Reader in psychiatry at the Institute of Psychiatry, Shepherd began his career with important work in psychopharmacology, helping to pioneer the technique of the randomized clinical trial (RCT).† In a pioneering article in the *Lancet* in 1955, Shepherd and David Lewis Davies (1911–1983), also of the Maudsley Hospital, performed an RCT on **reserpine**, finding it of some effectiveness in the treatment of anxious and depressed patients. Later, Shepherd played a role in organizing the British Medical Research Council Clinical Trials committee and served as its secretary and chair for 20 years. In 1968 he, Malcolm Lader (1936–)—professor of psychopharmacology at the Maudsley—and Richard Rodnight wrote *Clinical Psychopharmacology*, an early text. In the judgment of Shepherd's obituarist David Healy (1954–), writing in 2004 in Ban, ed., *Reflections on Twentieth-Century Psychopharmacology,* "This early [epidemiological] work led to a huge literature with which many prominent names have been associated such as . . . **Gerald Klerman** and **Myrna Weissman** in the United States. The epidemiological catchment areas studies in the United States were directly descended from the original Shepherd studies" (p. 578).

Later, as professor of epidemiological psychiatry, Shepherd did significant work on London, ascertaining from a sample of general practices that psychiatric morbidity was really quite common in the population and that the great majority of it never entered the mental-health system. He and co-workers published these findings in a book

---

* Technically, the last drug marketed as an "SSRI" was Lundbeck's escitalopram (patented in 1990 and launched in the United States in 2002 by Forest as Lexapro). Yet, it is merely an isomer, or mirror-image, of citalopram.

† The RCT was first proposed by Sir Austin Bradford Hill (1897–1991), professor of medical statistics at the London School of Hygiene and Tropical Medicine, and was carried out by Hill and Marc Daniels in trials on the chemotherapy of pulmonary tuberculosis beginning in 1948, the results of which were described in 1952 in the *British Medical Journal*.

that established psychiatric epidemiology in Britain, *Psychiatric Illness in General Practice* (1966). To train family doctors better to cope with psychiatric problems, Shepherd helped found at the Maudsley the General Practice Research Unit, which, as his colleague at the Maudsley David Goldberg (1934–) put it, "formed a nursery for a whole generation of young social psychiatrists" (*Psychological Medicine*, 1995, p. 1110). He cofounded the journal *Psychological Medicine* and was famously involved in a debate with Mogens Schou about the therapeutic efficacy of **lithium**, in which Shepherd greatly disbelieved. Sheperd was not the most amiable of men, although undoubtedly brilliant, and David Goldberg later said of the experience of working with him, "Sometimes I simply couldn't stay awake in his ward rounds because his manner with patients was so unpleasant that I found consciousness was no longer possible. I learnt to stick closely beside him and go into a deep delta sleep during those ward rounds but he never looked at me and so I think I was never discovered."

SLATER, ELIOT TREVOR OAKESHOTT (1904–1983). One of the founders of psychiatric genetics, Slater was born in London, his father a schoolmaster and his mother, Violet Oakeshott Slater, a painter. He studied medicine at Cambridge, then in 1927–1930 was a house officer at St. George's Hospital in London. After a brief stint at the West End Hospital for Nervous Diseases, in 1931 he went to the **Maudsley Hospital,** where he would remain in various capacities (director of the branch called the Sutton Emergency Hospital in Sutton, Surrey, during the war) until 1946. At the Maudsley, **Aubrey Lewis** guided Slater toward genetics. In 1946, Slater shifted to the National Hospital at Queen Square in London as physician in psychological medicine until his retirement in 1964, after which his various appointments were honorary in nature. Between 1959 and 1969, he was director of the MRC Psychiatric Genetics Unit at the Maudsley.

During the tenure of a Rockefeller Fellowship in 1934–1935, he was able to study genetics in Berlin and at the German Psychiatric Research Institute in Munich, which furthered his lifelong interest in twin studies as the mechanism of research in psychiatric genetics. Once back at the Maudsley, he began interviewing twin pairs, to see, when one twin had a major psychiatric illness, how often the co-twin acquired it as well. In 1936, he wrote on the inheritance of manic-depressive insanity in the *Proceedings of the Royal Society of Medicine*. Slater's book *Psychotic and Neurotic Illnesses in Twins* (1953) is one of the landmarks in psychiatric genetics. He amplified his research in *The Genetics of Mental Disorders*, published in 1971. On the basis of his wartime experience at Sutton Emergency Hospital, in 1944 he and **William Sargant** published *An Introduction to Physical Methods of Treatment in Psychiatry*, describing such procedures as **insulin coma** and **electroconvulsive therapy**. In 1954, led by **Willi Mayer-Gross**, Slater and Martin Roth wrote *Clinical Psychiatry*, probably the most influential textbook of psychiatry since **Kraepelin's**. Slater is also known for a battle with the Washington University in **St. Louis school**, chiefly **Samuel Guze**, about the nature of "hysteria," which Slater on the basis of his experiences at the neurologically oriented National Hospital thought an artifact (Guze said it was an inherited illness). *See* Slater's "Hysteria 311" in the *Journal of Mental Science* in 1961. His main conceptual notion, beginning in 1958 in the *Acta Genetica et Statistica Medica*, was a "monogenic" theory of schizophrenia, arguing that the illness was caused by one gene.

SLEEP DISORDERS. Insomnia is the most common sleep disorder. For its treatment, *see* **BARBITURATES; BENZODIAZEPINES.** *See also* **NARCOLEPSY; REM (RAPID EYE MOVEMENT) SLEEP.**

SNYDER, SOLOMON H. (1938–). A pioneer of the study of brain receptors and the binding of psychiatric drugs to them, Snyder was born in Washington, D.C., his father a cryptographer for the National Security Agency. After earning his M.D. at Georgetown University in 1962, between 1963 and 1965 he worked in the laboratory of pharmacologist Julius Axelrod (1912–) at the **National Institute of Mental Health,** where he acquired basic knowledge of molecular biology. Still intent upon becoming a psychiatrist, in 1965 he began training at Johns Hopkins University while lecturing there in the department of pharmacology. Snyder remained at Hopkins with his primary appointment in pharmacology, yet seeing psychiatric patients and supervising residents.

From the late 1960s on, Snyder and co-workers in his laboratory made a number of important discoveries that opened up the field of receptorology. In 1972, wishing to do something to help out in the nation's "war on drugs," they tried to find the target of opiates in the brain using binding approaches (attempting to find a "ligand," or radiolabeled drug, that binds to a given receptor). In 1973 Snyder and Candace Pert (1946–) discovered the opiate receptor (in research published in the *Proceedings of the National Academy of Sciences*), and shortly thereafter the two of them and others were able to identify agonists and antagonists of the receptor (in work published in 1973 in *Science*). Given that the properties of the opiate receptor "seemed very much like those of neurotransmitter receptors," as Synder later said, "we employed similar reversible ligand binding techniques to identify receptors for most of the major neurotransmitters in the brain, including those for dopamine [1975], alpha adrenergic [1976], . . . and serotonin [1975]." Julius Axelrod said of this work, "He revolutionized the field by using radioactive ligands of high specific activity to measure the binding constants of ligands to receptors. The grind and bind approach. . . . The whole field of receptorology exploded" (Healy, *Psychopharmacologists,* I, p. 42). His work on nitric oxide as a neurotransmitter, culminating in an article in *Science* in 1992 on "nitric oxide as a mediator of penile erection," helped lead to the drug sildenafil (Viagra) for erectile dysfunction.

SOCIOPATHY. *See* **CONDUCT DISORDER; CRIMINALITY AND PSYCHIATRY; PERSONALITY DISORDERS: Partridge** (1930).

SOMATIZATION. *See* **HYSTERIA-PSYCHOSOMATIC-SOMATIZATION** (1924 and after).

SOMATOFORM DISORDERS. *See* **HYSTERIA-PSYCHOSOMATIC-SOMATIZATION: *DSM-III*** (1980).

SPITZER, ROBERT L. (1932–). The architect of ***DSM-III,*** which completely revised psychiatric diagnosis in the United States and worldwide, Spitzer was born in White Plains, New York, and earned his M.D. in 1957 from New York University School of Medicine. He trained in psychiatry (1958–1961) at the New York State Psychiatric Institute (affiliated with the department of psychiatry of Columbia University), during which time he also completed a training program in psychoanalysis. (In later years, he came to regard psychoanalysis with great skepticism and as an obstacle to the development of an empirically based psychiatry.) In 1961, he became a research fellow in the biometrics research department, headed by Joseph Zubin (1900–1990), a research psychologist who in the mid-1950s had founded the biometrics department at "PI," and who stimulated Spitzer's interest in measurement. In 1968, Spitzer served as a consultant to the Committee on Nomenclature and Statistics of the American Psychiatric Association as they prepared ***DSM-II***. In 1973, he led the successful effort to remove homosexuality as a diagnosis from successive printings of the *DSM-II*. (*See* **HOMOSEXUALITY AND PSYCHIATRY**). In 1974, Spitzer became head of the Task Force that produced ***DSM-III***, and in this connection, in 1978 he co-authored the Research Diagnostic Criteria with **Eli Robins** (*see* **St. Louis school; *DSM***). Shortly after the appearance of *DSM-III* in 1980, Spitzer became chair of the work group to revise that document, his wife Janet B. W. Williams functioning as text editor; the product of that committee, ***DSM-III-R***, was published in 1987. Because of the enormous impact of *DSM-III* and its successors worldwide, Spitzer emerges as one of the most influential figures in the history of late-twentieth-century psychiatry. In an interesting demonstration of the frequent gap between real influence and official attainment, his name is not even listed in the 18th edition of *American Men and Women of Science* (1992).

STROEMGREN, ERIK (1909–1993). (*See also* **PSYCHIATRIC GENETICS**.) Pioneer of psychiatric epidemiology and of lithium treatment, Strömgren was born in Copenhagen, his parents Swedes who had spent 6 years in Germany before moving to Denmark. His father was a professor of astronomy at the University of Copenhagen (also president of the Danish Academy of Sciences), his mother a distinguished dentist. After gaining his M.D. in Copenhagen in 1934, he interned first at Vordingbord psychiatric hospital near the island of Bornholm, then at the local general hospital on Bornholm island, an isolated area that he thought would be perfect for a genetic-epidemiological study. In the course of making more than a thousand home visits, he realized that the great majority of Bornholmers with psychiatric symptoms had never come into contact of any kind with psychiatry. Later Strömgren said, "The existence of this large number of undiagnosed and mostly untreated mentally disordered human beings seemed to me to constitute one of the most important problems of psychiatry" (Shepherd, *Psychiatrists*, p. 155).

In 1935, Strömgren traveled to Germany for a 3-week visit to the German Psychiatric Research Institute (DFA) in Munich to study research basics with psychiatric geneticists Ernst Rüdin (1874–1952), Hans Luxenburger (1894–1976), Franz Kallmann (1897–1965) and Bruno Schulz (1901–1954). His Bornholm research eventuated in his 1938 doctoral thesis, *Contributions to Psychiatric Genetics on the Basis of an Island Population* (*Beiträge zur psychiatrischen Erblehre, auf Grund von Untersuchungen an einer Inselbevölkerung*), which carried out the first comprehensive population study using modern techniques, calculating prevalence rates and inquiring about family history; it is now recognized as a classic in psychiatric epidemiology.

During the Second World War, Strömgren was an assistant of August Wimmer (*see* **PSYCHOSIS: EMERGENCE: psychogenic psychosis** [1916]) at the university hospital in Copenhagen, then in 1942 became acting director of the big psychiatric hospital in Roskilde, moving on a year later to the Aarhus psychiatric hospital in Risskov, of which he became chief in 1945 and simultaneously professor of psychiatry at Aarhus University. At the psychiatric hospital, he set out to develop a research institute similar to the one in Munich. Central to this plan was moving to Aarhus a national register of psychiatric patients founded in Copenhagen in the late 1920s at the Institute of Human Genetics. Strömgren used this to monitor all current psychiatric admissions in Denmark. His *Contributions to Psychiatric Epidemiology and Genetics* (1968) summarized his ideas about "reactive psychoses" and "schizophreniform psychoses" as well as his findings on schizophrenia from twin studies. During the years, Strömgren also worked as a consultant for the World Health Organization in Geneva and in Copenhagen. Scientifically, Strömgren is known for his work on the psychogenic psychoses (*see* **PSYCHOSIS: EMERGENCE: psychogenic psychosis** [1974]), for supporting Mogen Schou's work on **lithium** treatment of manic-depressive illness, and above all for making the Danish National Case Register "a research instrument of extraordinary significance for population genetics," as Strömgren's biographer Heinz Häfner put it (in *Nervenärzte*, edited by Hans Schliack). *See also* the obituary by Aksel Bertelsen and Irving Gottesman in *Neurology, Psychiatry and Brain Research* (1994).

SUBSTANCE ABUSE. Before the middle of the nineteenth century, the main substance capable of being abused was alcohol. With the rise of such anesthetic gases as ether (first used medically in 1846), of injectable opiate narcotics (after the introduction of the hypodermic method for administering a drug by Alexander Wood [1817–1884] of Edinburgh in 1853), and with the advent of such psychoactive drugs as the **barbiturates**, the number of substances capable of abuse became legion. As **Emil Kraepelin** warned in the fifth edition of his textbook in 1896, "A psychic illness quite similar to alcoholism and still increasing with terrifying rapidity is addiction to morphine, as we have learned in recent decades. And with morphine as well we generally see the combined paralyzing and agitating effects of the poison on the brain" (p. 44). Thus, almost from the beginning, psychiatry recognized the concept of substance abuse. What has changed during the years, however, is the balance between the discipline's assessment of personal dependency vs. social harm.

Although there had been much medical writing on substance abuse before the Second World War, the contemporary narrative begins with the first edition of ***DSM*** in 1952, where "drug addiction" was an aspect of "sociopathic personality disturbance." No further detail was supplied.

After a 1964 meeting of the Expert Committee on Addiction-Producing Drugs of the World Health Organization that recommended replacing "addiction" and "habituation" with the concept of "drug dependence," ***DSM-II*** in 1968 recognized "drug dependence"; there followed a long list of compounds, including *Cannabis sativa* (marihuana) and amphetamines, upon which one could become dependent. Alcohol and tobacco were exempted. To make a diagnosis of dependency, evidence was required of "habitual use or a clear sense of need for the drug." Withdrawal symptoms, it was stressed in the *Manual* were not the gold standard of the diagnosis, because "they may be entirely absent when cocaine or marihuana are withdrawn" (p. 45).

DSM-III in 1980 introduced a quite different note: the concept of "substance use disorders." The emphasis was upon "behavioral changes" rather than dependency, upon putting the search for drugs high on one's list of priorities to the disadvantage of other kinds of behavior. Thus, to qualify for a diagnosis of "substance abuse,"one would have to show (1) a pattern of "pathological use," as manifest in criminal behavior, car accidents, or drug-seeking behavior; and (2) "impairment in social or occupational functioning" caused by the abuse. Also recognized in the *Manual* was "substance dependence," a more pharmacological than social measure of a substance-use disorder, including tolerance (steadily increasing doses) and withdrawal symptoms. Alcohol and tobacco were no longer exempt. The brain consequences of addiction were considered in a section on "substance-induced organic mental disorders," variants of which continued in subsequent editions.

DSM-III-R in 1987 changed relatively little in this, except to call the group of diagnoses "psychoactive substance use disorders." The distinction between behavior ("substance abuse") and dependency symptoms such as withdrawal was upheld, though a good deal of behavior such as organizing one's day around drug-seeking was shifted into the dependency category.

DSM-IV in 1994 called the relevant category "substance-related disorders," grouping the potential drugs of abuse into an ever-widening list that now had 11 categories. This edition put some starch into the abuse vs. dependence dichotomy—so strong in 1980—that *DSM-III-R* had muddied a bit: Dependence meant "a pattern of repeated self-administration that usually results in tolerance, withdrawal, and compulsive drug-taking behavior." Abuse meant behavioral issues resulting in trouble for the abuser or for society ("a maladaptive pattern of substance use"). This edition broke the discussion down into "dependence" (meaning continued use despite problems), "abuse" (social, legal problems), "intoxication" (brain effects), and "withdrawal."

DSM-IV set a considerably lower threshold of what would be considered "abuse": Though *DSM-III-R* had insisted that one of two criteria should be met (continued use despite problems, or in dangerous situations), *DSM-IV* would accept one out of any four criteria in order to award the diagnosis. Basically, the kinds of problems one might have were split in the *Manual* into three separate categories, and it was said that significant issues in any one of these gives a patient the diagnosis.

If there is a central trend in the meandering that psychiatry's approach to substance abuse has taken during the years, it is an ever-growing impatience with compounds that people ingest for pleasure. Even though nicotine, alcohol, and the barbiturates are all substances capable of damaging their users—and the world about them—the level at which the whistle is blown is vastly lower in *DSM-IV* than in the days of Emil Kraepelin. (*See also* **ALCOHOLISM; NATIONAL INSTITUTE OF MENTAL HEALTH**.)

SULLIVAN, HARRY STACK (1892–1949). An advocate of psychotherapy for schizophrenic patients and of "interpersonal theory," Sullivan was born in Norwich, New York. He earned his M.D. from the Chicago College of Medicine and Surgery in 1917, trained in psychoanalysis in 1917–1918, then spent the next few years either in military service or caring for veterans. Between 1923 and 1930, he was director of clinical research at the Sheppard and Enoch Pratt Hospital in Baltimore, where he ran a small unit designed to treat schizophrenic patients with a modified version of psychoanalysis. Between 1930 and 1939, he was in private practice in New York, thereafter in Washington, D.C., until his death.

During his Washington years, Sullivan was influenced by **Adolf Meyer**'s belief that psychiatric symptoms represent a pathological reaction to personal circumstances. Sullivan is associated with "interpersonal" approaches to psychiatry, to schizophrenia in particular. As he explained in the *American Journal of Psychiatry* in 1931, "Schizophrenia is meaningful only in an interpersonal context; its characteristics can only be established by a study of the interrelation of the schizophrenic with schizophrenic, less schizophrenic, and non-schizophrenic others" (p. 523). As for treatment, Sullivan said, "[The patients] must be activated by a well-integrated purpose of helping in the re-development or development *de novo* of self-esteem as an individual attractive to others" (p. 531).

Sullivan emphasized a form of what was being called "milieu therapy" (*see* **PSYCHOTHERAPY: "milieu therapy"** [from 1925]), an innovative approach to schizophrenia that was also being applied in other psychoanalytically oriented private clinics in those years, such as the **Menninger** Clinic, Chestnut Lodge in Rockville, Maryland (where Frieda Fromm-Reichmann [1889–1957] was the lead psychiatrist), and the Austen Riggs Center in Stockbridge, Massachusetts. As Sullivan explained in his *Conceptions of Modern Psychiatry* (1940), there were two forms of schizophrenia, one an organic brain disease leading to deterioration, the other "a disorder of living, not of the organic substrate." Several of his main publications appeared only posthumously, including *The Interpersonal Theory of Psychiatry* (1953).

SYNAPSE. This is the gap between two neurons, where the nerve impulse is transmitted by a chemical **neurotransmitter**, such as acetylcholine. Molecules of the neurotransmitter are released into the synapse by the end bulb (axon terminal) of the presynaptic neuron to bind to receptors on the surface of the postsynaptic neuron on the far side of the synapse. The neurotransmitter is then reabsorbed into the presynaptic neuron in a process known as "transport," or "reuptake."

The term "synapse" was coined by London neurophysiologist Charles Scott Sherrington (1857–1952) in 1897 in an article in Michael Foster's (1836–1907) *Text-Book of Physiology*; Sherrington hypothesized that a functional connection must exist between nerve cells, one that he initially called a "synapsis" (from the Greek "to clasp"), but that quickly morphed into synapse. Evidence for the chemical transmission of the nerve impulse was clinched by the Graz professor of pharmacology Otto Loewi (1873–1961) in 1921 in an epochal article on "vagus material" (Vagusstoff) that he wrote in *Pflügers Archive for Physiology* (*Pflügers Archiv für die gesamte Physiologie*), "On Humoral Transmission as the Mechanism of the Heart Nerves" (Über humorale Übertragbarkeit der Herznervenwirkung"). Loewi later conceded that the "Vagusstoff" must be acetylcholine, the physiological action of which had been discovered by his friend, the London physiologist Henry Hallett Dale (1875–1961), and discussed in 1914 in the *Journal of Pharmacology and Experimental Therapeutics*. For his achievement, Loewi won a Nobel Prize in 1936.

T

TARDIVE DYSKINESIA. A dyskinesia is an involuntary movement; tardive means that its onset is delayed. Tardive dyskinesia (TD) refers to an iatrogenic "extrapyramidal" disorder caused by the long-term administration of antipsychotic drugs. (*See* **EXTRAPYRAMIDAL SIDE EFFECTS [EPS]**.)

The mechanism of TD is still obscure, but it may be related to hypersensitivity of the "postsynaptic" (downstream) D2 dopamine receptors in the basal ganglia (as opposed to neuroleptic-induced **Parkinson's** disease, which is caused by a shortage of dopamine).

Extrapyramidal side effects of various kinds may be induced by antipsychotics. Some of the side effects include symptoms of Parkinson's disease, such as akinesia (inability to move) and tremor. But the extrapyramidal symptoms of TD, involving hypermotility of the muscles as in a chorea, are almost the opposite of those of neuroleptic-induced Parkinsonism. TD causes involuntary movements of the tongue and jaw in particular, especially lip-smacking and tongue-protrusion, and sometimes dyskinesias of the trunk and extremities as well. More than half of the cases remit after medication is discontinued, but some do not, and TD is among the more visible side effects of some of the classic antipsychotics such as haloperidol (trade name Haldol; developed by the Janssen company, introduced in Europe in 1959 and in the American market by McNeil Laboratories in 1967), or Smith Kline & French's trifluoperazine, marketed as Stelazine in 1958. (Newer "atypical" antipsychotics such as Sandoz's clozapine [Clozaril, introduced in the American market in 1990] and Lilly's olanzapine [Zyprexa, marketed 1996] have less Parkinsonism, and clozapine may be used to suppress TD; that is why they are called atypical.)

TD was first described in 1957 by Matthias Schönecker, on staff at a hospital in Essen-Brobeck, in *The Psychiatrist* (*Der Nervenarzt*) under the title "A Strange Kind of Oral Syndrome in Chlorpromazine Therapy" ("Ein eigentümliches Syndrom im oralen Bereich bei Megaphenapplikation"). The symptoms of lip-smacking struck him because they continued well after stopping the treatment. Jean Sigwald (1903–) and co-authors at the Brousse Psychiatric Hospital in Paris then characterized TD more fully in 1959 in the *Revue neurologique*, calling it "dyskinetic-hypertonic syndrome," especially "facial-buccal-lingual-pharyngeal dyskinesia" (p. 557). The term "TD" itself was coined in 1964 in the *Acta Psychiatrica Scandinavica* by Arild Faurbye (1907–1983), a psychiatrist at St. Hans Psychiatric Hospital in Roskilde, Denmark, and co-workers: "Tardive dyskinesia is first and foremost characterized by the occurrence of dyskinetic movements, besides that tremor and autonomic symptoms may occur, and the syndrome is often combined with [a] syndrome of rigidity" (p. 12). TD did not, however, loom prominently in the eyes of clinicians until the report of a joint task force in 1973 of the Food and Drug Administration and the American College of Neuropsychopharmacology, led by neurologist Daniel Tarsy of the Boston University medical school, and published in the *American Journal of Psychiatry*.

Simultaneously, George E. Crane (1912–) had been warning about TD since 1968 when he was at the **National Institute of Mental Health.** As he wrote in a supplement of the *American Journal of Psychiatry*, "The frequency of this syndrome in samples of chronic patients appears to be considerable" (p. 41). In a 1973 article in *Science* on "late, unanticipated effects of neuroleptics," Crane said, "Many physicians are still unaware of this problem or seem to be completely unconcerned about it, although tardive dyskinesia has become a common sight in all wards of hospitals where drugs are administered routinely for long periods of time" (p. 127). By this time, Crane was research director of the Spring Grove State Hospital in Baltimore.

The diagnosis TD entered the *DSM* system only in the fourth edition of the *Manual* in 1994 alongside the other "medication-induced movement disorders." They were put in the category of disorders "provided for further study."

TAVISTOCK CLINIC, LONDON. After the First World War, there was enormous interest in Britain in the treatment of such "functional nervous disorders" as the shell shock cases. (*See* **POSTTRAUMATIC STRESS DISORDER.**) In 1920, Hugh Crichton-Miller (1877–1959), a neurologist who even before the war had opened a private nervous clinic, took the lead in founding a clinic based on the principles of psychoanalysis to serve individuals who could not afford private psychotherapy. (The services of the consulting staff, as often was the case in British hospitals in those days, were unpaid.) The clinic was named after its original location in Tavistock Square in the Bloomsbury district of London. Although it moved in 1932 to nearby Malet Place near University College (and after 1965 to Belsize Lane), the name Tavistock, or affectionately "The Tavi," became ineradicably associated with psychoanalysis and social psychiatry. Crichton-Miller stepped down in 1933, succeeded by John Rawlings Rees (1890–1969), who became chief of army psychiatry during the Second World War.

After the war, the Tavi became influential in spreading theories of group therapy developed in part at Northfield Military Hospital near Birmingham by Tom Main (1911–1990). Wilfred R. Bion (1897–1979) and John Rickman (1891–1951) of the Tavi had also served briefly at Northfield; they described their group-therapy techniques in an article in the *Lancet* in 1943 and after the war contributed these experiences to the budding group therapy movement at the Tavi. (*See* **PSYCHOTHERAPY: therapeutic community**, [from 1939]). (Tom Main went on to become the director of the Cassell Hospital, another center of psychotherapy innovation.)

In 1946 a sister body, the Tavistock Institute of Human Relations, was set up to do research and training especially in social and industrial relations. As psychiatry historian Tom Harrison has written, "Northfield was . . . part of a much wider series of social-psychological innovations, much of which was taken up by the Tavistock Institute of Human Relations. It is through this organisation that many of the ideas were developed and broadcast to a wider audience. Their focus, however, moved away from psychiatry and mental illness to preventative work, particularly in industry" (*Bion, Rickman, Foulkes and the Northfield Experiments*, 2000, p. 268).

In 1948, the Tavistock Clinic joined the National Health Service. After the war, the clinic established units for adult psychiatry (under John Derg ["Jock"] Sutherland [1905–1991]) and for child psychiatry (called the Department for Children and Parents), under **John Bowlby**, known for his work on "attachment theory." The Tavi, with its interest in psychoanalysis, family affairs, and group relations, was said to represent in England the counter-pole to the **Maudsley Hospital,** with its interest in epidemiology, quantitative research, and postgraduate training. Henry Victor Dicks (1900–1977), head of the marital unit at the clinic, said in his history, *Fifty Years of the Tavistock Clinic* (1970), that "Since its inception in 1920 the Tavistock has steadfastly represented and emphasized the psychodynamic aspects of psychiatry, and stood for 'whole-person' medicine *vis-à-vis* the trend of the times concerned increasingly with laboratory research and physico-chemical theories of health and disease" (pp. 298–299).

TOURETTE'S SYNDROME (TS). TS is an organic brain disease involving unrhythmical muscle tics, involuntary coprolalia (swearing), and obsessive-compulsive behavior, among other symptoms. In 1885, Paris psychiatrist–neurologist Georges Gilles de la Tourette (1857–1904), then an assistant of **Jean-Martin Charcot** at the **Salpêtrière hospice,** described in the *Revue neurologique* several cases of what he called "ticcing disease" (la maladie des tics); the patient in the article with the most characteristic symptoms was a noblewoman, the Marquise de Dampierre (1799–1884), whose disorder psychiatrist Jean-Marc-Gaspard Itard (1774–1838)—who was famous for treating "the wild boy of the Aveyron"—had already chronicled and was well-known. Gilles based his own account on the version that Itard had published in the *Archives générales de la médecine* in 1825. In addition to her ticcing and strange compulsions, the lady was known in Parisian circles for shouting out spontaneously such imprecations as "shit" and "fucking pig." In one of his clinical lectures in 1886, Charcot named the disorder after Gilles: "the ticcing disease of Gilles de la Tourette." Later, the grab bag of different symptoms the disorder often entails became known as Tourette's syndrome.

Psychoanalytic efforts to understand TS were touched off by Budapest psychoanalyst Sandor Ferenczi in 1921 (1873–1933), when he argued in the *International Journal of Psychoanalysis* that tics resulted from the repressed desire to masturbate and that they represented "stereotyped equivalents of masturbation." Of later psychoanalytic efforts to improve on this formulation, most influential was that of Margaret S. Mahler (1897–1985), a child psychiatrist and psychoanalyst at Columbia University, beginning in 1943 in the *Psychiatric Quarterly* (a paper written with psychiatrist Leo Rangell [1913–], who was training at the New York Psychoanalytic Institute). She believed that, although the illness might have an organic substrate, it occurred only in children with repressed familial conflicts. She argued that ticcers were "highly narcissistic individuals, who invest an undue amount of attention in their own bodies and who are unable to retain stimuli or irritations without immediate defensive enervation."

In 1954, Johann Ludwig Clauss, a staff psychiatrist at a mental hospital in Berlin-Lichtenberg, and Karl Balthasar (qualified 1927), director of the neuropathology laboratory at a municipal hospital in Berlin-Lichtenberg, rather silently opened a new era by finding lesions in the basal ganglia of TS patients. They concluded on the basis of pathological anatomy that TS was an independent syndrome sui generis, not a chronic variant of Chorea minor. (Clauss had first presented some of these findings in 1943 at a meeting of the Berlin Neurological Society.) Their article, published in the *Archiv für Psychiatrie und Nervenkrankheiten*—and, of course, in German—was scarcely noticed in the United States.

In 1961, Jean-Noel Seignot (graduated in medicine in 1953), a psychiatrist at the spa in Boulogne-sur-Mer, France, showed in the *Annales médico-psychologiques* that TS responded well to the antipsychotic drug haloperidol (introduced in France in 1960 by the Janssen Le Brun company). "The effect of R. 1625 [haloperidol] is in fact remarkable, because the daily number of tics, which was formerly around a thousand, has been reduced to a handful" (p. 579).

With the licensing of haloperidol in the United States in 1967, New York psychiatrist Arthur K. Shapiro (1923–1995) at Montefiore Hospital and his wife, psychologist Elaine Shapiro, began a sustained drive to encourage the use of such antipsychotics as haloperidol in preference to psychoanalytic therapy for TS. Their first publication appeared in the *British Journal of Psychiatry* in 1968, "rejected by every major American psychiatric journal," in the words of Tourette-syndrome historian Howard Kushner. The Shapiros were instrumental in the formation of the precursor organization of the Tourette Syndrome Association later that year in New York.

TRANSFERENCE. Among the earliest concepts in psychoanalysis, transference surfaced before psychoanalysis as a system had even jelled in Freud's mind. In 1895 in *Studies in Hysteria* (*Studien über Hysterie*), Freud said that patients who "transfer" their attitudes toward another person onto the analyst himself are erecting obstacles to therapy: "Transference [Übertragung] to the physician occurs through a false linkage." At first, Freud was merely annoyed at this sort of nuisance—patients who recalled the barely conscious wish to kiss a male acquaintance now wanting to kiss Freud himself and feeling so embarrassed about it that they were unable to free-associate properly in the analytic session. But then Freud began to realize it was therapeutic "to motivate the patient to reveal situations where apparently personal issues involving a third person coincide with the physician." By the end of the analysis, the patients come to understand that this kind of transference is an illusion and it dissolves, he said (*Gesammelte Werke*, I, pp. 308–310).

Later, Freud came to see transference as inevitable and one of the basic therapeutic mechanisms of analysis. In a paper on "The Dynamics of Transference" ("Zur Dynamik der Übertragung"), published in 1912 in the *Central Journal of Psychoanalysis* (*Zentralblatt für Psychoanalyse*), he described the positive transference of the patient to the physician (fine feelings, manners) and the negative transference (sexual desire). Both had to be worked through. "This battle between doctor and patient, between intellect and the world of desire, between recognizing something and wanting to act on it, is carried out almost exclusively among the phenomena of transference. It is on this battlefield that victory must be won, the sign of which is a lasting recovery from neurosis" (*Gesammelte Werke*, VIII, p. 374).

TUKE FAMILY. An important dynasty of English psychiatrists and philanthropists.

William Tuke (1732–1822), a Quaker grocer in York, England, was moved by the circumstances under which a friend had died in the York County Asylum to propose in 1792 to the Society of Friends (Quakers) in Yorkshire the need for revolutionizing the treatment of the insane. The community thereupon resolved to build a 30-bed institution for the treatment of insane persons "on humane and enlightened principles." The York Retreat, as it was named, opened in 1796. (*See* **MORAL TREATMENT.**)

Henry Tuke (1755–1814) was the eldest son of William Tuke and took over the family business in York.

Samuel Tuke (1784–1857) was a son of Henry and grandson of William. Despite his interest in medicine, he remained in the family business. Yet, during the years he occupied himself with scholarship in the area of mental illness and the treatment of the insane, writing in 1813 a *Description of the Retreat*, and again in 1846 a *Review of the Early History of the Retreat*. Psychiatry historians Richard Hunter and Ida Macalpine have said that the "pioneer work" of these three generations of Tukes "opened a new chapter in the history of the insane because of the avowed aim to accord them the dignity and status of sick human beings, and to substitute self-restraint based on self-esteem . . . for the debasing and brutalising coercion and restraint [of the previous regimen]" (*300 Years*, p. 687). (Samuel Tuke's wife, Priscilla, was the daugher of James Hack.)

Daniel Hack Tuke (1827–1895) was a son of Samuel and great-grandson of William. Born in York, Hack Tuke became interested in the operation of the Retreat and decided to study medicine, qualifying in 1852 after studying at St. Bartholomew's Hospital in London (and gaining an M.D. degree at Heidelberg University the following year). He was made physician to the Retreat and lecturer on mental diseases at the school of medicine in York. In 1858, he and (Sir) John Charles Bucknill (1817–1897) published their *Manual of Psychological Medicine*, a work that kept its place in several successive editions as the principal text in the field. In his *Illustrations of the Influence of the Mind Upon the Body in Health and Disease, Designed to Elucidate the Action of the Imagination* (1872), he introduced the concept of "psycho-therapeutics," noting "the remarkable influence which the mind exerts upon any organ or tissue to which the attention is directed, to the exclusion of other ideas" (p. 393). This represents an early statement of the mechanism of suggestion.

After living in the port of Falmouth for a number of years because of his tuberculosis, Hack Tuke moved in 1875 to London, opening a private practice in psychiatry and from 1892 onward lecturing on mental diseases at Charing Cross Hospital. In the view of his biographer in *Munk's Roll*, "his greatest achievement was his publication of the *Dictionary of Psychological Medicine*" in 1892, which established him as one of the chief authorities of the day.

There was a second, apparently unrelated, line of Tukes who also made a name for themselves in mental medicine:

Edward Francis Tuke (ca. 1776–1846), from Bristol and also a Quaker, founded Manor House, a "private lunatic asylum," in Chiswick, a suburb of London.

Thomas Harrington Tuke (1826–1888), son of Edward Francis, took charge in 1846 of the family clinic, going on then to become himself a prominent psychiatrist. In 1858, he wrote a much-cited article in the *Journal of Mental Science* on hydrotherapy in insanity; he was said to have introduced nasal feeding of the insane (given that food refusal was quite common in asylum patients). He married the second daughter of **John Conolly**, the psychiatrist who introduced "no restraint" to England.

Known subsequently as "Chiswick House," the 35-bed sanatorium continued for decades in the hands of two psychiatrist sons of Harrington Tuke, Thomas Seymour Tuke (ca. 1856–?) and Charles Molesworth Tuke (1857–1925); it was administered in the early 1920s by the latter, who had qualified in 1881.

U

UNCONSCIOUS. *See* **ID.**

UNITARY PSYCHOSIS (from 1822). (*See also* **PSYCHOSIS: EMERGENCE.**) At the biological level, the concept probably originates with Parisian physician Antoine-Laurent-Jessé Bayle (1799–1858) in his work on what was recognized much later as cerebral syphilis (it was his 1822 doctoral dissertation, *Research on Mental Illness* (*Recherches sur les maladies mentales*). Bayle did not realize he was dealing with **neurosyphilis**; he noted only the thickening and adhesiveness of the meninges of the brain caused by some kind of inflammation, or meningitis. He was the first to see brain pathology in those paralysis patients who also had the symptoms of mental illness ("délire monomaniaque" was, for example, the first stage in the progression of symptoms). Bayle said "that chronic arachnitis exists and that it is the cause of a mental derangement with symptoms." Only later was it discovered that these pathological changes in the meninges of the brain ("arachnitis") were the result of neurosyphilis. The discovery of organicity in mental symptoms opened up the possibility that mental illness was just brain disease, and thus that there was really only one cause of madness.

Joseph Guislain (1797–1860), professor of psychiatry at the University of Ghent in Belgium, argued in his *Treatise on Phrenopathies* (*Traité sur les phrénopathies*, 1833) that there was just one basic form of mental illness, phrenopathy, but that it could take various forms such as mania and melancholia, one clinical picture dissolving into another.

This concept influenced a number of German writers, including Heinrich Neumann (1814–1884), then director of a private asylum in Pöpelwitz near Breslau (later professor of psychiatry in Breslau), who proposed in his 1859 *Textbook of Psychiatry* (*Lehrbuch der Psychiatrie*) that only one form of insanity existed, which he called simply "madness" (Irresein, later baptized Einheitspsychose), rather than the 48 that Heinroth had postulated. (*See* **GERMAN "ROMANTIC" PSYCHIATRY.**) Refining the work of earlier authors, who also had believed vaguely in a single process of madness, Neumann said that it went through stages: psychosis (Wahnsinn), marked by delusions and hallucinations; confusion (Verwirrtheit), marked by loosening of associations; dementia, marked by the collapse of mentation (p. 167). If applied not to all psychoses but to today's schizophrenia, Neumann's staging has a prescient quality.

Meanwhile in France, Jules Falret (1824–1902), the son of **Jean-Pierre Falret**, was arguing in a major paper in 1866, published in the *Annales Médico-psychologiques*, that "emotional insanity" (Pinel's manie sans délire; *see* **PSYCHOSIS: EMERGENCE**) did not exist and that "in psychological medicine there is no such thing as an isolated lesion of the sentiments or instincts without a simultaneous disturbance of the intellectual faculties" (p. 386). He said that his father had taken this view since 1819.

The debate in the nineteenth century reached a provisional end as **Wilhelm Griesinger**, in the influential second edition of his textbook, *The Pathology and Treatment of Mental Illnesses* (*Die Pathologie und Therapie der psychischen Krankheiten*)

(1861), took an agnostic position, saying that "a classification of mental illnesses on the basis on their nature, i.e. according to the anatomical brain changes at their core, is at present not possible; rather, because the entire class of mental illnesses is constructed only on the basis of symptoms, we are able to indicate their various forms only on the basis of different complexes of symptoms" (p. 211).

As the nosology of **Emil Kraepelin** came to rule the roost, the notion of a unitary psychosis seemed increasingly implausible.

In 1958, **Karl Menninger** revived the concept of "unitary psychosis," at least in a philosophical sense. Drawing upon the psychoanalytic tradition of uninterest in nosology, Menninger said, "Suppose that instead of putting so much emphasis on different kinds of illness we tried to think of all mental illness as being essentially the same in quality, and differing, rather, quantitatively." He wrote in the *Bulletin of the Menninger Clinic* that "the natural 'class' in psychiatry must be either the disturbed individual or all mankind in trouble." This article became the locus classicus for many years of the disbelievers in systematic classification.

During the years, the advocates of nosology see-sawed back and forth against the advocates of unitary disease. In 2000 psychiatrist Herbert Y. Meltzer (1921–) of Vanderbilt University School of Medicine argued in *Biological Psychiatry* that schizophrenia and manic-depressive illness ("bipolar disorder") seemed to have common genetic roots, "provid[ing] additional support for the unitary model of these disorders, the so-called Einheitspsychose of Griesinger" (p. 172).

V

VIENNA: PSYCHIATRY IN (since 1870). For a mid-sized European capital, Vienna had an extraordinary succession of well-known and highly productive academic psychiatrists. As for nonacademics: Many other famous Viennese researchers, such as **Sigmund Freud** and Paul Federn (1871–1950)—who later pioneered the treatment of schizophrenia with psychoanalysis—were Jewish and did not receive full (Ordinary) professorships, although their contributions had an international impact.

Theodor Meynert began the series of academic psychiatrists. A student of neuroanatomy under pathology professor Karl von Rokitansky (1804–1878), in 1865 Meynert achieved his Habilitation in central nervous system structure, having already been appointed as staff physician at the newly built Lower Austrian Asylum in Vienna. In 1868, he received permission to lecture in psychiatry as well and in 1870, at Rokitansky's urging, Meynert became director of the psychiatric clinic (clinic in the sense of teaching medical students) in the asylum. In 1873, he received a professorship, the first for Vienna, in psychiatry.

The plot thickens in Vienna a bit because 2 years later, in 1875, a second psychiatric clinic was set up for Meynert in the General Hospital (Allgemeines Krankenhaus), following the intense mutual dislike between Meynert and the director of the Lower Austrian Asylum. Max Leidesdorf (1816–1889), the proprietor of an exclusive private nervous clinic, followed Meynert in the asylum-clinic. Vienna now had two psychiatry professors, a situation that was not ended until 1911. Meynert retained his post as professor of psychiatry at the clinic in the General Hospital until his death in 1892.

At the psychiatric clinic of the General Hospital, Meynert was followed by **Richard von Krafft-Ebing** in the years from 1892 to 1902, then between 1902 and 1928 by **Julius Wagner von Jauregg** (usually written as Wagner-Jauregg). Between 1928 and 1945, Otto Pötzl (1877–1962) was professor of psychiatry. He encouraged Manfred Sakel's research on **insulin coma** treatment. He is remembered for having quickly embraced the Nazi regime. After the war, in the years 1945–1949, Otto Kauders (1893–1949) held the chair, and between 1949 and 1969 it was held by Hans Hoff (1897–1969). Driven into emigration into 1938, Hoff was active in the mental hygiene movement after he received the chair.

After Hoff, the chair was split between neurology and psychiatry. Holding the psychiatry chair from 1971 to 1991 was Peter Berner (1924–), whose two major contributions were his follow-up study of paranoiac patients, published in 1965 as *Paranoiac Syndrome* (*Das paranoische Syndrom*), and his system of "multiaxial classification," or polydiagnosis, in which a computerized database shows which large diagnostic systems may illuminate a patient's particular set of symptoms; this was published with co-workers in 1982 in the *Psychiatry Journal of the University of Ottawa*.

In 1873, psychiatrist Heinrich Obersteiner (1847–1922) became professor of neuropathology, founding in 1882 the world-famous Vienna Neurological Institute (Neurologisches Institut). In 1919, the institute was taken over by his pupil, the neurologist Otto Marburg (1874–1948), who simultaneously became professor of neurology.

Vienna had numerous internationally known psychoanalysts, and the membership list of the Vienna Psychoanalytic Society reads almost like a list of household names, **Sigmund Freud** being of course the most famous. Yet, having international followings as well were Otto Fenichel (1897–1946), who is remembered for his theories of neurosis; Heinz Hartmann (1894–1970), the founder of modern psychoanalytic "ego" psychology; Margaret S. Mahler (1897–1985), who as an emigrée became one of America's foremost child psychiatrists; and Otto Rank (Rosenfeld) (1884–1939), a lay analyst known for his 1924 work on *Birth Trauma* (*Das Trauma der Geburt*).

As for Viennese psychiatrists who were not psychoanalysts (and who never became Ordinary professors), several deserve special mention. Erwin Stengel (1902–1973) later became famous in England. Having worked as an assistant under Wagner-Jauregg and Pötzl, Stengel acquired an international reputation only after his emigration in 1938 to London; after re-doing his medical studies, he landed at the **Maudsley Hospital**, ultimately becoming professor of psychiatry in Sheffield in 1956. In 1958, Stengel wrote an influential study of *Attempted Suicide*. (He had earlier studied psychoanalysis, which he viewed as "the God that failed," and attempted to reconcile it with neuropsychiatry.)

Bernhard Dattner (1887–1952) and Josef Gerstmann (1887–1969), by contrast, ended up in New York. Dattner, an eclectic figure who had studied psychoanalysis but was expert in the treatment of neurosyphilis, emigrated in 1938 and was appointed at New York University.

Gerstmann had habilitated in Vienna in 1921 in psychiatry and neurology and had been chief psychiatrist at the Maria-Theresien-Schlössel in Vienna, an important private nervous clinic. He emigrated to England in 1938, thence to Springfield State Hospital in Maryland, and to a number of consulting posts in New York City. He is known for describing Gerstmann syndrome, a loss of visual recognition of the finger (among other symptoms) associated with a specific brain lesion; he brought this forth in 1924 in the *Vienna Clinical Weekly* (*Wiener Klinische Wochenschrift*). Gerstmann's wife, Martha, recalls that, when Wagner-Jauregg received the Nobel Prize in 1927, Wagner presented a copy of Gerstmann's book on the treatment of neurosyphilis to the King of Sweden. (**Max Fink**, himself born in Vienna, said of this: "There was a mentor!")

A decided non-fan of psychoanalysis was Josef Berze (1866–1957), for many years director of the Vienna city asylum "Am Steinhof," who described "primary insufficiency of psychic activity" in schizophrenia in a 1914 book of that title.

Finally, the most distinguished neuroscientist to emerge from early-twentieth-century Vienna was Constantin von Economo (1876–1931), the Count (Freiherr) of San Serff. From a noble Greek family, von Economo had grown up in Trieste, then studied medicine in Vienna, where he remained. In 1906, he became an assistant of Wagner-Jauregg in the psychiatric clinic and dedicated himself to pathbreaking research both in basic neuroscience (the neurophysiology of swallowing) and in clinical medicine: he acquired world fame with his discovery of the "encephalitis lethargica," announced in the *Vienna Clinical Weekly* (*Wiener Klinische Wochenschrift*) in 1917. Shortly before his death, he opened a brain research institute attached to the psychiatric clinic.

Why a city such as Vienna should have become such a center of psychiatric thinking is unclear. Some scholars, mindful of the city's failure to regain its former status after the Second World War, argue that Vienna's prominence was owing to the presence of a large number of Jewish clinicians and scientists; this is signficant because at that time, Jewish homes were more focused on book learning and scholarship than non-Jewish homes. Yet, the distinguished professors, such as Krafft-Ebing and Wagner-Jauregg, were non-Jewish. It is certainly not true that Vienna owed its luminosity mainly to psychoanalysis because Wagner-Jauregg, Leidesdorf, Berze, Sakel, and others had no interest in Freud's ideas. The most likely explanation is the presence of the University of Vienna, liberally funded by the state, that late in the eighteenth century began to build a distinguished medical faculty and academic hospital system, remaining a magnet for talent until the forced union with Germany in 1938. Readers may consult Erna Lesky's book, *The Vienna Medical School of the 19th Century* (German original *Die Wiener Medizinische Schule im 19. Jahrhundert*, 1978).

On other Viennese:

Aichhorn. *See* **PSYCHOTHERAPY: milieu therapy** (1925).
Asperger. *See* **AUTISM.**
Bettelheim. *See* **PSYCHOTHERAPY: milieu therapy** (1944).
Bierer. *See* **PSYCHOTHERAPY: therapeutic community** (1939).
Deutsch. *See* **WOMEN IN PSYCHIATRY: Helene Deutsch.**
Feuchtersleben. *See* **PSYCHOSIS: EMERGENCE** (1845).
Freud, Anna. *See* **FREUD, ANNA.**
Klein. *See* **KLEIN, MELANIE.**
Kohut. *See* **FREUDIAN PSYCHOTHERAPY: TECHNIQUE** (1971).
Leidesdorf. *See* **DEPRESSION: EMERGENCE: hypochondria** (1860).
Moreno-Lewy. *See* **PSYCHOTHERAPY: group psychotherapy** (1911).
Sakel. *See* **INSULIN COMA THERAPY** (1930).
Schilder. *See* **SCHILDER, PAUL FERDINAND.**
Steinberg. *See* **WOMEN IN PSYCHIATRY: Hannah Steinberg.**
Stekel. *See* **FREUDIAN PSYCHOTHERAPY: TECHNIQUE: Stekel** (1919).
Stransky. *See* **SCHIZOPHRENIA: EMERGENCE: Stransky's intrapsychic ataxia** (1903).

W-Z

WAGNER VON JAUREGG, JULIUS (pronounced VAAG-ner fon YOW-Reg) (1857–1940). Initiator of the malarial-fever cure for **neurosyphilis**, Wagner was born in a small town in Upper Austria, into the family of a provincial bureaucrat. (His father, Adolf Johann Wagner, added the suffix "von Jauregg" after his ennoblement in 1883.) The name, however, is usually given simply as Wagner-Jauregg, or Wagner. In 1880, Wagner graduated in medicine from the University of Vienna, and after a brief period of training in internal medicine he became a resident (Assistent)—despite minimal interest in psychiatry—in the psychiatric clinic of the Vienna asylum under Leidesdorf. (*See* **VIENNA.**) Habilitated in psychiatry and nervous diseases in 1885, in 1889 he was called as **Richard von Krafft-Ebing**'s successor to the chair of psychiatry in Graz, then in 1893 received one of the psychiatry chairs in Vienna. In 1902, after Krafft-Ebing's death, Wagner took over the psychiatry chair in the General Hospital (the two chairs—the asylum and the hospital—were unified in 1911). Wagner remained the professor of psychiatry in Vienna until his emeriting in 1928.

In scientific terms, Wagner is remembered as one of the earliest researchers to revive the recommendation of thyroid preparations for the treatment of endemic cretinism, a common cause of **mental retardation** in those days. This was a subject of continuous interest to him from the beginning of his scientific career onward, because the inhabitants of the mountainous areas around Graz had diets chronically deficient in iodine. Of greater impact worldwide, in a series of articles in 1918–1919 in the *Psychiatry and Neurology Weekly* (*Psychiatrisch-neurologische Wochenschrift*), Wagner described the malarial-fever cure for neurosyphilis ("progressive paralysis") that he had initiated in 1917. (He had been experimenting with fever cures of various kinds for psychosis since 1887.) Neurosyphilis thus became the first treatable brain disease causing major psychiatric symptoms, and the fever-cure represents the beginning of the physical therapies in psychiatry. (*See* **CONVULSIVE THERAPIES: CHEMICAL; DEEP-SLEEP THERAPY; ELECTROCONVULSIVE THERAPY; INSULIN COMA THERAPY.**) Wagner received a Nobel Prize for this work in 1927. He remained hostile to psychoanalysis all his life and drove increasing numbers of its adepts out of his clinic. Wagner blighted his historical reputation by permitting himself to be enrolled in the Nazi Party after the union of Austria with Hitler's Germany in 1938.

WEISSMAN, MYRNA (1935–). An investigator who shaped the field of psychiatric epidemiology, Weissman was born in Boston into the family of Samuel Milgram, a small businessman, and Jeanette Milgram, a housewife. With a master's degree in social work from the University of Pennsylvania in 1958, she started out as a social worker at the clinical center of the National Institutes of Health, moving to New Haven, Connecticut, in 1967 to work at Yale's clinical psychopharmacology research unit on the New Haven-Boston Collaborative Depression Research Project, led by **Gerald Klerman**. (*See* **PSYCHOTHERAPY: interpersonal therapy**.) In 1974, she received a Ph.D. from Yale University in epidemiology and chronic diseases, and from 1975 to 1987 she served at Yale as professor of psychiatry and epidemiology. In 1987, she became professor of epidemiology in psychiatry at Columbia University and chief of the department of clinical-genetic epidemiology at the New York State Psychiatric Institute.

At Yale, she was principal investigator of research undertaken in 1975–1976 on the epidemiology of depression in New Haven, Connecticut, published in the *Archives of General Psychiatry* in 1981. She led an epidemiological study of suicidal ideation in panic disorder, published in 1989 in the *New England Journal of Medicine*. In the 1990s, Weissman was chief investigator of a large international study of the epidemiology of major depression and bipolar disorder, some results from which appeared in 1996 in the *Journal of the American Medical Association*. As well, together with her late husband **Gerald L. Klerman** and others, she wrote *A Comprehensive Guide to Interpersonal Psychotherapy*, which appeared in 1984. Among her other books might be mentioned, with co-author British psychiatrist Eugene Paykel (1934–), *The Depressed Woman: A Study of Social Relationships* (1974).

WERNICKE–KLEIST–LEONHARD PATHWAY (from 1900). The central theme in this pathway is classifying psychotic illness not on the basis of outcome, as Kraepelin did, but on the basis of hypothetical underlying neurological impairment or common family history. The pathway had the effect of significantly narrowing the diagnosis schizophrenia and of differentiating a number of schizophrenia-like illnesses and cyclical illnesses—of which Kleist and Leonhard enumerated at least 26 varieties—that may be differentially responsive to treatment.

Wernicke's "sejunction" theory (1900). Carl Wernicke (1848–1905), a student of Heinrich Neumann's (1814–1884) in Breslau, became in 1885 Neumann's successor to the chair of psychiatry and neurology in Breslau. Wernicke had already established a large name for himself with his discovery in 1874 of the sensory speech center in the temporal lobe. This finding alerted Wernicke all the more to the importance of neurology in understanding behavior and led him to an elaborate hypothesis—later scorned by **Karl Jaspers** as "brain mythology"—about the underlying brain mechanisms of psychiatric illness. In his textbook of clinical lectures in 1900 (*Grundriss der Psychiatrie in klinischen Vorlesungen*), Wernicke postulated a "sejunction"—or loosening of the continuity of the association fibers—as the underlying source of psychosis. As he told the medical students, "We shall indicate this process of loosening [Loslösung] with the appropriate term of sejunction, and we cannot avoid seeing in it an [organic] defect, an interruption of continuity, which must correspond to the failure of certain association connections" (p. 109 of the 2nd ed., 1906). Wernicke asserted that "disorientation is the fundamental symptom of all psychoses," best diagnosed clinically by the patient's expression of "perplexity" (Ratlosigkeit) (p. 210). In 1904, Wernicke became professor of psychiatry in Halle. His contribution to the pathway was really his gift for careful observation.

Karl Kleist's cycloid psychoses (1879–1960). Kleist was briefly an assistant of Wernicke's in Halle before the latter's death in 1905. Kleist shared Wernicke's biases both about brain pathology (about half of Kleist's lifetime writing was neurological in nature) and about psychopathology. Kleist set out to devise "psychic disease systems"; in 1908–1909 he studied with neurologist Ludwig Edinger (1855–1918) in Frankfurt and with **Alois Alzheimer** in Munich; he wrote his Habilitation thesis with Gustav

Specht (1860–1940) in Erlangen, beginning to study systematically the chronic psychoses. In 1920, he became professor of psychiatry in Frankfurt and head of the City Psychiatric Clinic. Here, he founded the Frankfurt Research Institute for Brain Pathology and Psychopathology (Frankfurter Forschungsstelle für Gehirnpathologie und Psychopathologie).

Kleist held a deep animus against the stark **Kraepelinian** division between **manic-depressive illness** and **schizophrenia** and sought to identify separate illness entities in the borderland between the two large diagnoses. It was Kleist's idea that all these separate disease entities could, in theory at least, be localized in the brain. As early as 1911, Kleist devised a set of diagnoses regarding motility, running from "hyperkinetic motility psychosis" to stupor ("akinetic motility psychosis"); motility means involving motor symptoms (*see* his article in the *Zeitschrift für die gesamte Neurologie und Psychiatrie*, 1911).

By 1921, Kleist had proposed a group of recurrent "sudden, fully-formed constitutional psychoses" (autochthone konstitutionelle Psychosen) different from Kraepelin's manic-depressive illness; the group of psychoses were nondeteriorating, with a stable clinical picture over time, and included principally periodic mania, periodic melancholia, and some circular psychoses. (Kleist used the term "degeneration" as a synonym for constitutional, meaning predisposed; many were demonstrably hereditary. He summarized his work in 1921 in the *Zeitschrift für die gesamte Neurologie und Psychiatrie*.)

In 1926, Kleist suggested the concept of the "cycloid degeneration psychoses" in the *Archive for Psychiatry and Nervous Diseases* (*Archiv für Psychiatrie und Nervenkrankheiten*) to characterize a wide variety of mental phenomena that circled between two poles (but were not Kraepelin's manic-depressive illness). There were basically two kinds: the confusional psychoses that alternated between agitated confusion and stupor, and the motility psychoses that alternated between hyperkinesis and akinesis. In further work, he identified several other cyclic psychoses.

Of the three members of the pathway, it was only Kleist who made a big issue of underlying neurological impairment; Wernicke was more interested in hypothesized brain communication; Leonhard in genetics. (English-speaking readers will find a clear explanation of Kleist's and Leonhard's classifications in an article by Gottfried Teichmann of the University of Würzburg—a center sympathetic to the Wernicke–Kleist–Leonhard pathway—in *Psychopathology*, published in 1990.)

Frankfurt psychiatrist Edda Neele (1910–) was part of the Kleist team, and she analyzed all patients with "cycloid" psychoses to come through the Frankfurt clinic between 1938 and 1942. Her 1949 monograph, *The Phase-like Psychoses According to Presentation and Family History* (*Die phasischen Psychosen nach ihrem Erscheinungs-und Erbbild*), summing up this research provided evidence that Kleist's disease categories did correspond in part to natural genotypes. (She is, on the basis of this work, apparently the first woman to have written a Habilitation in Germany in psychiatry.) Neele used Kleist's concepts "one-pole" and "two-pole" disorders ("einpolige und zweipolige Erkrankungen").

In 1953, Kleist introduced the terminological refinement of calling circular psychoses either "unipolar" or "bipolar" (for the group of psychoses that he called "Phasophrenien") in the *Monatsschrift für Psychiatrie und Neurologie*. This later became a fundamental terminological bulwark of the ***DSM*** system.

In sum, Kleist's contribution to the pathway was to construct diseases from Wernicke's syndromes and then attempt to validate them in follow-up studies. Besides the Kraepelinian schizophrenia and manic-depressive illness, Kleist distinguished a number of "grey-area psychoses" (Randpsychosen) having a good outcome.

Karl Leonhard's endogenous psychoses (1957). Leonhard continued Kleist's efforts to identify "good-outcome" (gutartige) psychoses.

Karl Leonhard (1904–1988) joined Kleist at the Frankfurt City Psychiatric Clinic in 1936, and in 1937 produced his own monograph on anxiety-depression among older patients (*Involutive und idiopathische Angstdepression*). It was this work on the genetics of catatonia, cycloid psychoses, and paranoid schizophrenia that led to the startling new synthesis of all bipolar and psychotic phenomena that Leonhard achieved in 1957: *The Classification of Endogenous Psychoses* (*Die Aufteilung der endogenen Psychosen*)—published as he was still professor of psychiatry at Erfurt (the year in which he left to become professor of psychiatry at the Charité Hospital of the Humboldt University in East Berlin). Leonhard was fundamentally in agreement with Kraepelin's move up from syndromes to "actual diseases" in the form of manic-depressive illness and dementia praecox. "Unfortunately," he said in a lecture in Leipzig in 1957, "this progress was achieved with a terrible simplification of the clinical realities."

To better refine upon Kraepelin, Leonhard distilled the Wernicke–Kleist teachings into three great groups of "endogenous psychoses": (1) the affective, or phasic, psychoses ("bipolar" distinguished from "monopolar"); "phasic" means either mania or depression; (2) the cycloid psychoses (which include motility psychosis); and (3) the schizophrenic psychoses, which Leonhard divided into "systematic" (meaning that the symptoms underwent no marked change once established) and the nonsystematic psychoses (meaning fluctuating severity and symptom picture). The system is notable for rehabilitating the term "melancholia," Leonhard's "pure melancholia" being distinct from his "pure depressions" of various kinds.

In formulating these subtypes, Leonhard first began with chronic patients, then validated the subtypes in patients at earlier stages of illness. As Gabor Ungvari commented in 1993, "His diagnoses imply prognostic prediction, that is, they are true life-time diagnoses. This 'backward' direction of his classification system enabled Leonhard to identify the most persistent signs and symptoms as characteristics of a particular subtype during its natural history" (*Biological Psychiatry*, 1993, p. 750).

Frank Fish of Edinburgh University gave the following account of the schizophrenias in the Leonhard system in *Psychiatric Quarterly* (1964): Among the systematic psychoses were the systematic paraphrenias (including seven subforms), the hebephrenias (four subforms), and the systematic catatonias (six subforms). Leonhard divided the nonsystematic psychoses into affect-laden paraphrenia (widely considered to be the diagnosis of the mathematician John Nash in the book and movie *A Beautiful Mind*); cataphasia (which Leonhard had once called schizophasia); and periodic catatonia. Affect-laden paraphrenia, as the term suggests, was characterized by a high affective loading of the symptoms ("bitter" complaints about persecution, "enthusiasm" about grandiose delusions); cataphasia by a breakdown of speech and thought while the patients otherwise continued to behave more or less rationally; periodic catatonia by its shift-like course, with alternating stupor and excitement.

"The Leonhard system is not easy to use," noted Fish in a touch of understatement. In fact, the system called for very careful observation of the patients and the ability to discern small differences among the subcategories, many of which blended into one another. Yet, the alert clinician might find that the effort repayed itself, for the main groups of psychoses had quite different prognoses: the systematic ones being poor, the nonsystematic rather better. Even more interesting, after the introduction of **chlorpromazine** and the other phenothiazine antipsychotics in 1952, the nonsystematic psychoses turned out highly responsive to drug treatment, whereas the systematic psychoses responded scarcely at all. Christian Astrup (1921–1989) discovered this in research he did at Gaustad Hospital in Oslo, Norway, where he was later joined by Frank Fish. Astrup's initial findings appeared in the *Acta Psychiatrica Scandinavica* in 1959, where, using a five-illness model of the Leonhard scheme, he found that chronic schizophrenics with "slight paranoid defects" responded well, those with "systematic catatonias" poorly; Fish then published additional cases in *L'Encéphale* in 1964. These findings, once widely overlooked in the psychiatric literature, are being rexamined attentively today. (Astrup's work on conditional reflexes in the Leonhard-style psychoses was published as *Schizophrenia: Conditional Reflex Studies* in 1962.)

For a comprehensive assessment of the ideas of this pathway, and the evidence that gives them at least some credence, the reader may consult the book edited by Würzburg University psychiatry professor Helmut Beckmann (1940–), *Endogenous Psychoses: Leonhard's Impact on Psychiatry* (1995).

The diagnoses of the Wernicke–Kleist–Leonhard pathway have made almost no impact on ***DSM***-style U.S. psychiatry. Yet, they have had a small echo in the World Health Organization's *International Classification of Diseases*, tenth edition (*ICD-10*), which describes "acute polymorphic psychotic disorder without symptoms of schizophrenia" (F23.0) and will accept either **Valentin Magnan**'s bouffée délirante or non-schizophrenic "cycloid psychosis" in fulfilment of the diagnosis.

WERNICKE–KORSAKOFF SYNDROME. Wernicke and Korsakoff are two very familiar eponyms that only recently have been joined. First: Korsakoff. There is a Korsakoff syndrome, also referred to as Korsakoff psychosis, that the Russian psychiatrist Sergei S. Korsakoff (1853–1900) discovered in 1887. (*See* **DEMENTIA: Korsakoff** [1887].) The syndrome refers mainly to memory loss about time and space, confabulation, and polyneuritis. (The personality is preserved.) It is caused by a deficiency of the vitamin thiamine and typically is seen in chronic alcoholism.

There is also a Wernicke's disease: In 1881, Breslau psychiatry professor Carl Wernicke (1848–1905) described in his neurology textbook (*Lehrbuch der Gehirnkrankheiten*) a disease that he called "acute, hemorrhagic polioencephalitis superior," meaning that the histopathology resembled that of poliomyelitis in the spine, yet it was situated in the brain and was clinically characterized by limited eye movement, ataxic gait, and disorientation. The three cases he discussed in his textbook had quickly ended fatally. Two of the three had been heavy drinkers. This was the first description of what became known as "Wernicke's disease," a sometimes fatal form of necrosis (death) of brain tissue.

In retrospect, it is clear that the basic pathology of the acute form of Wernicke's disease is lesions involving the limbic lobe, especially the mammillary bodies, and other areas of the brain as well, caused by deficiency of thiamine—and typically seen in severe alcoholics who are poorly nourished.

As stated above, 6 years after Wernicke, in 1887 Korsakoff described in a Russian journal a syndrome involving memory loss and polyneuritis. Although Korsakoff did not know it at the time, what he was portraying represented the chronic version of Wernicke's disease, in which a prominent symptom is also memory loss.

Suspicion began to grow that these two memory-loss diseases were the same. In 1904, psychiatry professor Karl Bonhoeffer (1868–1948), then at **Heidelberg,** noted in the *Allgemeine Zeitschrift für Psychiatrie* how closely the clinical picture of Korsakoff's syndrome resembled Wernicke's disease, though he did not assert that they were the same disease.

In 1947, Hugh Edward de Wardener (M.B. 1939), in the department of medicine in St. Thomas's Hospital, and Bernard Lennox (M.B. 1936), a lecturer in morbid anatomy at the Postgraduate Medical School of the University of London, both of whom had been held prisoner-of-war in Singapore by the Japanese under what must have been appalling conditions, attributed Wernicke's disease to thiamine deficiency (in an article in the *Lancet* on "Cerebral Beriberi (Wernicke's Encephalopathy: Review of 52 Cases in a Singapore Prisoner-of-War Hospital"). Rather tongue-in-cheek the authors noted, "An opportunity for placing a large number of healthy adults simultaneously on a standardised deficient diet and observing the results over a period of years is one which the many workers on the vitamin-B complex must have coveted" (p. 11).

It was Harvard neurologist Raymond Adams (1911–), together with his longtime collaborator Maurice Victor (1920–), later professor of neurology at Case Western University in Cleveland, who put the two diseases together. In 1961, in an article in the *American Journal of Clinical Nutrition,* they confirmed the role of thiamine deficiency in Wernicke's disease—without citing the De Wardener–Lennox contribution—and noted that "Korsakoff's psychosis and alcoholic dementia or pseudoparesis are the common psychic manifestations of Wernicke's disease," also attributable, at least in part, "to a deficiency of thiamine" (p. 394). Then, in their book *The Wernicke-Korsakoff Syndrome* (1971), Victor and Adams, together with George H. Collins (1927–), demonstrated that Korsakoff's psychosis (or dementia) and Wernicke's disease were the same disease. In their textbook *Principles of Neurology* (1977), Adams and Victor said succinctly: "Stated in another way, Korsakoff's psychosis is the psychic manifestation of Wernicke's disease" (quote from second edition, 1981, p. 704).

WIKLER, ABRAHAM (1910–1981). The first American psychiatrist to construct a bridge to psychopharmacology, Wikler was born in New York City, earned his M.D. in 1935 from the Long Island College of Medicine, and trained in psychiatry at the United States Public Health Service hospital in St. Louis, Missouri. In 1940, he took a research position at the Lexington Narcotics Hospital of the Public Health Service (opened in 1935 and known as the "Narcotic Farm") in Lexington, Kentucky. In 1948, in the *American Journal of Psychiatry,* he suggested that environmental cues were important in the relapsing of heroin addicts, thus initiating a large research agenda on cue reactivity and addiction. In 1952, Wikler became the chief of the psychiatric section of the hospital (which in 1942 had started accepting neuropsychiatric patients). In 1967, the hospital was placed under the **National Institute of Mental Health** and designated a clinical research center. Here, Wikler founded what was to become the intramural research program of the National Institute on Drug Abuse (the hospital itself was transferred to the Bureau of Prisons in 1974). Between 1947 and 1962, Wikler lectured in psychiatry at the University of Cincinnati, thereafter in psychiatry and pharmacology at the University of Louisville. He is known in addiction research for calling attention to craving and abstinence as conditioned rather than primarily pharmacological phenomena and for writing in 1957 one of the first textbooks of psychopharmacology, *The Relation of Psychiatry to Psychopharmacology*. **Joel Elkes** later said of Wikler's contribution to psychopharmacology, "His work on dependence and addiction was a model of rigor and clarity, but from the vantage point of someone working both at the bench and in the clinic, he saw, long before most of us, the true dimensions of our field" (Elkes, *Psychopharmacology*, 1995, p. 101).

WING, JOHN (1923–). One of the key figures in social psychiatry at the **Maudsley Hospital**, Wing received his M.D. and Ph.D. from University College London. After serving in the Royal Navy during the Second World War, he joined the Institute of Psychiatry at the Maudsley and from 1965 to 1989 was director of the MRC Social Psychiatry Unit there. From 1989 to 1994, he headed the research unit of the Royal College of Physicians.

Under John Wing's supervision, in January 1965 the Social Psychiatry Unit launched the Camberwell Register (initiated in 1964 by Lorna Wing), which was to become a storehouse of information on the uptake of psychiatric services by in- and outpatients (Camberwell is a London district). Further, the Social Psychiatry Unit turned to the social and psychological circumstances under which patients with schizophrenia relapse; specially unfavorable for the prognosis is exposure to high levels of "expressed emotion" within families, meaning emotional over-involvement from which patients withdraw. To measure the psychopathology of schizophrenia, in 1961 Wing published in the *Journal of Mental Science*, "A Simple and Reliable Subclassification of Chronic Schizophrenia." This began the research that eventuated in a 1967 article by Wing and other members of his group in the *British Journal of Psychiatry* (the new title of the *Journal of Mental Science*) on "measuring and classifying 'present psychiatric state.'" An earlier draft of this had formed the basis of the World Health Organization's international pilot study of schizophrenia, launched in 1965. In 1970, Wing and sociologist George William Brown (1930–), a professor at the Social Research Unit of Bedford College, University of London, wrote a widely cited study, *Institutionalism and Schizophrenia*, showing the vulnerability of schizophrenics to an understimulating environment, whether in an institution or outside. Simultaneously in 1970, he co-authored with London psychiatrist Edward H. Hare (1917–1996) a standard textbook, *Psychiatric Epidemiology*.

WINOKUR, GEORGE (pronounced WIN-o-ker) (1925–1996). An important student of the genetics of mood disorders, Winokur was born in Philadelphia, received his M.D. from the University of Maryland in 1947, and trained in psychiatry from 1948 to 1950 at the Seton Institute in Baltimore. Winokur came to Washington University in **St. Louis** in 1951 as an instructor in the psychiatry department and remained there until becoming chair of psychiatry in 1971 at the University of Iowa. At Iowa, as

Raymond Crowe (1942–) puts it, "He built a department based on the Washington University model: psychiatry was a medical science founded on empirical data, not opinion and anecdote" (obituary, *Psychiatric Genetics*, 1998, p. 128). Winokur became known for his efforts to put psychiatric genetics on a sound empirical footing, and in 1969 he published a landmark book, *Manic Depressive Illness*. Beginning in 1974, in an article in *International Pharmacopsychiatry*, he distinguished among "pure" depression (someone with an affective disorder in the family), "spectrum" depression (someone with any disorder in the family), and "sporadic" depression (no mental illness in the family). Out of Winokur's work with Ming T. Tsuang (1931–), who had come with Winokur from St. Louis to Iowa, came in 1996 the *Natural History of Mania, Depression and Schizophrenia*, based on the Iowa "follow-up" study. Winokur is also known for his work with Guze and Robins on the "St. Louis criteria," **Feighner** being first author.

WOMEN IN PSYCHIATRY. Several of the women involved with psychoanalysis, such as **Anna Freud** and **Melanie Klein**, are familiar figures. Yet, the lives of many other women who also made distinguished contributions to the fields of psychoanalysis, psychiatry, and psychopharmacology are relatively unknown. Here follows a partial list, one that could be considerably expanded.

Marie Asberg (1938–). Pioneer investigator in psychopharmacology, Asberg graduated in medicine in 1965 at the Karolinska Institutet in Stockholm. She trained in psychiatry at the "KI," becoming associate professor of psychiatry there in 1975, then professor of psychiatry in 1982, chair of the department of psychiatry in 1985, and chair of the department of clinical neuroscience in 1993. Asberg is associated with several important discoveries in biological psychiatry. Based on the finding of other Swedish researchers that, at the same dose, there are large genetically determined differences in blood levels of the antidepressant drug nortriptyline from patient to patient, in 1971 she discovered, along with co-workers, and published in the *British Medical Journal*, that the patients with higher blood levels tended to develop side effects. As she later put it, "The high concentrations were not only unpleasant for the patient, but also made them less likely to recover from their depression." This was an early contribution to pharmacogenetics. She then became interested in the relationship between levels of the neurotransmitter serotonin and depression, and by chance in 1976 made a quite important discovery: that depressed patients with low levels of a metabolite of serotonin (called 5-HIAA, or 5-hydroxy-indole-acetic acid) in their spinal fluid were much more likely to attempt suicide than equally depressed patients with a high level of the serotonin metabolite. Bearing the name of two co-investigators as well, this work was published in the *Archives of General Psychiatry*. She is, however, best known for a psychiatric rating scale for depression that she and English psychiatrist Stuart Montgomery published in 1979 in the *British Journal of Psychiatry* and called the Montgomery–Asberg Rating Scale for Depression, or MADRS, which became standard in treatment studies all over the world.

Lauretta Bender (1897–1987). An early student of the biological approach in child psychiatry, Bender was born in Butte, Montana, into a lawyer's family. After studying neuropathology in Europe, in 1926 she graduated with an M.D. from the University of Iowa. She trained in psychiatry at the Boston Psychopathic Hospital, then in 1929–1930 was a research associate at the Phipps Clinic at Johns Hopkins

University. In 1930, she came on staff in the psychiatric department of Bellevue Hospital in New York City, becoming in 1934 the psychiatrist in charge of the children's service, where she remained until becoming in 1956 director of research of the new children's unit at Creedmoor State Hospital. As well, from 1941 to 1958 she was professor of psychiatry at the New York University College of Medicine, and after 1959, she was professor at the College of Physicians and Surgeons of Columbia University. In 1974, she moved to Annapolis, where she taught at the University of Maryland until her death.

Bender is best known for her studies of childhood schizophrenia, for which she introduced in 1934 the Bender Visual Motor Gestalt Test and in 1938 described it in a book of that title. She soon became convinced that schizophrenia was an organic condition and during the years introduced a variety of biological approaches to it, controversial at the time because she shunned such concepts as "schizophrenogenic mother." Her influential 1956 book, *Psychopathology of Children with Organic Brain Disorders*, extended the "organic" concept to include childhood schizophrenia. In 1961, she became president of the Society of Biological Psychiatry. She had followed psychiatrist **Paul Schilder** to New York in 1930 and married him in 1936 after his divorce; Schilder was killed in 1940 in a traffic accident, leaving her with three small children.

Paula Jean Clayton (1934–). One of the best-known members of the **St. Louis school**—and the first woman to chair a department of psychiatry in the United States—Clayton was born in St. Louis, Missouri, and earned her M.D. at Washington University in 1960. After training in psychiatry at Washington University, she joined the department in 1965, becoming full professor in 1976. In 1980, she became head of the department of psychiatry at the University of Minnesota, where she served until her retirement in 1999. In 1965, she and **George Winokur** wrote in *Comprehensive Psychiatry* a definitive paper on mania, and during the years she and other members of the St. Louis school laid the basis for studying the genetics of mania and other affective disorders. Beginning in 1968, she undertook, in an article in the *American Journal of Psychiatry*, what turned out to be a lifelong study of bereavement, initially in widows, later in children and others. She was also interested in the mortality of patients with mood disorders, and in 2002, together with Jules Angst of Zurich's university psychiatric hospital and other researchers, she published in the *Journal of Affective Disorders* a landmark 38-year follow-up study of such patients.

Helene Rosenbach Deutsch (1884–1982). Celebrated for applying psychoanalytic concepts to the lives of women, Helene Rosenbach was born in Przemysl, Galicia, Austria (later Poland), into a prominent lawyer's family. She finished her medical studies at the University of **Vienna** in 1912, then trained in psychiatry under **Julius Wagner von Jauregg** at the university clinic until 1919, becoming the first woman to serve as an assistant (albeit without the formal title) in that clinic. In 1918–1919, she did a training analysis with **Sigmund Freud** and quickly became part of his inner circle. In 1924, based on her experience with the Berlin psychoanalytic institute 1 year previously, she became founding director of the new training institute of the Vienna Psychoanalytic Society. In 1912, she married Felix Deutsch (1884–1964) (who later became Freud's personal physician), and in 1935 Helene Deutsch and her son emigrated to the United States, followed by Felix a year later. The family settled in Boston, where Helene Deutsch joined the teaching staff of the Boston Psychoanalytic Institute; she was president of the Boston Psychoanalytic Society from 1939 to 1941.

She is known for her psychoanalytic explorations of various phases of the life cycle of women, writing in 1925 *Zur Psychoanalyse der weiblichen Sexualfunktionen* (translated into English in 1991 as *Psychoanalysis of the Sexual Functions of Women*) and then *The Psychology of Women: A Psychoanalytic Interpretation* (2 vols., 1944–1945). She is also remembered for having postulated a kind of "as if" personality style in accounting for what she believed was a female tendency to be "imitatively suggestible," as her biographer Paul Roazen puts it. Given that Boston then was a stronghold of psychoanalysis, she supervised training analyses of many later influential figures in American psychiatry, including John C. Whitehorn (1894–1973), later head of the Phipps Clinic at Johns Hopkins University (from 1941 to 1960), and Erich Lindemann (1900–1974), who succeeded Stanley Cobb (1887–1968) as head of psychiatry at Massachusetts General Hospital. (On Lindemann, *see* **BARBITURATES: narcotherapy; POSTTRAUMATIC STRESS DISORDER: acute grief** [1944].)

Charmian Elkes (1919–1995). Responsible for one of the earliest controlled clinical trials in psychopharmacology, Elkes was born in London, the daughter of Aleck Bourne, a noted gynecologist. She read medicine at King's College Hospital, graduating in 1942. The following year, she married **Joel Elkes** and followed him to Birmingham, where she first worked as a family physician, then from 1949 to 1952 trained in psychiatry at All Saints Hospital; she served there as senior medical officer until 1957. In 1957, she and her husband moved to the United States. Joining the intramural program of the **National Institute of Mental Health** in 1959—and then as a staff psychiatrist at Johns Hopkins Medical School—from 1960 to 1968 she developed a pioneering program to train mental health counselors. Later, she was founding chief of psychiatry at a hospital in Columbia, Maryland, until her retirement in 1978.

In Birmingham, from 1945 until 1951, she and Joel were involved in drug trials for schizophrenic catatonia; then, from 1952 to 1954, in Birmingham at the Winson Green Hospital, she led the first controlled trial of **chlorpromazine**, publishing the results together with her husband in 1954 in the *British Medical Journal*. (It was a crossover study, using the patients as their "own controls" by shifting them on and off placebo at various points during the trial.) She also ran a controlled trial of the Rauwolfia alkaloids including **reserpine** at the All Saints Hospital on chronic psychotic patients, noting that "The change in ward atmosphere brought about by reserpine is striking" (*Journal of Mental Science*, 1957, p. 473).

Barbara Fish (1920–). A pioneer of pharmacotherapy in child psychiatry, especially in childhood schizophrenia, Fish was born in New York, her father an engineer, and graduated with an M.D. from New York University in 1945. A student of Lauretta Bender (*see above*), she trained in pediatrics and psychiatry at Bellevue Hospital, then served during the 1950s in various hospital and university appointments in New York. In 1960, she became psychiatrist in charge of the children's service of the psychiatry division of Bellevue, and in 1972 she became professor of psychiatry at the University of California in Los Angeles, where she was emerited in 1991.

She was a prominent student of the neurological antecedents of childhood schizophrenia, and as an investigator in the Children's Psychopharmacological Research Unit of the New York University School of Medicine, she helped to open up the pharmacotherapy of the illness. She is especially known for the first long-term follow-up study of the children of schizophrenic mothers—following some of them to age 30—which she began at Bellevue Hospital in 1952. On the basis of early neurological development, she was able to predict which adults would develop schizotypal (schizophrenia-like) traits. *See* among other publications her article in the *American Journal of Psychiatry* in 1962. As one biographer says, "Her conception of schizophrenia as a neurobiological disorder met with hostility from the psychiatric community in the 1950s, when notions of castrating mothers and bungled toilet training were more popular as explanations for mental illnesses" (Halcomb, *Women Making It*, p. 216).

Karen Horney (pronounced HORN-eye) (1885–1952). The initiator of feminist psychoanalysis, Horney was born Karen Danielsen in the wealthy Hamburg suburb of Blankenese, the daughter of a socially prominent sea captain's family. She began medical studies first at Freiburg—where she was one of the first female medical students, then completed her state exam in Berlin in 1911 (having married in Berlin a fellow Freiburg student, Oscar Horney [1882–1948]). In 1911, she joined the newly founded (1910) Berlin Psychoanalytic Institute. She quickly had two daughters, then received her M.D. degree in 1915. After training in psychiatry (she had earlier undergone some psychoanalytic sessions, either for training or for personal therapy), she served in a military hospital during the First World War, and in 1919 opened a psychoanalytic private practice in the suburb of Zehlendorf. In 1920, she commenced a training analysis with Hanns Sachs (1881–1947) and later became director of training of the institute.

As early as 1923 she began publishing on what became for her lifelong themes, such as the psychology of femininity and women's sexuality and relationship to men; *see* particularly an article on the "female castration complex" in the *International Journal of Medical Psychoanalysis* (*Internationale Zeitschrift für* [*ärztliche*] *Psychoanalyse*) (the adjective "medical" was removed from the German title in 1920). In 1932, she emigrated to the United States as director of training of fellow Berliner Franz Alexander's just-founded Chicago Institute of Psychoanalysis. Two years later, in 1934, she moved to New York to teach at the New School for Social Research and open a private practice. Because she ended up denying such theories as "penis envy"—believing women's problems are much more a consequence of their oppression—some observers have hesitated even to call her a psychoanalyst (she never knew Freud and owed little to the Vienna circle). Indeed, the radical nature of her views about the constancy of change in the personality led to her expulsion, together with a like-minded group, in 1941 from the New York Psychoanalytic Institute, whereupon she organized her own Association for the Advancement of Psychoanalysis and an associated teaching institute.

As a member of the "second generation" of analysts following Freud, Horney adopted a number of unconventional views, particularly in regard to women. She saw "women's neuroses" more as a product of women's position in the culture than of psychic development. She saw personality change as constant and ongoing rather than being cast in concrete at the end of infantile development. Among her books, translated in numerous languages and continuously reprinted, are *The Neurotic Personality of Our Time* (1937)—a book that rejected many of the key concepts of psychoanalysis—*New Ways in Psychoanalysis* (1939), and *Our Inner Conflicts, A Constructive Theory of*

Neurosis (1945). Her collected essays, published posthumously in 1967 as *Feminine Psychology*, were influential in feminist theory.

Eve Johnstone (1944–). An innovator in biological studies of schizophrenia, Johnstone grew up in Glasgow, her father a dental surgeon, and read medicine at the University of Glasgow (M.B. in 1967). From 1968 to 1972, she trained in psychiatry in various Glasgow hospitals, then began lecturing at the university. Early in her medical studies, she became curious about patients with schizophrenia: "I was fascinated by them. I could not believe that so little was known about this disease which so cruelly transformed, and indeed destroyed people who were the age that I was then." From 1974 to 1989, at the instigation of **Timothy Crow**, she served as a member of the scientific staff of the Medical Research Council's clinical research center at Northwick Park Hospital in Harrow. In 1989, she returned to Scotland as chair of psychiatry at the University of Edinburgh.

In 1976, with the MRC group at Harrow, she led the first team to discover brain abnormalities in schizophrenia with the aid of computerized tomography. (*See* **NEUROIMAGING; SCHIZOPHRENIA: RECENT CONCEPTS** [1976].) Published in the *Lancet*, this was the first finding of structural change in schizophrenia involving controls. It was in 1976 as well that Johnstone published an important but little noted paper in *Psychopharmacologia* on biochemical predictors of response to the antidepressant drug phenelzine (slow "acetylators" of the drug do better because they keep more of it on board). This was one of the first papers to identify a "polymorphic," meaning probably genetic, marker of drug response in psychopharmacology. In other work, Johnstone and colleagues did a controlled trial of real vs. sham ECT, discovering the real version to be more effective (reported in the *Lancet* in 1980). In research published in the *British Journal of Psychiatry* in 1986, she, Crow, and others determined that schizophrenic patients treated early with antipsychotics had a better prognosis, a finding that turned out to be of much interest.

Veronica Murphy Pennington (1894–1986). A pioneer psychopharmacologist, she was born in Lansing, Iowa, and graduated with an M.D. from the University of Iowa in 1919 as the only woman in her class. After training in psychiatry at state hospitals in Cherokee, Iowa, and Peter, Minnesota, in 1928 she founded with her husband, Dr. Elree Pennington, a private psychiatric sanatorium in South Bend, Indiana, which they maintained until 1943. After further service at state hospitals in Indiana, Georgia, and Texas, in the mid-1950s she became senior staff psychiatrist at Whitfield Hospital in Mississippi. From that vantage point, she became part of the U.S. delegation to the Second World Congress of Psychiatry in Zurich in 1957, giving a paper on her various controlled trials, which had begun with **reserpine** in 1954 and **chlorpromazine** in 1955. At Whitfield, she further studied a whole series of drugs, the results of which endorsed some innovative combination therapies (which shortly, and perhaps unjustly, were to go out of style). (*See* her article in the *American Journal of Psychiatry*, 1962, summarizing this work, beginning with trials of reserpine in 1953 and continued through the 1950s with a host of antipsychotic agents.) She told the Congress that she had abandoned **electroconvulsive therapy**: "I now believe chemotherapy to be the most efficacious and safest treatment for neuropsychiatric patients" (Kline, *Frontiers*, p. 166).

In the 1960s, Pennington shifted to the Veterans Administration hospital in Jackson, Mississippi, where she became part of the network of VA hospital trialists studying psychoactive drugs. Also in the 1960s, she authored or co-authored several key articles on psychotropic compounds just being introduced, especially a 1966 article in the *Journal of the American Medical Association* on the differential effect of various drugs in depression, which she co-wrote with John Overall (1929–), a psychologist–statistician at the University of Texas Medical Branch at Galveston (who had just moved there from a VA hospital in Kansas), and Leo Hollister (1920–2000) at the Veterans Administration hospital in Palo Alto, California.*

Judith Livant Rapoport (1933–). A pioneer of biological child psychiatry, Rapoport was born in New York City, her parents Louis and Minna Livant Rapoport. She graduated with an M.D. from Harvard University in 1959, then trained in psychiatry at the Massachusetts Mental Health Center in Boston and at **St. Elizabeths Hospital** in Washington, D.C. After a postdoctoral fellowship at the Karolinska Hospital in Stockholm, in 1964 she became a **National Institute of Mental Health** fellow in child psychiatry at Children's Hospital in Washington and remained associated with NIMH for the remainder of her career, serving simultaneously as a lecturer (later professor) in pediatric psychiatry at Georgetown University in Washington. In 1984, she became chief of the child psychiatry branch of NIMH's division of intramural (meaning on-campus) research programs.

Rapoport is known for her bestselling book, *The Boy Who Couldn't Stop Washing* (1989), which placed **obsessive-compulsive disorder** (OCD) for children on the map. She and her group developed the first animal model for studying OCD. This work gave research on OCD a scientific basis and raised awareness of the disorder, so that currently there are about 500 treatment clinics specifically for OCD across the United States. She also helped found the discipline of pediatric psychopharmacology and in general was an early investigator of biological aspects of severe childhood psychiatric disorders, studied with magnetic resonance imaging.

Hannah Steinberg (ca. 1926–). A pioneer of experimental psychopharmacology, Steinberg was born in Vienna; her father was a lawyer who practiced only briefly, thereafter helping Hannah's mother in her wholesale pelt business. Hannah Steinberg came to London in 1939 in a Kindertransport—child Holocaust survivors who were brought by the British Jewish Refugee Committee, without their parents, out of Austria, Germany, Poland, and Czechoslovakia to Great Britain. After finishing high school in Putney, in 1948 she earned an undergraduate psychology degree at University College London (UCL), going on to a Ph.D. in the subject in 1954. After a postdoctoral fellowship in psychology, she began lecturing in psychopharmacology at UCL, where in 1970 she became professor of psychopharmacology, the first such professorship in the world. (She was emerited in 1989.)

Working with Ruth Rushton and Michael Besser, she showed in 1963 in the *British Journal of Pharmacology* that—as she put it later—"combinations of amphetamines and a barbiturate could induce spectacular hyperactivity in rodents. It was much greater than

* Hollister and Overall were among the most prominent of the early psychopharmacologists; it was in these years that they were developing computer-assisted assessment of patients. In 1962, Overall and Donald R. Gorham (1903–) at the Veterans Administration Central Neuropsychiatric Research laboratory, proposed the Brief Psychiatric Rating Scale [BPRS] in *Psychological Reports*, a test of psychopathology.

any activity obtainable with any dose of the separate drugs and also greater than the sum of the activity induced by the separate ingredient drugs. We also showed comparable effects in volunteers." (*See* **ANTIDEPRESSANT: first-generation antidepressants.**) On the basis of this and similar research on the drug clenbuterol and the **benzodiazepines**, she received a lifetime achievement award from the British Association of Psychopharmacology that stated, "Only now are we beginning to realise that Hannah was tapping into the effects of drug combinations on neuronal second messenger systems, or beyond, and that understanding the interactions of drugs with receptors is merely the first step in explaining their effects on behaviour." Steinberg's later research on the positive effects on mood of regular exercise also aroused a good deal of interest (*see European Psychologist*, 1998).

Bibliographic Essay

The following essay mentions some of the main resources for conducting research in the history of psychiatry.

There are several standard works that one must simply have at one's side. Essential in the study of disease history is German E. Berrios's great work, *The History of Mental Symptoms: Descriptive Psychopathology since the Nineteenth Century* (Cambridge, UK: Cambridge University Press, 1996). Necessary for navigating in psychopharmacology is Lundbeck Institute, *Psychotropics 2002/2003* (Denmark: Lundbeck Institute, 2003). For general reference, see John G. Howells and M. Livia Osborn, *A Reference Companion to the History of Abnormal Psychology*, 2 vols. (Westport, CT: Greenwood, 1984). A useful scholarly overview is German Berrios and Roy Porter (Eds.), *A History of Clinical Psychiatry: The Origin and History of Psychiatric Disorders* (London: Athlone, 1995). For a global bird's-eye view, one might consult John Howells (Ed.), *World History of Psychiatry* (New York: Brunner/Mazel, 1975). On the history of psychiatry in the twentieth century, *see* Hugh Freeman (Ed.), *A Century of Psychiatry*, 2 vols. (London: Mosby-Wolfe, 1999). For a scholarly overview of the entire modern history of psychiatry, *see* Edward Shorter, *A History of Psychiatry from the Era of the Asylum to the Age of Prozac* (New York: John Wiley & Sons, 1997). An uneven reference work with heavy emphasis on psychoanalysis is Benjamin B. Wolman (Ed.), *International Encyclopedia of Psychiatry, Psychology, Psychoanalysis & Neurology*, 12 vols. (New York: Van Nostrand, ca. 1977).

Among other reading on international themes: On the history of psychopharmacology, for a basic narrative *see* Walter Sneader, *Drug Discovery: The Evolution of Modern Medicines* (Chichester, UK: John Wiley & Sons, 1985); for a scholarly account of the evolution of the field to the 1950s, *see* Matthias M. Weber, *Die Entwicklung der Psychopharmakologie im Zeitalter der naturwissenschaftlichen Medizin: Ideengeschichte eines psychiatrischen Therapiesystems* (Munich: Urban & Vogel, 1999); on the social history of psychopharmacology, essential reading is David Healy, *The Antidepressant Era* (Cambridge, MA: Harvard University Press, 1997); and Healy, *The Creation of Psychopharmacology* (Cambridge, MA: Harvard University Press, 2002). Important source reading in this area is Healy's three-volume collection of interviews, *The Psychopharmacologists* (London, 1996–2000; Chapman and Hall published vols. 1–2; Arnold, vol. 3). Short autobiographical accounts of the lives of leading psychopharmacologists may be found in Thomas Ban, David Healy, and Edward Shorter (Eds.), *The Rise of Psychopharmacology* (Budapest: Animula, 1998); *The Triumph of Psychopharmacology* (2000); and *From Psychopharmacology to Neuropsychopharmacology in the 1980s* (2002). A general kind of reference work on the history of psychopharmacology, including as well further autobiographies, is Thomas Ban, David Healy, and Edward Shorter, eds., *Reflections on Twentieth-Century Psychopharmacology* (Budapest: Animula, 2004).

For systematic comparisons of national systems of mental-health care, *see* K. Pandy, *Die Irrenfürsorge in Europa: Eine vergleichende Studie* (Berlin: Reimer, 1908); and World Health Organization, *Atlas: Country Profiles of Mental Health Resources, 2001* (Geneva: WHO, 2001). An illuminating cross-national look at European psychiatry is offered in a contemporary document from 1938: Katherine Angel et al. (Eds.), *European Psychiatry on the Eve of War: Aubrey Lewis, the Maudsley Hospital, and the Rockefeller Foundation in the 1930s* (London: Wellcome Trust Centre for the History of Medicine at UCL, 2003).

GERMANY AND GERMAN-SPEAKING EUROPE

Although the Germans have done poorly at writing histories of their psychiatry, the sources are formidable. For biography, Theodor Kirchhoff's *Deutsche Irrenärzte: Einzelbilder Ihres Lebens und Wirkens*, 2 vols. (Berlin: Springer, 1921–1924) is the point of departure. Essential is Alma Kreuter's magnificent historical bibliography of the work of almost all German academic psychiatrists, *Deutschsprachige Neurologen und Psychiater: ein biographisch-bibliographisches Lexikon von den Vorläufern bis zur Mitte des 20. Jahrhunderts*, 3 vols. (Munich: Saur, 1996). For more recent biographical accounts see, Kurt Kolle (Ed.), *Grosse Nervenärzte*, 3 vols. (Stuttgart: Thieme, 1963 and after). This series is updated in Hans Schliack and Hanns Hippius (Eds.), *Nervenärzte: Biographien* (Stuttgart: Thieme, 1998). A comprehensive view of academic psychiatry, considering all German-speaking universities, may be found in Hans-Heinz Eulner, *Die Entwicklung der medizinischen Spezialfächer an den Universitäten des deutschen Sprachgebietes* (Stuttgart: Enke, 1970), pp. 670–680. Heinz-Peter Schmiedebach's *Psychiatrie und Psychologie im Widerstreit: Die Auseinandersetzung in der Berliner medicinisch-psychologischen Gesellschaft (1867–1899)* (Husum: Matthiesen, 1986) contains useful biographical information on the members. For information on psychiatrists in German-speaking countries after the Second World War, *see* Who's Who International Red Series, *Who's Who in Medicine*, 5th ed. (Zurich: Who's Who Verlag, 1981).

There are few useful national histories of German psychiatry, although a tremendous literature exists for the Nazi period (listed in the following bibliography). *See*, however, Michael Schmidt-Degenhard, *Melancholie und Depression* (Stuttgart: Kohlhammer, 1983); and Werner Leibbrand and Annemarie Wettley, *Der Wahnsinn: Geschichte der abendländischen Psychopathologie* (Freiburg: Alber, 1961). Especially to be recommended for its scholarly thoroughness and archivally based research is Eric J. Engstrom, *Clinical Psychiatry in Imperial Germany: A History of Psychiatric Practice* (Ithaca, NY: Cornell University Press, 2004).

On the history of psychiatry in Switzerland, *see* Thomas Haenel, *Zur Geschichte der Psychiatrie: Gedanken zur allgemeinen und Basler Psychiatriegeschichte* (Basel: Birkhäuser, 1982); and Christian Müller, *Vom Tollhaus zum Psychozentrum* (Hürtgenwald: Pressler, 1993). Markus Schär's brilliant history of suicide in Zurich must be mentioned: *Seelennöte der Untertanen: Selbstmord, Melancholie und Religion im Alten Zürich, 1500–1800* (Zurich: Chronos, 1985).

On the history of psychiatry in Austria, the focus is mainly on psychoanalysis. As an entry point to this enormous literature, see Peter Gay, *Freud: A Life for Our Time* (New York: Norton, 1988). Two especially fine collective biographies are Elke Mühlleitner, *Biographisches Lexikon der Psychoanalyse* (Tübingen: Diskord, 1992), which concerns exclusively the members of the Vienna Psychoanalytic Society; and Uwe Henrik Peters, *Psychiatrie im Exil: die Emigration der dynamischen Psychiatrie aus Deutschland, 1933–1939* (Düsseldorf: Kupka, 1992), which also considers the emigré Austrians, despite the title. For a classic scholarly account of the history of psychiatry at the University of Vienna, *see* relevant parts of Erna Lesky, *Die Wiener Medizinische Schule im 19. Jahrhundert* (Graz: Böhlau, 1978).

As for psychiatric dictionaries, a useful one is Christian Müller (Ed.), *Lexikon der Psychiatrie* (Berlin: Springer, 1973).

FRANCE

The biographical resources for studing the history of psychiatry in France are more limited than for Germany. Essential is Pierre Morel, *Dictionnaire biographique de la psychiatrie* (Paris: Les Empêcheurs de penser en rond, 1996); biographies of the well-known figures in French psychiatry may be found in René Semelaigne, *Les pionniers de la psychiatrie française avant et après Pinel,* 2 vols. (Paris: Baillière, 1930–1932). A fundamental source for the history of French psychiatry—with comparisons to the rest of Europe—is Paul Sérieux, *L'Assistance des aliénés en France, en Allemagne, en Italie et en Suisse* (Paris: Imprimerie municipale, 1903).

For an overview of the history of (mainly) French psychiatry, *see* Pierre Pichot, *A Century of Psychiatry* (Paris: Dacosta, 1983); and Jacques Postel and Claude Quetel, *Nouvelle histoire de la psychiatrie,* rev. ed. (Paris: Dunod, 2002).

An exceptionally detailed history of the French pharmaceutical industry is Alexandre Blondeau, *Histoire des laboratoires pharmaceutiques en France et de leurs médicaments,* 3 vols. (Paris: Cherche Midi, 1992–1998).

There are three useful French psychiatric dictionaries: Jean Thuillier, *La Folie: histoire et dictionnaire* (Paris: Laffont, 1996), which is partly a historical dictionary as well as containing Thuillier's own thoughts about the history of psychiatry; Jacques Postel, *Dictionnaire de psychiatrie et de psychopathologie clinique* (Paris: Larousse, 1993); and Antoine Porot, *Manuel alphabétique de psychiatrie,* 7th ed. (Paris: Presses universitaires de France, 1996).

As for special studies in the history of French psychiatry, the following may be mentioned: Dora B. Weiner, *Comprendre et soigner: Philippe Pinel (1745–1826): La médecine de l'esprit* (Paris: Fayard, 1999); Marcel Gauchet and Gladys Swain, *La pratique de l'esprit human: L'institution asilaire et la révolution démocratique* (Paris: Gallimard, 1980); Jan Goldstein, *Console and Classify: The French Psychiatry Profession in the Nineteenth Century* (New York: Cambridge University Press, 1987); Ruth Harris, *Murders and Madness: Medicine, Law, and Society in the fin de siècle* (Oxford: Clarendon, 1989); and Elisabeth Roudinesco, *Histoire de la psychanalyse en France,* 2 vols. (Paris: Seuil, 1986).

BRITAIN

What is lacking in Britain in the way of primary directories of the kind the Germans possess so amply is made up for by a number of excellent scholarly analyses.

In terms of discovering the details of personalities, the only accessible reference work is *"Munk's Roll": Lives of the Fellows of the Royal College of Physicians of London.* Volume IV covers those who died in the period 1826–1925; vol. V, continued to 1965; vol. VI, continued to 1975 and subsequent volumes for more recent years. For psychiatrists who became famous, the *Dictionary of National Biography* is a useful resource, yet few did.

British medical historians have covered the history of psychiatry better than in any other country. For an introduction *see* W. F. Bynum et al. (Eds.), *The Anatomy of Madness,* 3 vols. (London: Tavistock, 1985–1988). On behalf of the Royal College of Psychiatrists, German E. Berrios and Hugh Freeman have edited a two-volume work,

150 Years of British Psychiatry (London: Gaskell, 1991–1996). For volumes of interviews, see Greg Wilkinson (Ed.), *Talking About Psychiatry* (London: Gaskell, 1993); and Michael Shepherd (Ed.), *Psychiatrists on Psychiatry* (Cambridge, UK: Cambridge University Press, 1982)—the latter being more international in flavor. On eugenics, *see* Pauline M. H. Mazumdar, *Eugenics, Human Genetics and Human Failings: The Eugenics Society, its Sources and its Critics in Britain* (London: Routledge, 1992).

UNITED STATES

Psychiatrists' biographies may be found in American Psychiatric Association, *Biographical Directory of the Fellows & Members of the American Psychiatric Association* (New York: Bowker, 1963; there were subsequent editions of this, from various publishers, until 1989); *American Men & Women of Science*, many editions (New Providence, NJ: Bowker); and Martin Kaufman et al. (Eds.), *Dictionary of American Medical Biography*, 2 vols. (Westport, CT: Greenwood, 1984). A fundamental source is the state-by-state review of mental hospitals, including extensive material on their histories, in Henry M. Hurd, *The Institutional Care of the Insane in the United States and Canada*, 4 vols. (Baltimore: Johns Hopkins Press, 1916–1917). The foremost historian of American psychiatry is Gerald Grob, and the books of his most to recommend are *Mental Illness and American Society, 1875–1940* (Princeton, NJ: Princeton University Press, 1983); *From Asylum to Community: Mental Health Policy in Modern America* (Princeton, NJ: Princeton University Press, 1991); and *The Mad Among Us: A History of the Care of America's Mentally Ill* (New York: Free Press, 1994).

A psychiatric dictionary for the Anglo-Saxon world heavily weighted toward psychoanalysis is Robert Jean Campbell, *Psychiatric Dictionary*, 7th ed. (New York: Oxford, 1996).

The American Psychiatric Association has attempted to chart the history of the discipline in the United States in various volumes. *See* American Psychiatric Association, *One Hundred Years of American Psychiatry* (New York: Columbia University Press, 1944); Walter E. Barton, *History and Influence of the American Psychiatric Association* (Washington, DC: APA Press, 1987); and Roy W. Menninger and John C. Nemiah (Eds.), *American Psychiatry after World War II (1944–1994)* (Washington, DC: APA Press, 2000).

Bibliography

BOOKS ABOUT THE HISTORY OF PSYCHIATRIC ILLNESS

Bell, Rudolph M. (1985). *Holy Anorexia.* Chicago: University of Chicago Press.

Brumberg, Joan Jacobs. (1988). *Fasting Girls: The Emergence of Anorexia Nervosa as a Modern Disease.* Cambridge, MA: Harvard University Press.

Dean, Eric T., Jr. (1997). *Shook Over Hell: Post-Traumatic Stress, Vietnam, and the Civil War.* Cambridge, MA: Harvard University Press.

Fischer-Homberger, Esther. (1970). *Hypochondrie: Melancholie bis Neurose, Krankheiten und Zustandsbilder.* Berne: Huber.

Fischer-Homberger, Esther. (1975). *Die traumatische Neurose: Vom somatischen zum sozialen Leiden.* Berne: Huber.

Gilman, Sander L. (1985). *Difference and Pathology: Stereotypes of Sexuality, Race, and Madness.* Ithaca, NY: Cornell University Press.

Gilman, Sander L., et al. (1993). *Hysteria Beyond Freud.* Berkeley: University of California Press.

Gosling, F. G. (1987). *Before Freud: Neurasthenia and the American Medical Community, 1870–1910.* Urbana, IL: University of Illinois Press.

Habermas, Tilmann. (1994). *Zur Geschichte der Magersucht: Eine medizinpsychologische Rekonstruktion.* Frankfurt/M: Fischer Taschenbuch.

Hacking, Ian. (1995). *Rewriting the Soul: Multiple Personality and the Sciences of Memory.* Princeton: Princeton University Press.

Jamison, Kay Redfield. (1993). *Touched with Fire: Manic-Depressive Illness and the Artistic Temperament.* New York: Free Press.

Kushner, Howard I. (1989). *Self-Destruction in the Promised Land: A Psychocultural Biology of American Suicide.* New Brunswick, NJ: Rutgers University Press.

Kushner, Howard I. (1999). *A Cursing Brain? The Histories of Tourette Syndrome.* Cambridge, MA: Harvard University Press.

Lipowski, Z. J. (1980). *Delirium: Acute Brain Failure in Man.* Springfield: Charles C Thomas. *See* section on history of delirium.

López Piñero, José M. (1983). *Historical Origins of the Concept of Neurosis.* Cambridge, UK: Cambridge University Press.

Lucire, Yolande. (2003). *Constructing RSI: Belief and Desire.* Sydney: University of New South Wales Press. *See* section on history of Repetitive Strain Injury.

MacDonald, Michael. (1981). *Mystical Bedlam: Madness, Anxiety, and Healing in Seventeenth-Century England.* Cambridge, UK: Cambridge University Press.

MacDonald, Michael, & Murphy, Terence R. (1990). *Sleepless Souls: Suicide in Early Modern England.* Oxford, UK: Clarendon Press.

Micale, Mark S. (1995). *Approaching Hysteria: Disease and Its Interpretations.* Princeton: Princeton University Press.

Micale Mark S., & Lerner, Paul (Eds.), (2001). *Traumatic Pasts: History, Psychiatry, and Trauma in the Modern Age, 1870–1930.* Cambridge, UK: Cambridge University Press.

Oppenheim, Janet. (1991). *"Shattered Nerves": Doctors, Patients, and Depression in Victorian England.* New York: Oxford University Press.

Radkau, Joachim. (1998). *Das Zeitalter der Nervosität: Deutschland zwischen Bismarck und Hitler.* Munich: Hanser.

Shephard, Ben. (2000). *A War of Nerves: Soldiers and Psychiatrists in the Twentieth Century.* Cambridge, MA: Harvard University Press.

Shorter, Edward. (1992). *From Paralysis to Fatigue: A History of Psychosomatic Illness in the Modern Era.* New York: Free Press.

Shorter, Edward. (1994). *From the Mind into the Body: the Cultural Origins of Psychosomatic Symptoms.* New York: Free Press.

Showalter, Elaine. (1985). *The Female Malady: Women, Madness, and English Culture, 1830–1980.* New York: Pantheon.

Showalter, Elaine. (1997). *Hystories: Hysterical Epidemics and Modern Culture.* New York: Columbia University Press.

Temkin, Owsei. (1971). *The Falling Sickness: A History of Epilepsy from the Greeks to the Beginnings of Modern Neurology,* rev. ed. Baltimore: Johns Hopkins University Press.

Torrey, E. Fuller. (1980). *Schizophrenia and Civilization.* New York: Aronson.

Torrey, E. Fuller, & Miller, Judy. (2001). *The Invisible Plague: The Rise of Mental Illness from 1750 to the Present.* New Brunswick, NJ: Rutgers University Press.

Trimble, Michael R. (1981). *Post-Traumatic Neurosis: From Railway Spine to Whiplash.* Chichester, UK: Wiley.

Vandereycken, Walter, & van Deth, Ron. (1994). *From Fasting Saints to Anorexic Girls: The History of Self-Starvation.* New York: New York University Press.

Warren, Carol A. B. (1987). *Madwives: Schizophrenic Women in the 1950s.* New Brunswick, NJ: Rutgers University Press.

Wessely, Simon, Hotopf, Matthew, & Sharpe, Michael. (1998). *Chronic Fatigue and Its Syndromes.* Oxford, UK: Oxford University Press. *See* section on history of the disorder.

Young, Allan. (1995). *The Harmony of Illusions: Inventing Post-Traumatic Stress Disorder.* Princeton: Princeton University Press.

PSYCHIATRISTS: AUTOBIOGRAPHIES AND BIOGRAPHIES

Baruk, Henri. (1976). *Des hommes comme nous: Mémoires d'un neuropsychiatre.* Paris: Laffont.

Black, Shirley B. (1995). *An 18th Century Mad-Doctor: William Perfect of West Malling* Sevenoaks, UK: Darenth Valley Publications.

Bromberg, Walter. (1982). *Psychiatry Between the Wars, 1918–1945: A Recollection.* Westport, CT: Greenwood.

Robeson Burr, Anna. (1929). *Weir Mitchell: His Life and Letters.* New York: Duffield.

Clervoy, Patrick. (1997). *Henri Ey, 1900–1977: Cinquante ans de psychiatrie en France.* Paris: Institut Synthélabo.

Collie, Michael. (1988). *Henry Maudsley: Victorian Psychiatrist: A Bibliographical Study.* Winchester, UK: St. Paul's Biographies.

Ellenberger, Henri F. (1970). *The Discovery of the Unconscious: The History and Evolution of Dynamic Psychiatry.* New York: Basic Books. Pierre Janet, Sigmund Freud, Alfred Adler, Carl Gustav Jung.

Finger, Stanley. (2000). *Minds Behind the Brain: A History of the Pioneers and Their Discoveries.* New York: Oxford University Press. A history of neuroscience, told as biography.

Forel, Auguste. (1968). *Briefe, Correspondance, 1864–1927.* Berne: Huber.

Friedman, Lawrence J. (1990). *Menninger: The Family and the Clinic.* Lawrence, KS: University Press of Kansas.

Frigessi, Delia, Giacanelli, Ferruccio, & Mangoni, Luisa. (Eds.) (1995). *Cesare Lombroso: Delitto, Genio, Follia: Scritti scelti.* Turin: Bollati.

Gay, Peter. (1988). *Freud: A Life for Our Time.* New York: Norton.

Gilman, Sander L. (1993). *The Case of Sigmund Freud: Medicine and Identity at the Fin de Siècle.* Baltimore: Johns Hopkins University Press.

Goetz, Christopher G., Bonduelle, Michel, & Gelfand, Toby. (1995). *Charcot: Constructing Neurology.* New York: Oxford University Press.

Hirschmüller, Albrecht. (1978). *Physiologie und Psychoanalyse in Leben und Werk Josef Breuers.* Berne: Huber.

Hirschmüller, Albrecht. (1991). *Freuds Begegnung mit der Psychiatrie: Von der Hirnmythologie zur Neurosenlehre.* Tübingen: Diskord.

Hoche, Alfred E. (1936). *Jahresringe: Innenansicht eines Menschenlebens.* Munich: Lehmann.

Kraepelin, Emil. (1983). *Lebenserinnerungen.* Berlin: Springer.

Lanczik, Mario. (1988). *Der Breslauer Psychiater Carl Wernicke.* Sigmaringen: Thorbecke.

Lomax, Montagu. (1921). *The Experiences of an Asylum Doctor.* London: Allen and Unwin.

Müller, Max. (1982). *Erinnerungen: Erlebte Psychiatriegeschichte, 1920–1960.* Berlin: Springer.

Neumärker, K.-J. (1990). *Karl Bonhoeffer: Leben und Werk eines deutschen Psychiaters.* Berlin: Springer.

Oosterhuis, Harry. (2000). *Stepchildren of Nature: Krafft-Ebing, Psychiatry, and the Making of Sexual Identity.* Chicago: University of Chicago Press.

Palem, Robert M. (1997). *Henri Ey: Psychiatre et philosophe.* Paris: Éditions Rive Droite.

Parker, Beulah. (1987). *The Evolution of a Psychiatrist: Memoirs of a Woman Doctor.* New Haven: Yale University Press.

Pigeaud, Jackie. (2001). *Aux portes de la psychiatrie: Pinel, l'ancien et le moderne.* Paris: Aubier.

Pongratz, Ludwig J. (Ed.) (1977). *Psychiatrie in Selbstdarstellungen.* Berne: Huber. Walter von Baeyer, Lothar B. Kalinowsky, Jakob Klaesi, Roland Kuhn, Karl Leonhard, Jakob Wyrsch, and so forth.

Roazen, Paul. (1984). *Freud and His Followers.* New York: New York University Press.

Rollin, Henry R. (1990). *Festina Lente: A Psychiatric Odyssey.* London: British Medical Journal.

Satzinger, Helga. (1998). *Die Geschichte der genetisch orientierten Hirnforschung von Cécile und Oskar Vogt in der Zeit von 1895 bis ca. 1927.* Stuttgart: Deutscher Apotheker Verlag.

Schimmelpenning, Gustav W. (1990). *Alfred Erich Hoche.* Göttingen: Vandenhoeck & Ruprecht.

Sulloway, Frank J. (1979). *Freud: Biologist of the Mind: Beyond the Psychoanalytic Legend.* New York: Basic Books.

Thuillier, Jean. (1999). *Ten Years That Changed the Face of Mental Illness.* London: Dunitz. Autobiography.

Weber, Matthias M. (1993). *Ernst Rüdin: Eine kritische Biographie.* Berlin: Springer.

White, William A. (1933). *Forty Years of Psychiatry.* New York: Nervous and Mental Disease Publishing Company.

Whitrow, Magda. (1993). *Julius Wagner-Jauregg (1857–1940).* London: Smith-Gordon.

HISTORIES OF INSTITUTIONS

Andrews, Jonathan, Briggs, Asa, Porter, Roy, Tucker, Penny, & Waddington, Keir. (1997). *The History of Bethlem.* London: Routlege.

Crammer, John. (1990). *Asylum History: Buckinghamshire County Pauper Lunatic Asylum—St. John's.* London: Gaskell.

Digby, Anne. (1985). *Madness, Morality and Medicine: A Study of the York Retreat, 1796–1914.* Cambridge, UK: Cambridge University Press.

Dowdall, George W. (1996). *The Eclipse of the State Mental Hospital: Policy, Stigma, and Organization.* Albany: State University of New York Press.

Fallon, Brian A., & Gorman, Jack M. (Eds.). (1998). *The New York State Psychiatric Institute: American Psychiatry at the Centennial.* New York: NYSPI.

Fox, Richard W. (1978). *So Far Disordered in Mind: Insanity in California, 1870–1930.* Berkeley: University of California Press.

Goldberg, Ann. (1999). *Sex, Religion, and the Making of Modern Madness: The Eberbach Asylum and German Society, 1815-1849.* New York: Oxford University Press.

Harrison, Tom. (2000). *Bion, Rickman, Foulkes and the Northfield Experiments: Advancing on a Different Front.* London: Kingsley.

Hunter, Richard, & Macalpine, Ida. (1974). *Psychiatry for the Poor: 1851 Colney Hatch Asylum-Friern Hospital 1973: A Medical and Social History.* London: Dawson.

Jones, Kathleen. (1993). *Asylums and After: A Revised History of the Mental Health Services: From the Early 18th Century to the 1990s.* London: Athlone.

Keating, Peter. (1993). *La science du mal: L'institution de la psychiatrie au Québec, 1800–1914.* Montreal: Boréal.

Kolb, Lawrence C., & Roizin, Leon. (1993). *The First Psychiatric Institute.* Washington, DC: American Psychiatric Press. New York State Psychiatric Institute.

Lippi, Donatella. (1996). *San Salvi: Storia di un Manicomio.* Florence: Olschki.

Lunbeck, Elizabeth. (1994). *The Psychiatric Persuasion: Knowledge, Gender, and Power in Modern America.* Princeton: Princeton University Press. About the Boston Psychopathic Hospital around the time of the First World War.

MacKenzie, Charlotte. (1992). *Psychiatry for the Rich: A History of Ticehurst Private Asylum, 1792–1917.* London: Routledge.

McCandless, Peter. (1996). *Moonlight, Magnolias, and Madness: Insanity in South Carolina from the Colonial Period to the Progressive Era.* Chapel Hill: University of North Carolina Press.

McGovern, Constance M. (1985). *Masters of Madness: Social Origins of the American Psychiatric Profession.* Hanover, NH: New England University Press.

Noll, Steven. (1995). *Feeble-Minded in Our Midst: Institutions for the Mentally Retarded in the South, 1900–1940.* Chapel Hill: University of North Carolina Press.

Pantozzi, Giuseppe. (1989). *Gli spazi della follia: Storia della psichiatria nel Tirolo e nel Trentino, 1830–1942.* Trent, Italy: Centro Studi "M.H. Erickson."

Parry-Jones, William. (1972). *The Trade in Lunacy: A Study of Private Madhouses in England in the Eighteenth and Nineteenth Centuries.* London: Routledge.

Reaume, Geoffrey. (2000). *Remembrance of Patients Past: Patient Life at the Toronto Hospital for the Insane, 1870–1940.* Toronto: Oxford University Press.

Rothman, David J. (1980). *Conscience and Convenience: The Asylum and its Alternatives in Progressive America.* Boston: Little, Brown.

Rothman, David J. (1990). *The Discovery of the Asylum: Social Order and Disorder in the New Republic*, rev. ed. Boston: Little, Brown.

Shortt, S. E. D. (1986). *Victorian Lunacy: Richard M. Bucke and the Practice of Late Nineteenth-Century Psychiatry.* Cambridge, UK: Cambridge University Press.

Simmons, Harvey G. (1982). *From Asylum to Welfare.* Toronto: National Institute on Mental Retardation. Institutions for the Mentally Retarded in Ontario.

Stohl, Alfred. (2000). *Der Narrenturm oder die dunkle Seite der Wissenschaft.* Vienna: Böhlau.

Sutton, S. B. (1986). *Crossroads in Psychiatry: A History of the McLean Hospital.* Washington, DC: American Psychiatric Press.

Tomes, Nancy. (1984). *A Generous Confidence: Thomas Story Kirkbride and the Art of Asylum-keeping, 1840–1883.* Cambridge, UK: Cambridge University Press.

Turner, Trevor H. (1992). *A Diagnostic Analysis of the Casebooks of Ticehurst House Asylum, 1845–1890.* Cambridge, UK: Cambridge University Press.

Warsh, Cheryl Krasnick. (1989). *Moments of Unreason: The Practice of Canadian Psychiatry and the Homewood Retreat, 1883–1923.* Montreal: McGill-Queen's University Press.

PSYCHIATRY AND SOCIETY

Bayer, Ronald. (1987). *Homosexuality and American Psychiatry: The Politics of Diagnosis.* Princeton: Princeton University Press.

Dörner, Klaus. (1969). *Bürger und Irre.* Frankfurt/M: Europäische Verlagsanstalt.

Guarnieri, Patrizia. (1993). *A Case of Child Murder: Law and Science in Nineteenth-Century Tuscany.* Cambridge, UK: Polity Press.

Horwitz, Allan V. (2002). *Creating Mental Illness.* Chicago: University of Chicago Press.

Kirk, Stuart A., & Kutchins, Herb. (1992). *The Selling of DSM: The Rhetoric of Science in Psychiatry.* New York: Aldine.

Lewis, Milton. (1988). *Managing Madness: Psychiatry and Society in Australia, 1788–1980.* Canberra: Australian Government Publishing Service.

Micale, Mark S. & Porter, Roy (Eds.). (1994). *Discovering the History of Psychiatry.* New York: Oxford University Press.

Porter, Roy. (1987). *Mind-Forg'd Manacles: A History of Madness in England from the Restoration to the Regency.* Cambridge, MA: Harvard University Press.

Radkau, Joachim. (1998). *Das Zeitalter der Nervosität: Deutschland zwischen Bismarck und Hitler.* Munich: Hanser.

Roelcke, Volker. (1999). *Krankheit und Kulturkritik: Psychiatrische Gesellschaftsdeutungen im bürgerlichen Zeitalter (1790–1914).* Frankfurt/M: Campus.

Rosario, Vernon A. (Ed.) (1997). *Science and Homosexualities.* New York: Routledge.

Shorter, Edward. (2000). *The Kennedy Family and the Story of Mental Retardation.* Philadelphia: Temple University Press.

Trent, James W., Jr. (1994). *Inventing the Feeble Mind: The History of Mental Retardation in the United States.* Berkeley: University of California Press.

HISTORY OF THERAPEUTICS IN PSYCHIATRY

Ayd, Frank J., & Blackwell, Barry. (Eds.) (1984). *Discoveries in Biological Psychiatry.* Baltimore: Ayd Medical Communications.

Braslow, Joel. (1997). *Mental Ills and Bodily Cures: Psychiatric Treatment in the First Half of the Twentieth Century.* Berkeley: University of California Press.

Healy, David. (1997). *The Antidepressant Era.* Cambridge, MA: Harvard University Press.

Healy, David. (2002). *The Creation of Psychopharmacology.* Cambridge, MA: Harvard University Press.

Healy, David. (2004). *Let Them Eat Prozac.* New York: New York University Press.

Pressman, Jack D. (1998). *Last Resort: Psychosurgery and the Limits of Medicine.* Cambridge, UK: Cambridge University Press.

Smith, Mickey C. (1985). *Small Comfort: A History of the Minor Tranquilizers.* New York: Praeger.

Valenstein, Elliot S. (1986). *Great and Desperate Cures: The Rise and Decline of Psychosurgery and Other Radical Treatments for Mental Illness.* New York: Basic Books.

PSYCHIATRY, EUGENICS, THIRD REICH, HOLOCAUST

Aly, Götz (Ed.) (1989). *Aktion T4, 1939–1945: Die 'Euthanasie'-Zentrale in der Tiergartenstrasse 4.* Berlin: Hentrich.

Aly, Götz. (1995). *"Endlösung": Völkerverschiebung und der Mord an den europäischen Juden.* Frankfurt/M.: Fischer.

Bock, Gisela. (1986). *Zwangssterilisation im Nationalsozialismus: Studien zur Rassenpolitik und Frauenpolitik.* Opladen: Westdeutscher Verlag.

Broberg, Gunnar, & Roll-Hansen, Nils (Eds.) (1996). *Eugenics and the Welfare State.* East Lansing: Michigan State University Press.

Burleigh, Michael. (1994). *Death and Deliverance: "Euthanasia" in Germany, c. 1900–1945* Cambridge, UK: Cambridge University Press.

Cocks, Geoffrey. (1985). *Psychotherapy in the Third Reich: The Göring Institute.* New York: Oxford University Press.

Dowbiggin, Ian. (1991). *Inheriting Madness: Professionalization and Psychiatric Knowledge in Nineteenth-Century France.* Berkeley: University of California Press.

Dowbiggin, Ian. (1997). *Keeping America Sane: Psychiatry and Eugenics in the United States and Canada, 1880–1940.* Ithaca: Cornell University Press.

Faulstich, Heinz. (1993). *Von der Irrenfürsorge zur "Euthanasie": Geschichte der badischen Psychiatrie bis 1945.* Freiburg i. B.: Lambertus.

Faulstich, Heinz. (1998). *Hungersterben in der Psychiatrie, 1914–1949: Mit einer Topographie der NS-Psychiatrie.* Freiburg i. B.: Lambertus.

Finzen, Asmus. (1996). *Massenmord ohne Schuldgefühl: Die Tötung psychisch Kranker und geistig Behinderter auf dem Dienstweg.* Bonn: das Narrenschiff im Psychiatrie-Verlag.

Glass, James M. (1997). *"Life Unworthy of Life": Racial Phobia and Mass Murder in Hitler's Germany.* New York: Basic Books.

Harwood, Jonathan. (1993). *Styles of Scientific Thought: The German Genetics Community, 1900-1933.* Chicago: University of Chicago Press.

Kevles, Daniel J. (1985). *In the Name of Eugenics: Genetics and the Uses of Human Heredity.* Berkeley: University of California Press.

Kühl, Stefan. (1994). *The Nazi Connection: Eugenics, American Racism, and German National Socialism.* New York: Oxford University Press.

Larson, Edward J. (1995). *Sex, Race, and Science: Eugenics in the Deep South.* Baltimore: Johns Hopkins University Press.

Lockot, Regine. (1985). *Erinnern und Durcharbeiten: Zur Geschichte der Psychoanalyse und Psychotherapie im Nationalsozialismus.* Frankfurt/M: Fischer Taschenbuch.

Lockot, Regine. (1994). *Die Reinigung der Psychoanalyse: Die Deutsche Psychoanalytische Gesellschaft im Spiegel von Dokumenten und Zeitzeugen (1933–1951).* Tübingen: Diskord.

Macrakis, Kristie. (1993). *Surviving the Swastika: Scientific Research in Nazi Germany.* New York: Oxford University Press.

Mazumdar, Pauline M. H. (1992). *Eugenics, Human Genetics and Human Failings: The Genetic Society, its Sources and its Critics in Britain.* London: Routledge.

McLaren, Angus. (1990). *Our Own Master Race: Eugenics in Canada: 1885–1945.* Toronto: McClelland & Stewart.

Pick, Daniel. (1989). *Faces of Degeneration: A European Disorder, c. 1848–c. 1918.* New York: Cambridge University Press.

Proctor, Robert N. (1988). *Racial Hygiene: Medicine under the Nazis.* Cambridge, MA: Harvard University Press.

Reilly, Philip R. (1991). *The Surgical Solution: A History of Involuntary Sterilization in the United States.* Baltimore: Johns Hopkins University Press.

Schmuhl, Hans-Walter. (1992). *Rassenhygiene, Nationalsozialismus, Euthanasie: Von der Verhütung zur Vernichtung "lebensunwerten Lebens," 1890–1945.* Göttingen: Vandenhoeck & Ruprecht.

Weindling, Paul. (1989). *Health, Race and German Politics Between National Unification and Nazism, 1870–1945.* Cambridge, UK: Cambridge University Press.

Weingart, Peter. (1988). *Rasse, Blut und Gene: Geschichte der Eugenik und Rassenhygiene in Deutschland.* Frankfurt/M: Suhrkamp.

Index

Note: Page numbers in boldface type indicate the location of main dictionary entries.

Index

Printed and bound in the UK by
CPI Antony Rowe, Eastbourne

The manufacturer's authorised representative in the EU for product safety is Oxford University Press España S.A. of El Parque Empresarial San Fernando de Henares, Avenida de Castilla, 2 - 28830 Madrid (www.oup.es/en or product.safety@oup.com). OUP España S.A. also acts as importer into Spain of products made by the manufacturer.
Printed and bound by CPI Group (UK) Ltd, Croydon, CR0 4YY
15/09/2026
02217439-0001